McGraw-Hill's
DAT

McGraw-Hill's
DAT

Thomas Evangelist
Wendy Hanks

New York   Chicago   San Francisco   Lisbon   London   Madrid   Mexico City
Milan   New Delhi   San Juan   Seoul   Singapore   Sydney   Toronto

1 2 3 4 5 6 7 8 9 10 QDB/QDB 1 9 8 7 6 5 4 3 2

ISBN   978-0-07-178797-0   (book and CD set)
MHID   0-07-178797-6   (book and CD set)

ISBN   978-0-07-178794-9   (book for set)
MHID   0-07-178794-1   (book for set)

e-ISBN 978-0-07-178795-6
e-MHID   0-07-178795-X

Library of Congress Control Number   2012931066

DAT® is a registered trademark of the American Dental Association, which was
not involved in the production of, and does not endorse, this product.

Interior artwork by Cenveo Publisher Services

McGraw-Hill products are available at special quantity discounts to use as
premiums and sales promotions or for use in corporate training programs.
To contact a representative, please e-mail us at bulksales@mcgraw-hill.com.

This book is printed on acid-free paper.

Many thanks to the students I taught and coached during the 2010–11 school year; to Yevgeniy Genchanok for his invaluable help; and to Mike, Boris, and Billy—my three favorite dentists.
—Thomas Evangelist

I'd like to thank my family—Kim, Isabella, and Noah—for their support.
—Wendy Hanks

Contents

How to Use This Book xi

PART I: GETTING STARTED

Chapter 1   Introducing the DAT 3

Chapter 2   General Test-Taking Strategies 7

PART II: DAT DIAGNOSTIC TEST

Chapter 3   Sample DAT Test and Answers 13

PART III: NATURAL SCIENCES

Biology

Chapter 4   The Cell and Molecular Biology 125

Chapter 5   The Diversity of Life 153

Chapter 6   Structure and Function of Systems 167

Chapter 7   Developmental Biology 211

Chapter 8   Genetics 215

Chapter 9   Evolution, Ecology, and Behavior 231

General Chemistry

Chapter 10   Atomic and Molecular Structure 240

Chapter 11   The Periodic Table and Periodic Trends 252

Chapter 12 Bonding 257

Chapter 13 Gases, Liquids, and Solids 273

Chapter 14 Moles and Stoichiometry 286

Chapter 15 Solution Chemistry 293

Chapter 16 Chemical Kinetics and Equilibrium 301

Chapter 17 Thermodynamics and Thermochemistry 309

Chapter 18 Acids and Bases 319

Chapter 19 Redox and Electrochemistry 328

Chapter 20 Nuclear Chemistry 333

Chapter 21 General and Organic Chemistry Laboratory Skills 339

Organic Chemistry

Chapter 22 The Basics: Nomenclature, Stereochemistry, Properties 348

Chapter 23 Reactions and Mechanisms 361

Chapter 24 Reactions of Major Functional Groups 373

Chapter 25 Aromaticity and Reactions of Benzene 386

Chapter 26 Spectrometric Methods 390

PART IV: PERCEPTUAL ABILITY

Chapter 27 Keyhole 409

Chapter 28 Top/Front/End Projection 413

Chapter 29 Angle Ranking 418

Chapter 30 **Paper Folding** 421

Chapter 31 **Cube Stacking** 427

Chapter 32 **Form Creation** 431

PART V: READING COMPREHENSION

Chapter 33 **Preparing for the Reading Comprehension Test** 439

Chapter 34 **Approaching Questions on the Reading Comprehension Test** 444

Chapter 35 **Reading Comprehension Practice** 449

PART VI: QUANTITATIVE REASONING

Chapter 36 **Mathematics: A Basic Review** 457

Chapter 37 **Algebra** 464

Chapter 38 **Geometry and Trigonometry** 470

Chapter 39 **Probability and Statistics** 480

How to Use This Book

Welcome to *McGraw-Hill's DAT*. You've made the decision to pursue a career in dentistry, you've studied hard, you've taken and passed difficult science courses, and now you must succeed on this very tough exam. We're here to help you.

This book has been created by a dedicated team of teachers and test-prep experts. Together, they have helped thousands of students score high on all kinds of exams, from rigorous science tests to difficult essay-writing assignments. They have pooled their knowledge, experience, and test-taking expertise to make this the most effective DAT preparation program available.

McGraw-Hill's DAT contains a wealth of features to help you do your best. In the months, weeks, or days before you take the test, you can substantially improve your chances of scoring high by using this book as follows:

➤ In Part I, you'll learn basic facts about the test, become familiar with the test format, and learn about the kinds of questions you're going to encounter. You'll also find important tips about pacing and guessing. In addition, you can review some basic test-taking strategies to keep in mind throughout all phases of the exam.

➤ In Part II, you can take a Sample Diagnostic Test. The questions on this test follow the DAT format and cover the same topics as the actual exam. When you finish the test, use the results to measure how well prepared you currently are to take the DAT. You can also use the results to decide which topics to focus on during the course of your review.

➤ In Parts III through VI, you can review every subject you must know for the DAT. These parts present detailed coverage of all tested topics in biology, general chemistry, organic chemistry, perceptual ability, reading comprehension, and quantitative reasoning. You will find valuable advice for tackling DAT questions in each particular topic area.

➤ On the enclosed CD-ROM, you'll find **two complete sample DATs** for practice. These tests present questions spanning the entire range of subjects you're likely to find on the DAT. Take the test under actual testing conditions: set aside the time you'll need to take the entire test at one sitting. Screen out distractions, and concentrate on doing your best. Of course, these practice tests can provide only an approximation of how well you will do on the actual DAT. However, if you approach them as you would the real test, they should give you a very good idea of how well you are prepared. After you take the tests, read through the explanations for each question, paying special attention to those you answered incorrectly or had to guess on. If necessary, go back and reread the corresponding sections in the subject reviews in this book.

Different people have different ways of preparing for a test like the DAT. You must find a preparation method that suits your schedule and your learning style. We have tried to make *McGraw-Hill's DAT* flexible enough for you to use in a way that works best for you, but to succeed on this rigorous exam, there's no substitute for serious, intensive review and study. The more time and effort you devote to preparing, the better your chances of achieving your DAT goals.

PART I
GETTING STARTED

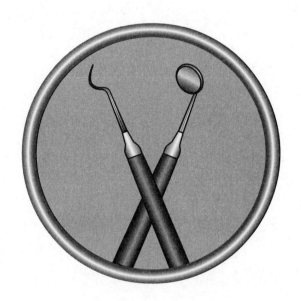

CHAPTER 1

Introducing the DAT

Read This Chapter to Learn About

➤ DAT Basics
➤ Where and When to Take the DAT
➤ The Format of the Test
➤ Scoring
➤ How Dental Schools Use DAT Scores
➤ Reporting Scores to Dental Schools

DAT BASICS

The Dental Admission Test (DAT) is a standardized exam that is used to assess applicants to dental schools. It is required as part of the admissions process by all U.S. dental schools and is taken by students in Canada as well. The test is created by the American Dental Association and administered at Prometric Test Centers in the United States and Canada.

The questions on the DAT are designed to measure your knowledge of science and problem-solving and critical thinking skills. Test sections assess your mastery of basic concepts in biology, general chemistry, and organic chemistry. Other sections test your ability to perceive spatial relations (perceptual ability) as well as reading comprehension and quantitative reasoning (math).

WHERE AND WHEN TO TAKE THE DAT

The DAT is given year-round at Prometric Test Centers, but you need to apply to the ADA first to take the test. First, obtain a DENTPIN, or dental personal identification number, from the ADA. You will then apply to take the DAT by filling out the electronic application. Both of these items are located on the ADA's Dental Admission Test page on the ADA website: http://www.ada.org/dat.aspx.

Once you've received your eligibility letter, you will be able to register to take the test, but choose a date for your test carefully if you don't want to pay a rescheduling fee later.

THE FORMAT OF THE TEST

The DAT consists of four separately timed sections. The test takes approximately five hours, including an optional tutorial at the beginning, a short rest break about halfway through the test, and an optional survey after the test. The four sections are always given in the same order. The following table shows the sections in order, with the number of questions and time allowed for each section. There are a total of 280 questions on the test.

Test Part	Sections	Time Limit	Number of Questions
Natural sciences		90 min.	
(Measures knowledge of the principles and concepts of biology, general chemistry, and organic chemistry.)			
	Biology		40
	General chemistry		30
	Organic chemistry		30
Perceptual ability		60 min.	
(Measures your skill at making conclusions based on your ability to perceive spatial relations.)			
	Keyhole		15
	Top/front/end projection		15
	Angle ranking		15
	Paper folding		15
	Cube stacking		15
	Form creation		15
Reading comprehension		60 min.	50
(Measures ability to comprehend, analyze, and interpret reading passages.)			
Quantitative reasoning		45 min.	40
(Measures skills in arithmetic processes and understanding of mathematical concepts and relationships.)			

The Perceptual Ability Test

In contrast to the other sections on the DAT, the Perceptual Ability Test (PAT) uniquely assesses your ability to comprehend, analyze, and mentally manipulate two- and three-dimensional objects. Superior spatial visualization skills are necessary for dental students and directly correlate to manual dexterity. A strong PAT score indicates that you have the mental agility necessary for success in the profession. Dental school admissions committees often consider PAT scores as the most significant score on the DAT. Since the types of questions presented on the PAT will most likely be unfamiliar to you, you should spend time preparing and practicing for the PAT. By learning certain strategies and methods for the different question types and practicing those strategies, you can significantly increase your score on this section of the DAT. These skills *can* be learned, and they can be honed with practice so that you can perform the tasks more quickly.

The Perceptual Ability Test consists of six different types of visual perception exercises, in which you will be required to imagine the manipulation of two- and three-dimensional objects. The six types of questions appear in this order: keyhole, top/front/end projection, angle ranking, paper folding, cube stacking, and form creation. The six types of questions are presented in separate sections within the PAT, but there are no breaks in between and the test is given as a whole. You may move back and forth between the sections as you like and allocate your time as you like.

SCORING

The four main parts of the DAT are the natural sciences, perceptual ability, reading comprehension, and quantitative reasoning. The natural sciences section covers biology (40 questions), general chemistry (30 questions), and organic chemistry (30 questions). The perceptual ability test is divided into six sections: keyhole, top/front/end projection, angle ranking, paper folding, cube stacking, and form creation; each of these includes 15 questions. Each correct answer contributes to a raw score. (Unlike some tests, there's no penalty on the DAT for guessing.) The raw score is then converted into a standard score based on the performance of all the test takers for that particular exam. If you received a raw score of, say, 30 on the biology section, your standard score might be 17.

After you finish the entire exam, you'll receive an unofficial score before leaving the testing center. For all tests taken in 2012 and onward, only standard scores will be given out. You'll receive a score for each of the individual tests you've just taken: biology, general chemistry, organic chemistry, perceptual ability, reading comprehension, and quantitative reasoning. You'll also receive two additional scores: the Total Science score is based on the three natural sciences tests, and the Academic Average is based on all the tests you've just taken except perceptual ability. The official scores for each of these eight standard scores are sent to the dental schools you've chosen.

The Perceptual Ability Test Scoring

While there are 90 questions on the Perceptual Ability Test, only 75 of them are scored; the remaining 15 questions are experimental questions that do not affect your score. These experimental questions are distributed randomly throughout the test, and you will not know which ones are the experimental questions. There is no penalty for a wrong answer, so be sure to answer every question on the test. Once the correct answers to the 75 scored questions are added up, your score is adjusted to a scale of 1 to 30. The national average score on the PAT is about 17. However, most dental schools have an average entrance score of 18 to 19, so that should be your minimum goal.

HOW DENTAL SCHOOLS USE DAT SCORES

Dental school admission committees emphasize that DAT scores are only one of several criteria that they consider when evaluating applicants. When making their decisions, they also consider students' college and university grades, recommendations, personal interviews, and involvement and participation in extracurricular or healthcare-related activities. If the committee members are unfamiliar with the college you attend, they may pay more attention than usual to your DAT scores.

There is no hard-and-fast rule about what schools consider to be an acceptable DAT score. Dental schools have their own judgments about a desirable DAT score. Contact the programs to which you are applying to gauge what score you will need to be competitive for admission.

REPORTING SCORES TO DENTAL SCHOOLS

Official transcripts of your DAT scores are sent to the institutions to which you requested your scores be reported on your application. Additional official transcripts can be requested for a fee online.

CHAPTER 2

General Test-Taking Strategies

Read This Chapter to Learn About

➤ General Strategies for Answering DAT Questions

➤ Coping with Exam Pressure

➤ Approaching Questions on the Perceptual Ability Test

GENERAL STRATEGIES FOR ANSWERING DAT QUESTIONS

Use the strategies described in this chapter to help you do your best on the DAT.

Take Advantage of the Multiple-Choice Format

All the questions on the DAT are in the multiple-choice format, which you have undoubtedly seen many times before. That means for every question, the correct answer is right in front of you. All you have to do is pick it out from the incorrect choices, or "distracters." Consequently, you can use the process of elimination to rule out incorrect answer choices. The more answers you rule out, the easier it is to make the right choice.

Answer Every Question

On the DAT, there is no penalty for choosing a wrong answer. Therefore, if you do not know the answer to a question, you have nothing to lose by guessing. So make sure that you answer every question. If time is running out and you still have not answered some questions, make sure to enter an answer for the questions you have not tackled.

With luck, you may be able to pick up a few extra points, even if your guesses are totally random.

Make Educated Guesses

What differentiates great test takers from merely good ones is the ability to guess in such a way as to maximize the chance of guessing correctly. The way to do this is to use the process of elimination. Before you guess, try to eliminate one or more of the answer choices. That way, you can make an educated guess, and you have a better chance of picking the correct answer. Odds of one out of two or one out of three are better than one out of five!

Go with Your Gut

In those cases where you are not 100 percent sure of the answer you are choosing, it is often best to go with your gut feeling and stick with your first answer. If you decide to change that answer and pick another one, you may well pick the wrong answer because you have overthought the problem. More often than not, if you know something about the subject, your first answer is likely to be the correct one.

Use the Writing Materials Provided

Don't bring scratch paper to the test site; you won't be able to write on your own paper. Instead, you'll be provided with writing materials with which you can jot down notes or make calculations. Don't be shy about asking the proctor for more writing materials if you need them.

COPING WITH EXAM PRESSURE

The following strategies will help you cope with exam pressure and make the most of the exam time.

Keep Track of the Time

Make sure that you are on track to answer all the questions within the time allowed. With so many questions to answer in a short time period, you are not going to have a lot of time to spare. Keep an eye on your watch. (Don't forget to bring one!)

Do not spend too much time on any one question. If you find yourself stuck for more than a minute or two on a question, then you should make your best guess and move on. If you have time left over at the end of the section, you can return to the question and review your answer. However, if time runs out, do not give the question another thought. Save your focus for the rest of the test.

Do Not Panic if Time Runs Out

If you pace yourself and keep track of your progress, you should not run out of time. If you do, however, do not panic. Because there is no guessing penalty and you have nothing to lose by doing so, enter answers to all of the remaining questions. If you are able to make educated guesses, you will probably be able to improve your score. Even random guesses may help you pick up a few points. In order to know how to handle this situation if it happens to you on the test, make sure you observe the time limits when you take the practice tests. Guessing well is a skill that comes with practice, so incorporate it into your preparation program.

If Time Permits, Review Questions You Were Unsure Of

If time permits, you may want to take advantage of the opportunity to review questions you were unsure of, or to check for careless mistakes. However, once you have completed an entire section, you cannot go back to it and make changes.

APPROACHING QUESTIONS ON THE PERCEPTUAL ABILITY TEST

When it comes to taking tests, knowing what to expect is half the battle. The PAT assesses a variety of visual perception skills, from comparison skills to higher-level analysis and manipulation skills. There are some general things you can do to prepare for this section, as well as the specific strategies presented in this book. For general practice, try the following:

➤ **Practice creative visualization.** When you are holding an object, look at it from various angles. What does your fork look like from each side?
➤ **Try origami.** Paper folding is just one section of the PAT with which a familiarity with origami might assist you. Your performance on form creation might also be significantly improved by practicing origami.
➤ **Play with alphabet blocks.** Your cube stacking performance might be improved by playing with blocks. Practice stacking the blocks in different ways and then seeing what faces show. Alphabet blocks can also help with form creation because you can practice predicting which letters will be adjacent to each other when the block is flat.
➤ **Work visual puzzles.** There are a number of visual puzzle books available that will exercise your mental ability to visualize objects in different ways.

Use the process of elimination on these questions to maximize your efficiency. When you look at the choices, you will probably be able to eliminate one or two very quickly, but if you try to do that in your head, you will forget which ones you eliminated and cause yourself to duplicate your efforts. The best way to keep track of which answer choices you want to eliminate is to use an answer grid. This is a simple chart like the one shown here:

	A	B	C	D	E
1	x		x	x	
2		x			x
3	x	x		x	

For question-specific strategies, read through and do all of the practice exercises in this book. Take the full-length practice test included in the book. Go to the ADA website and download the free practice material and work through that as well. Each of the six question types is unique and must be prepared for individually. The chapters in Part IV examine each type of perceptual ability question individually.

PART II

DAT DIAGNOSTIC TEST

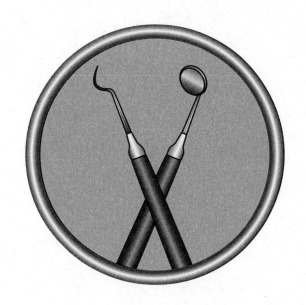

CHAPTER 3

Sample DAT Test and Answers

In This Section You Will Find

➤ A full-length DAT diagnostic test covering all subjects tested

➤ Hundreds of sample questions like the ones on the real exam

➤ Explanations in the answer key for every question

This chapter contains a complete, full-length DAT diagnostic test. It is designed to help you test your knowledge of each subject area and sharpen your test-taking skills. The questions are modeled on the questions in the real exam. They cover the same topics and are designed to be at the same level of difficulty. Explanations to each of the questions are given at the end of the test.

When you are finished with the test, carefully read the explanations for the answers, especially for any questions that you answered incorrectly. Identify any weak areas by determining the subjects in which you made the most errors. Then review the corresponding chapters in this book. If time permits, you may also want to review your stronger areas.

This practice test will help you gauge your test readiness if you treat it as an actual examination. Here are some hints on how to take the test under conditions similar to those of the actual exam:

➤ Find a time when you will not be interrupted.

➤ Complete the test in a single session, following the suggested time limits.

➤ If you run out of time on any section, take note of where you ended when time ran out. This will help you determine if you need to speed up your pace.

NATURAL SCIENCES

Directions: This section consists of **100 questions**. They cover biology (questions 1–40), general chemistry (41–70), and organic chemistry (71–100). You will have **90 minutes** to complete them.

1. A prokaryotic cell is most likely to
   A. have organelles
   B. be larger in size than a typical eukaryotic cell
   C. have a single loop of DNA
   D. be in domain Eukarya
   E. none of the above

2. Energy production in the cell is most associated with the
   A. Golgi apparatus
   B. cell membrane
   C. mitochondria
   D. lysosomes
   E. centriole

3. This part of the cell controls what enters and exits the cell:
   A. Golgi apparatus
   B. cell membrane
   C. mitochondria
   D. lysosomes
   E. centriole

4. Digestion within the cell occurs in the
   A. Golgi apparatus
   B. cell membrane
   C. mitochondria
   D. lysosomes
   E. centriole

5. This processes and packs materials in the cell.
   A. Golgi apparatus
   B. Cell membrane
   C. Mitochondria
   D. Lysosomes
   E. Centriole

6. This part of the cell is composed of microtubules.
   A. Golgi apparatus
   B. Cell membrane
   C. Mitochondria
   D. Lysosomes
   E. Centriole

7. Which of the following does not describe enzymes?
   A. Consumed in the reaction
   B. Made up of proteins
   C. Lowers activation energy
   D. Highly specific
   E. Contains an active site

8. Which of the following would least impact an organism's offspring negatively?
   A. Deletion
   B. Duplication
   C. Translocation
   D. Inversion
   E. Meiotic division

9. The electron transport chain in humans does not involve
   A. a proton pump
   B. rubisco
   C. the mitochondrial membrane
   D. NADH
   E. oxygen gas

10. Which of the following does not belong with the other four choices?
    A. Stroma
    B. Thylakoids
    C. Granum
    D. Mitochondria
    E. Chlorophyll

11. Which of the following is correctly sequenced?
    A. Metaphase I, anaphase I, prophase II
    B. Prophase I, telophase I, metaphase II
    C. Telophase II, anaphase II, daughter cells
    D. Anaphase I, telophase I, prophase II
    E. Anaphase II, telophase II, prophase II

12. Which of the following is true?
    A. Eukaryotes must be unicellular.
    B. Bacteria are eukaryotic.
    C. Archaea lack a nucleus.
    D. Viruses have a nucleus.
    E. None of the above is true.

13. Fungi
    A. can be uni- or multicellular
    B. can reproduce sexually or asexually
    C. contain a mycelium
    D. Only A and C are correct.
    E. Choices A, B, and C are correct.

14. Lag, logarithmic growth, stationary phase, and decline are terms best associated with
    A. viruses
    B. bacteria
    C. eukaryotes
    D. sickle cells
    E. yeasts

15. The one term below that is not associated with the other four is
    A. hyphae
    B. stamen
    C. anther
    D. carpel
    E. stigma

16. The nerve cell is least associated with
    A. myelin sheath
    B. node of Ranvier
    C. dendrite
    D. axon
    E. stomata

17. Sensorimotor coordination for complex muscle movement patterns and balance
    is best associated with the
    A. diencephalon
    B. brain stem
    C. spinal cord
    D. cerebrum
    E. cerebellum

18. Which one of the following bones is least associated with the other four?
    A. Maxilla
    B. Skull
    C. Mandible
    D. Sacrum
    E. Cranium

19. Which structure and hormone are correctly paired?
    A. Stomach: testosterone
    B. Ovary: gastrin
    C. Pancreas: FSH
    D. Small intestine: CCK
    E. Thymus: melatonin

20. Regarding the circulatory system:
    A. Veins have a method to prevent blood backflow.
    B. Capillaries connect arterioles and venules.
    C. Veins have a thicker wall than arteries.

D. None of the above choices are correct.

E. Choices A and B are correct.

21. Which choice below BEST demonstrates airflow into the body?
    A. Nasal cavity, then epiglottis, then trachea, larynx
    B. Pharynx, then trachea, then bronchus
    C. Alveoli, then trachea, then bronchiole
    D. Diaphragm, then glottis, then mouth
    E. Mouth, then pharynx, then alveoli, then bronchiole

22. Chemical digestion is better completed by
    A. gastric juices
    B. churning of the stomach
    C. teeth
    D. tongue
    E. peristalsis

23. The Bowman's capsule is best described as part of the
    A. kidney
    B. nephron
    C. bladder
    D. urethra
    E. urine

24. A tertiary line of defense by the immune system includes
    A. skin
    B. tears
    C. inflammation
    D. attack by the white blood cells
    E. production of memory B cells

25. During an average 30-day menstrual cycle
    A. progesterone levels will peak with LH levels
    B. estrogen levels will rise just once
    C. LH and FSH levels will peak together
    D. FSH and progesterone levels will peak together
    E. regressing corpus luteum will occur with higher levels of LH

26. The male reproductive system includes
    A. vas deferens
    B. seminal vesicle
    C. epididymis
    D. Choices A and C only are correct.
    E. Choices A, B, and C are correct.

27. During the gastrula stage of development
    A. an ectoderm layer forms
    B. a mesoderm layer forms

C. an endoderm layer forms

D. only the ectoderm and endoderm layers form

E. all of the layers form

28. The fluid-filled sac that protects the embryo and fetus is the

    A. placenta

    B. chorion

    C. allantois

    D. amnion

    E. yolk sac

29. Labor is triggered by

    A. HCG

    B. oxytocin

    C. estrogen

    D. progesterone

    E. FSH

30. A structural component of ribosomes is

    A. DNA

    B. RNA

    C. rRNA

    D. mRNA

    E. tRNA

31. Deoxyribose sugar in the nucleotide is part of

    A. DNA

    B. RNA

    C. rRNA

    D. mRNA

    E. tRNA

32. A, T, C, G are best associated with

    A. DNA

    B. RNA

    C. rRNA

    D. mRNA

    E. tRNA

33. Which of the following transfers amino acids to the ribosome?

    A. DNA

    B. RNA

    C. rRNA

    D. mRNA

    E. tRNA

34. The double helix is most associated with
   A. DNA
   B. RNA
   C. rRNA
   D. mRNA
   E. tRNA

35. Which of the following is not true regarding genes?
   A. Environmental factors can influence genes.
   B. Women will express a recessive trait with just one recessive allele.
   C. Color blindness is a sex-linked trait.
   D. Epistasis is when one gene influences the expression of another.
   E. A cross between two heterozygotes will have a 75% dominant genotype.

36. Almost all of our cells are specialized; they only express the genes pertinent to the function of the cell. This is called
   A. segregation
   B. codominance
   C. genotype
   D. differentiation
   E. phenotype

37. These account for the most energy in the food pyramid.
   A. Producers
   B. Herbivores
   C. Carnivores
   D. Humans
   E. None of the above

38. These are the link between photosynthetic organisms and carnivores.
   A. Producers
   B. Herbivores
   C. Carnivores
   D. Humans
   E. None of the above

39. Evolutionary evidence taken from the fossil record is best approached by the field of
   A. biogeography
   B. paleontology
   C. comparative anatomy
   D. comparative embryology
   E. molecular biology

40. A win-win situation for two organisms could include
   A. parasitism
   B. altruism
   C. competition

    D. extinction

    E. predation

41. H_2SO_4

    A. has a GFM of 98 g/mol

    B. is a diprotic acid

    C. will change red litmus paper to blue

    D. Choices A and B are correct.

    E. Choices B and C are correct.

42. When 32 grams of methane combust in air (assume STP conditions),

    A. 32 grams of carbon dioxide will be formed

    B. 2 moles of oxygen gas will react

    C. 36 grams of water will form

    D. 44.8 liters of carbon dioxide will form

    E. the reaction will be endothermic

43. Given glucose, molecular formula $C_6H_{12}O_6$,

    A. the empirical formula will have the same percent composition as the molecular formula

    B. the percent composition of the carbon atoms will be greater than that of the oxygen atoms

    C. only a nonpolar solvent can dissolve $C_6H_{12}O_6$

    D. the molecule is formed in cellular respiration

    E. its solubility decreases with an increase in temperature of the solvent

44. An equal mixture of the noble gases is in a sealed container. When a hole is poked in the container

    A. the element with atomic number 10 will leave the container at the fastest rate

    B. the element with the highest density will leave the container at the fastest rate

    C. the element with atomic number 2 will leave the container at the slowest rate

    D. Kr will leave the container faster than Ar will

    E. the element with the lowest density will have the lowest partial pressure remaining after 2 minutes

45. Which of the following is not consistent with the Kinetic Molecular Theory?

    A. Gas molecules need to have forces of attraction between them.

    B. Gas molecules need to be far apart.

    C. Gas molecules have perfectly elastic collisions.

    D. Gas molecules travel in a straight line, random motion.

    E. Gas molecules have an increase in average kinetic energy with an increase in temperature.

46. The ideal gas constant, R, has the units of

    A. $\dfrac{K \cdot atm}{mol \cdot L}$

    B. $\dfrac{L \cdot atm}{mol \cdot K}$

C. $\dfrac{L \cdot torr}{mol \cdot K}$

D. $\dfrac{L \cdot atm}{mol \cdot kJ}$

E. $\dfrac{L \cdot atm}{grams \cdot K}$

47. Which compound is not paired with the correct intermolecular force?
   A. Methane / dispersion forces
   B. HBr / dipoles
   C. Ammonia / dispersion
   D. NaCl / ionic bonds
   E. Carbon dioxide / dispersion forces

48. Which is expected to have the greatest boiling point?
   A. Ethanol
   B. Acetone
   C. Butane
   D. Water
   E. Salt water

49. A solid, liquid, and gas can exist at the same time at the
   A. normal boiling point
   B. freezing point
   C. critical point
   D. triple point
   E. flash point

50. When 58.5 grams of NaCl are dissolved in water to make 2.0 liters of solution,
   A. the freezing point of the water will be depressed
   B. the solution will be acidic
   C. the molarity of the solution will be 1.0 M
   D. Choices A and B are correct.
   E. Choices A and C are correct.

51. Which of the following aqueous reactants does not produce a precipitate?
   A. Sodium chloride and silver nitrate
   B. Lead iodide and magnesium chloride
   C. Lithium bromide and ammonium nitrate
   D. Silver nitrate and potassium iodide
   E. Calcium chloride and sodium carbonate

52. 50.0 grams of LiCl are dissolved to make 750 ml of solution. Then another 250 mL of water is added.
   A. The solubility of the salt will increase with an increase in temperature.
   B. The molarity of the original solution was 1.13 M.
   C. The molarity of the diluted solution will increase if water is allowed to evaporate.

D. None of the above are correct.

E. Choices A, B, and C are correct.

53. A weak, monoprotic acid has a Ka value of 1.5×10^{-5}. What is the pH of a 0.2 M solution of this acid?

A. 3.0×10^{-6}

B. 2.0

C. 2.76

D. 0.0017

E. 11.23

54. Which of the following is the result of hydrolysis?

A. NaCl will give a basic solution.

B. $NaC_2H_3O_2$ will give a basic solution.

C. LiCl will give an acidic solution.

D. H_2SO_4 will give a basic solution.

E. NH_4Cl will give a basic solution.

55. 0.0284 L of 0.18 M NaOH is diluted to make 0.0400 L of solution. If the new solution is titrated using 0.0249 L of HCl, what is the molarity of the HCl?

A. 0.18 M

B. 0.205 M

C. 0.005 M

D. 0.114 M

E. 0.1278 M

56. Given the reaction: heat + 2A(g) + 3B(g) $\leftrightarrow$ C(g) + D(g), to make more products we could shift the equilibrium by

A. removing A

B. adding D

C. decreasing the temperature

D. decreasing the pressure

E. removing C

57. Which of the following is a correct component when writing the relative rates for the reaction $N_2(g)$ + $3H_2(g)$ $\leftrightarrow$ $2NH_3(g)$?

A. $\dfrac{-(1)\Delta(N_2)}{(3)\Delta t}$

B. $\dfrac{+(1)\Delta(N_2)}{(2)\Delta t}$

C. $\dfrac{-(1)\Delta(H_2)}{(3)\Delta t}$

D. $\dfrac{+(1)\Delta(N_2)}{(1)\Delta t}$

E. $\dfrac{-(1)\Delta(NH_3)}{(2)\Delta t}$

58. A laboratory student records the following data for the reaction: $A + B \rightarrow C$.

Exp	[A]	[B]	Initial Rate (M/s)
1	0.020	0.010	2×10^{-5}
2	0.020	0.020	4×10^{-5}
3	0.020	0.040	8×10^{-4}
4	0.040	0.020	1.6×10^{-3}

The order of the reaction is best expressed by

A. $k[A]^2 [B]^1$
B. $k[A]^0 [B]^1$
C. $k[A]^2 [B]^2$
D. $k[A]^1 [B]^2$
E. $k[A]^2 [B]^0$

59. The following processes are observed taking place:

The raking up of leaves.
Hockey pucks scattered at a rink are placed into a bucket.
Two kids throw eggs at each other on Halloween.

Which of the above has a negative value for ΔS?

A. The raking up of leaves only
B. The raking up of leaves and two kids throw eggs at each other on Halloween only
C. Two kids throw eggs at each other on Halloween only
D. The raking up of leaves and hockey pucks scattered at a rink are placed into a bucket only
E. The raking up of leaves, the placing of pucks into a bucket, and the throwing of eggs

60. ΔH is best defined as

A. heat of reaction
B. potential energy of the products
C. activation energy
D. potential energy of the activated complex
E. potential energy of the reactants

61. $PE_{activated\ complex} - PE_{reactants}$ best defines

A. heat of reaction
B. potential energy of the products
C. activation energy
D. potential energy of the activated complex
E. potential energy of the reactants

62. Which of the following is needed to start a reaction?

A. Heat of reaction
B. Potential energy of the products

C. Activation energy

D. Potential energy of the activated complex

E. Potential energy of the reactants

63. Oxygen could have an oxidation number equal to
   A. +2 only
   B. 0 only
   C. −2 only
   D. +2 or 0 only
   E. +2, 0, or −2

64. Oxidation
   A. occurs at the cathode
   B. is the result of the loss of electrons
   C. results in a lower oxidation number
   D. None of the above are correct.
   E. A and C are the only correct choices.

65. $1s^2 2s^2 2p^6 3s^2 3p^6$ represents
   A. a chlorine atom only
   B. an argon atom only
   C. an argon ion only
   D. a bromine ion only
   E. an atom of argon or a potassium ion

66. The rules for orbital notation tell us all of the following except
   A. the l value of 1 signifies a p orbital
   B. the d orbital can have m_l of −2, −1, 0, 1, or 2
   C. the f orbital can hold 14 electrons
   D. m_s is restricted to a value of $+\dfrac{1}{2}$
   E. principal energy level 2 has possible l values of 0 and 1

67. Trigonal bipyramidal refers to the molecular geometry of
   A. PCl_5
   B. CH_4
   C. H_2O
   D. CO_2
   E. XeF_6

68. A student took note about the properties of a substance: purple solid, sublimes, terrible odor. This substance is most likely found in group
   A. 18
   B. 17
   C. 5
   D. 2
   E. 1

69. Which two elements are expected to have similar chemical properties?
A. Br and Ba
B. N and Ne
C. Ca and Sr
D. C and B
E. H and He

70. Which of the following is not true?
A. Alpha particles can pass through a thin sheet of gold foil.
B. Beta particles and electrons are the same in structure.
C. Gamma radiation and neutrons will not be deflected in an electric field.
D. Beta particles are heavier than alpha particles.
E. Elements with an atomic number of 84 or greater have an unstable nucleus.

71. An organic compound has the modifier *oxo* in its name. A possible functional group present could be a(n)
A. lactone
B. ether
C. alcohol
D. nitrile
E. aldehyde

72. trans-2,3-dichloro-2-butene can also be named using the letter
A. β
B. E
C. Z
D. S
E. R

73. Nonsuperimposable mirror image isomers is best related to
A. a fork
B. the letter T
C. a shoe
D. a cup
E. benzene

74. Which reaction entails a 100 percent inversion of configuration?
A. S_N2
B. S_N1
C. Markovnikov
D. Anti-Markovnikov
E. Zaitsef

75. Which rule dictates that the double bond forms so as to have as many R groups as possible attached to the C=C?
A. S_N2
B. S_N1
C. Markovnikov

D. Anti-Markovnikov

E. Zaitsef

76. Which rule dictates that the addition of HX adds the H atom to the carbon atom that already has a greater number of H atoms?

A. S_N2

B. S_N1

C. Markovnikov

D. Anti-Markovnikov

E. Zaitsef

77. The following reaction involves

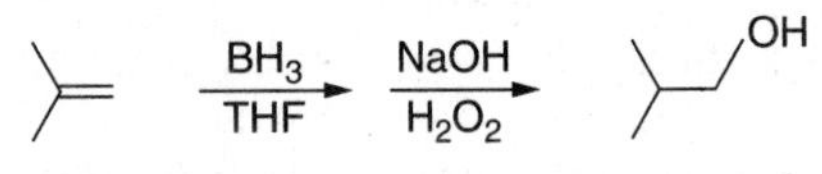

A. S_N2

B. S_N1

C. Markovnikov

D. anti-Markovnikov

E. Zaitsef

78. The following reaction involves

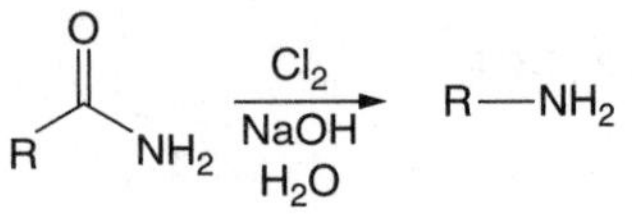

A. oxidation

B. reduction

C. Grignard

D. ozonolysis

E. Hofmann degradation

79. The following reaction involves

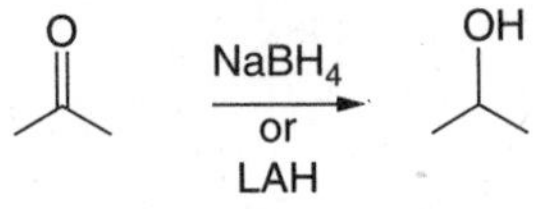

A. oxidation

B. reduction

C. Grignard

D. ozonolysis

E. Hofmann degradation

80. The following reaction involves

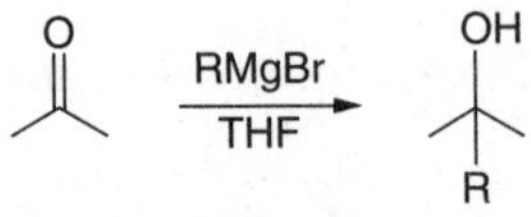

A. anti-Markovnikov

B. Markovnikov

C. Grignard

D. ozonolysis

E. Hofmann degradation

81. The following reaction involves

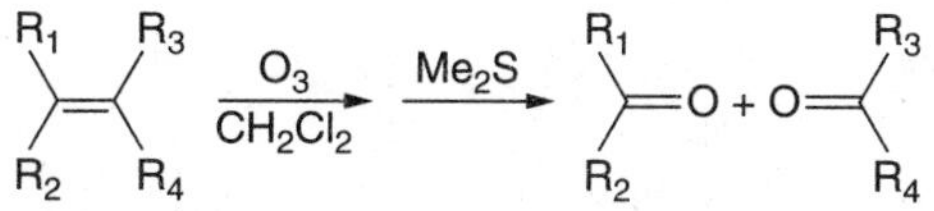

A. Zaitsef

B. reduction

C. Grignard

D. ozonolysis

E. Hofmann degradation

82. Benzene undergoes _____ and then is followed up with a reaction with H_2/cat. or Fe/HCl to yield aniline.

A. nitration

B. sulfonation

C. halogenation

D. Friedel-Crafts alkylation

E. esterification

83. Benzene undergoes _____ and then is followed up by a reaction of 1. Alkaline $KMnO_4$ / 2. H_2SO_4 to give benzoic acid.

A. nitration

B. sulfonation

C. halogenation

D. Friedel-Crafts alkylation

E. esterification

84. Benzene undergoes _____ followed up with a reaction with molten NaOH to yield phenol.

A. nitration

B. sulfonation or halogenation

C. hydrogenation

D. Friedel-Crafts alkylation

E. esterification

85. Reaction with benzene puts a deactivating ortho, para director on the benzene in

A. nitration

B. sulfonation

C. halogenation

D. Friedel-Crafts alkylation

E. esterification

86. Which of the following compounds will have an absorption maximum over 200 nm?
   A. Dimethyl ether only
   B. 1,3-butadiene only
   C. Ethyl benzene, dimethyl ether, and 1,3-butadiene
   D. Dimethyl ether and 1,3-butadiene only
   E. Ethyl benzene and 1,3-butadiene only

87. The mass spec of benzyl chloride will not have
   A. an M+ peak at 126 m/z
   B. an M+2 peak at 128 m/z
   C. a base ion of 91 m/z
   D. a significant peak at 77 m/z
   E. an M+2 peak that is about one-third the height of the M+ peak

88. Which of the following is not true about the spectra of 4-heptanone?
   A. There will be a strong, sharp peak at 1720 cm^{-1} in the IR.
   B. The HNMR will have peaks at a shift of 7.2 ppm.
   C. There will be four peaks in the 13C NMR.
   D. The mass spec will have two significant peaks at 43 and 71 m/z.
   E. The M+ peak will be at 114 m/z.

89. Looking at the following diagram, we see the various number of carbon atom environments for three different isomers of nitroaniline.

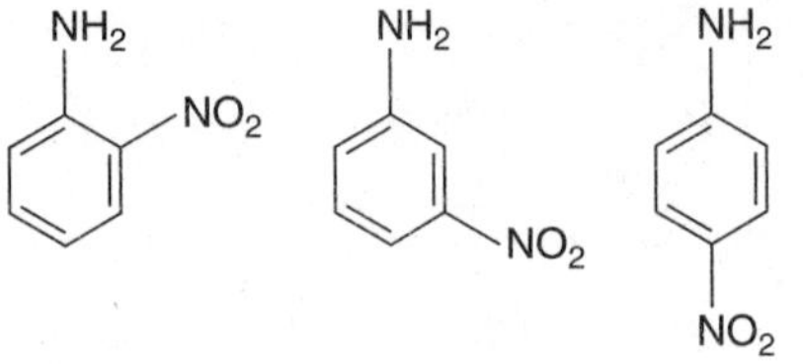

      I   II   III

   Which statement is true about the HNMR of these compounds?
   A. The ortho isomer will show five different sets of hydrogen atoms only.
   B. The meta isomer will show five different sets of hydrogen atoms only.
   C. The meta isomer will show five different sets of hydrogen atoms and the para isomer will show five different sets of hydrogen atom only.
   D. The ortho isomer will show five different sets of hydrogen atoms and the meta isomer will show five different sets of hydrogen atoms only.
   E. The ortho isomer will show five different sets of hydrogen atoms and the para isomer will show five different sets of hydrogen atom only.

90. The reaction 1,3-butadiene + cis-2-butene → 4,5-dimethyl-1-cyclohexene is best explained by
   A. Diels-Alder reaction to form an adduct
   B. keto-enol tautomerization
   C. esterification to form a lactone
   D. Cannizzaro reaction
   E. protonation-dehydration

91. The monochlorination of methane involves all of the steps below except
    A. Cl-Cl → 2Cl•
    B. 2Cl• → Cl-Cl
    C. CH_4 + Cl• → H-Cl + CH_3•
    D. CH_3• + Cl-Cl → CH_3Cl + Cl•
    E. 2H• → H-H

92. Which statement is not true regarding a molecule of cyclohexane?
    A. The flagpole hydrogen atoms will crowd each other in the boat conformation.
    B. The chair conformation will be most stable.
    C. A methyl group in the axial position will be more stable than a methyl group in the equatorial position.
    D. The half-chair conformation will require the most energy to overcome.
    E. Diaxial substituents will give rise to Van der Waals strain.

93. An organic molecule has four chiral centers. How many stereoisomers are possible for this compound?
    A. 4
    B. 8
    C. 16
    D. 32
    E. 64

94. Which of the following is expected to be the weakest acid?
    A. Propyne
    B. 1-propanol
    C. Propanoic acid
    D. Propanal
    E. 3-chloro-1propanol

95. The monobromination of propane
    A. will yield 1-bromopropane only
    B. will yield 2-bromopropane only
    C. involves a bromonium intermediate only
    D. will yield 1-bromopropane and 2-bromopropane only
    E. will yield 2-bromopropane and involves a bromonium intermediate only

96. Which of the following is not related to this diagram?

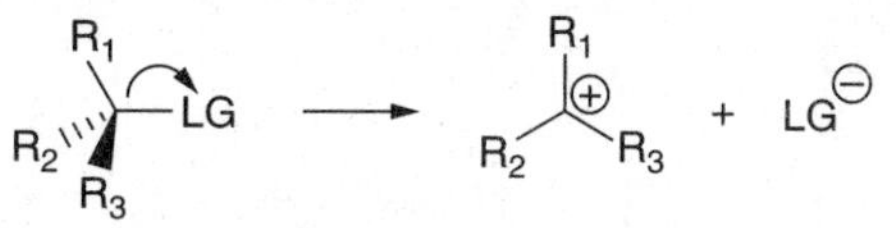

    A. Racemization
    B. Rate = k[reactant]
    C. Trigonal planar geometry
    D. Carbocation
    E. Bimolecular substitution

97. Which of the following groups is given the highest priority when determining the R/S configuration of a Fischer projection?

   A. H
   B. Methyl
   C. Ethyl
   D. Br
   E. OH

98. After the following reaction, what changes to the IR spectrum will be striking about the product as compared to the reactant?

   A. The appearance of overtones between 2000 and 1600 cm^{-1}
   B. The appearance of two strong sharp peaks at 770 and 700 cm^{-1}
   C. The appearance of a strong sharp peak at 1760 cm^{-1}
   D. The appearance of a strong, broad peak from 3600 to 3200 cm^{-1}
   E. The appearance of a moderate, sharp peak at 2250 cm^{-1}

99. How many degrees of unsaturation are there in

   A. 1
   B. 2
   C. 3
   D. 4
   E. 5

100. Tollen's silver mirror test will help to identify

   A. carboxylic acids
   B. ketones
   C. aldehydes
   D. amines
   E. tertiary alcohols

PERCEPTUAL ABILITY TEST

For this section you will have **60 minutes. There are six parts, each consisting of 15 questions.**

Part 1: Visualization

Questions 1–15

The visualization test involves matching a given object with the correct option in a group of apertures, or openings. A three-dimensional object is given, as shown to the left in the example below.

For each question, you are to choose which of the five apertures shown matches the given object. Imagine how the given object looks from any possible direction, not just from the direction that's shown. Then, picking from the five possible apertures outlined, choose the opening through which the given object could pass if the correct side were inserted first.

These are the conditions for each question:

➤ Before it passes through the aperture, the given object may face in any direction. (The side of the object that goes first through the opening may not be shown.)
➤ While the object goes through the aperture, it cannot be moved around and must pass completely through the opening. The aperture is always the exact shape of the corresponding outline of the object.
➤ The object and the apertures are drawn to the same scale. (An aperture might be the same shape as the given object but too small for the object to go through.) You can, however, judge any differences in size by eye.
➤ Parts of the given object that you can't see include no irregularities. Any symmetric indentations in the figure, however, are symmetric with any hidden part.
➤ There is only one correct choice.

Example (Do not mark the answer to this example on the answer sheet)

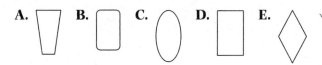

The correct answer is D since the object would pass through the aperture if the top or bottom side were introduced first.

Questions

1.

A. B.  C. D. E.

2.

A. 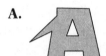 B.  C. D. E.

3.

A. B. C. D.  E.

4.

A. B.  C. D. E.

5.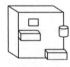

A.  B.  C.  D.  E.

6.

A. B.  C. D. E.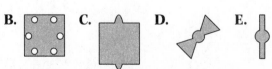

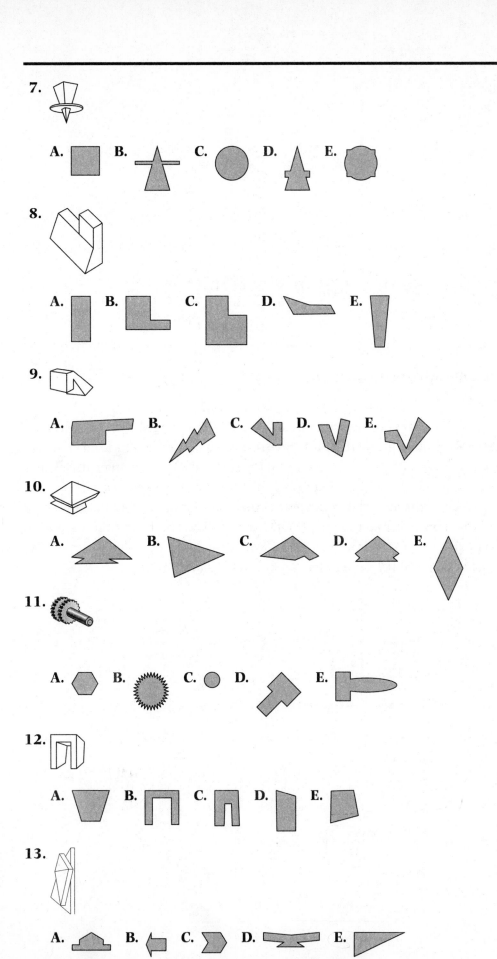

7.

A. B. C. D. E.

8.

A. B. C. D. E.

9.

A. B. C. D. E.

10.

A. B. C. D. E.

11.

A. B. C. D. E.

12.

A. B. C. D. E.

13.

A. B. C. D. E.

14.

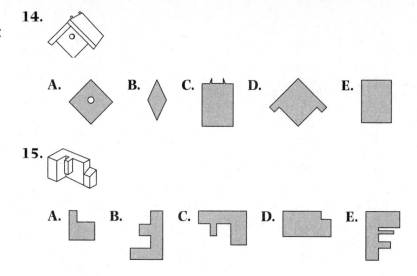

Part 2: Top/Front/End Projection

Questions 16–30

In this section you will choose a picture that represents a missing view of an object. As shown in the illustration below, there are three possible views given: top, front, and end. The views lack perspective—i.e., the points on the surface are seen along parallel lines of vision. The top view, shown in the upper left-hand corner, shows the view if you were looking down on the object. The front view, in the lower left-hand corner, shows how the object would be perceived from the front. The end view, the projection taken from the end perpendicular to the front view, is shown in the lower right-hand corner. The views are labeled accordingly and always appear in the same positions.

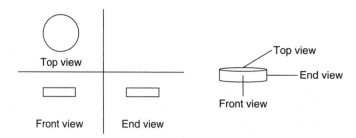

If there were a hole in the block, the views would look like this:

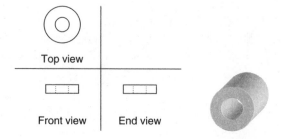

Note that lines that cannot be seen on the surface in some particular views are shown using dots in that view.

The questions in this section will show two of the three possible views. You will choose the correct missing view from the adjacent four options.

Example (Do not mark the answer to this example on the answer sheet)

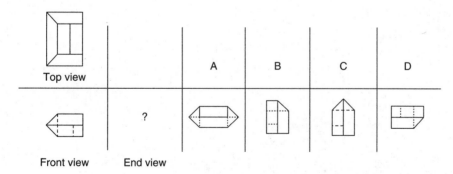

The front view shows that there is a small rectangle on top of the larger rectangle and that there are no holes. The end view shows that the figure is the same from that side, so the blocks must be cubes. The top view must show a cube on top of a cube, so the answer is **C**.

The missing side in the problems can be the top, front, or end view. The side you are to find is indicated by a question mark.

16. Choose the correct END VIEW.

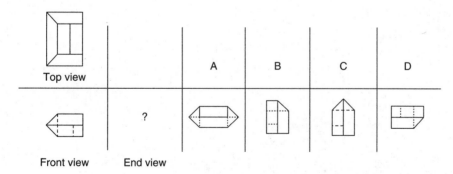

17. Choose the correct TOP VIEW.

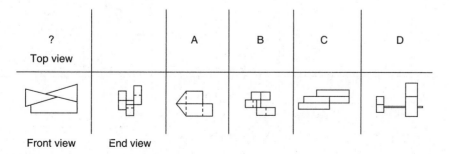

18. Choose the correct FRONT VIEW.

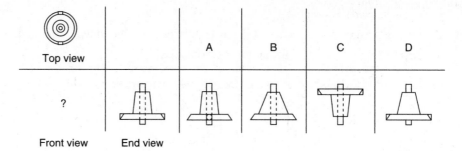

19. Choose the correct TOP VIEW.

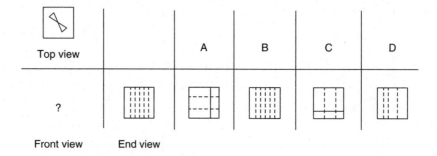

20. Choose the correct FRONT VIEW.

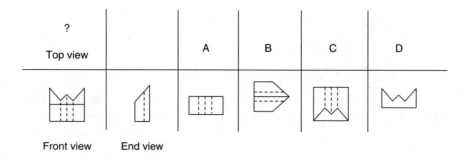

21. Choose the correct END VIEW.

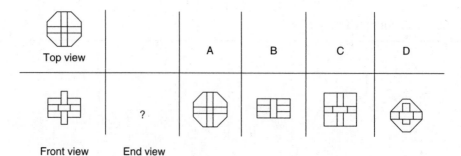

22. Choose the correct FRONT VIEW.

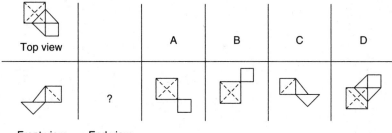

23. Choose the correct END VIEW.

24. Choose the correct END VIEW.

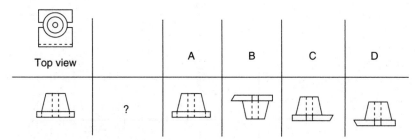

25. Choose the correct END VIEW.

26. Choose the correct FRONT VIEW.

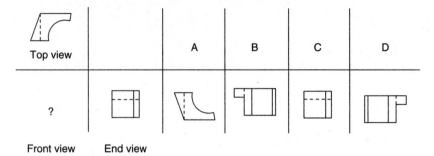

27. Choose the correct END VIEW.

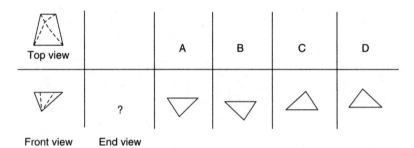

28. Choose the correct END VIEW.

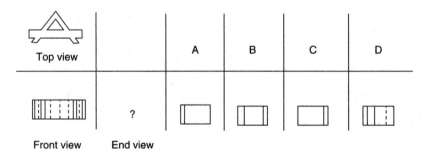

29. Choose the correct FRONT VIEW.

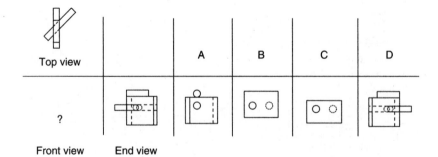

30. Choose the correct FRONT VIEW.

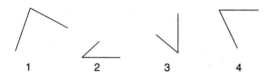

Part 3: Angle Ranking

Questions 31–45

In this section you will compare four *interior* angles and rank them according to size from *small* to *large*. Select the answer with the correct ranking.

Example (Do not mark the answer to this example on the answer sheet)

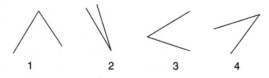

    A. 2-3-1-4
    B. 3-4-2-1
    C. 1-4-3-2
    D. 2-3-4-1

The correct ranking of the angles from small to large is 2-3-4-1; therefore, alternative D is correct. Now proceed to the questions, marking the correct alternative on your answer sheet.

31.

    A. 4-3-2-1
    B. 4-2-3-1
    C. 2-4-3-1
    D. 2-3-1-4

32.

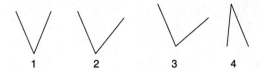

A. 4-1-3-2
B. 4-1-2-3
C. 1-4-2-3
D. 1-4-3-2

33.

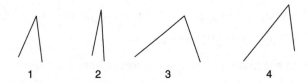

A. 2-1-4-3
B. 2-1-3-4
C. 1-2-3-4
D. 3-4-1-2

34.

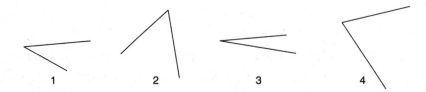

A. 2-4-1-3
B. 2-4-3-1
C. 3-1-4-2
D. 3-1-2-4

35.

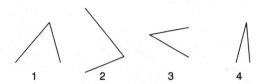

A. 2-1-3-4
B. 3-4-1-2
C. 4-3-1-2
D. 4-1-3-2

36.

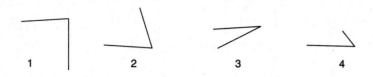

    1   2   3   4

    A. 4-3-2-1
    B. 3-4-2-1
    C. 3-4-1-2
    D. 4-3-1-2

37.

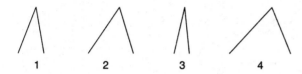

    1   2   3   4

    A. 3-1-2-4
    B. 3-1-4-2
    C. 1-3-2-4
    D. 3-2-1-4

38.

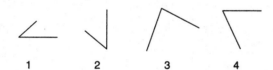

    1   2   3   4

    A. 1-2-3-4
    B. 2-1-3-4
    C. 1-2-4-3
    D. 2-1-3-4

39.

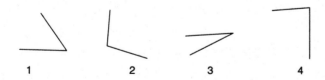

    1   2   3   4

    A. 3-2-1-4
    B. 2-4-1-3
    C. 3-1-2-4
    D. 3-1-4-2

40.

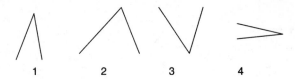

A. 1-4-3-2
B. 4-1-2-3
C. 4-1-3-2
D. 4-3-1-2

41.

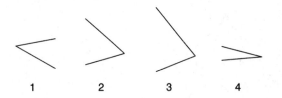

A. 4-1-3-2
B. 4-1-2-3
C. 4-2-1-3
D. 4-2-3-1

42.

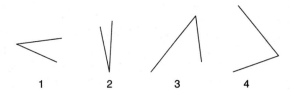

A. 2-3-1-4
B. 2-3-4-1
C. 2-1-3-4
D. 2-1-4-3

43.

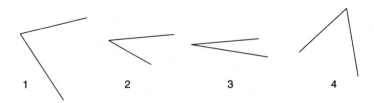

A. 2-3-1-4
B. 3-2-1-4
C. 2-3-4-1
D. 3-2-4-1

44.

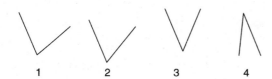

1   2   3   4

    A. 4-3-2-1
    B. 4-3-1-2
    C. 1-2-3-4
    D. 3-4-1-2

45.

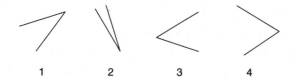

1   2   3   4

    A. 2-1-3-4
    B. 2-1-4-3
    C. 1-3-2-4
    D. 1-2-3-4

Part 4: Paper Folding

Questions 46–60

In this section, you will examine a flat square of paper that has been folded one or more times. A hole is punched into the paper after the last fold. You are to mentally unfold the paper and choose the answer that shows the position(s) of the hole(s) on the original square. There is only one correct answer for each question. The following rules apply:

➤ Broken lines show the original position of the paper.
➤ Solid lines indicate the position of the folded paper.
➤ The paper is never twisted or turned.
➤ The folded paper always stays within the margins of the original square.
➤ The paper may be folded one to three times.

Example (Do not mark the answer to this example on the answer sheet)

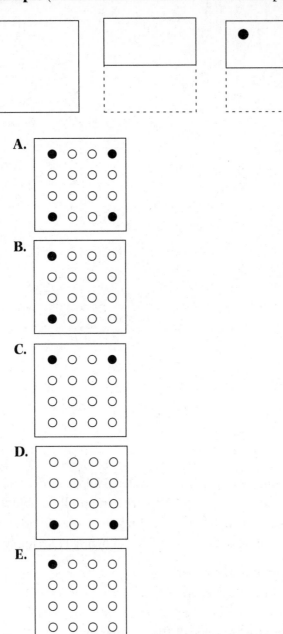

In the example, the first figure shows the original paper. The second figure shows the result of the fold. The third figure shows the position of the punched hole on the folded paper. When the paper is unfolded, the pattern of the holes on the original paper is shown in answer B. The answer has two holes on the top and bottom left since the paper was two thicknesses when punched in the top left.

46.

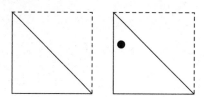

A.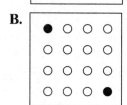

B.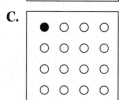

C.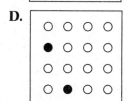

D.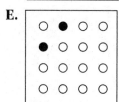

E.

47.

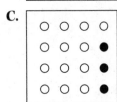

A.

B.

C.

D.

E.

48.

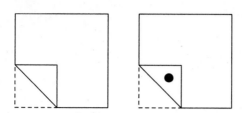

A.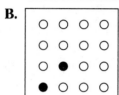

B.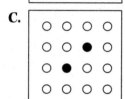

C.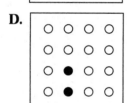

D.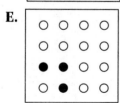

E.

49.

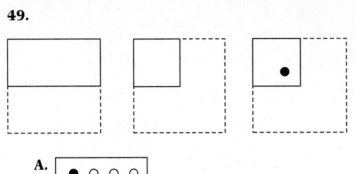

A.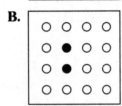

B.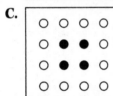

C.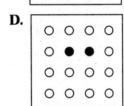

D.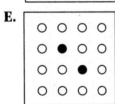

E.

50.

A.

B.

C.

D.

E.

51.

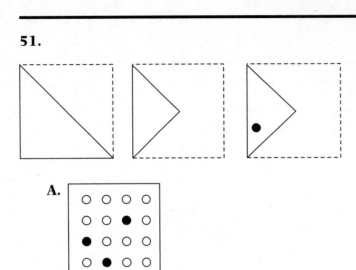

A.

B.

C.

D.

E.

52.

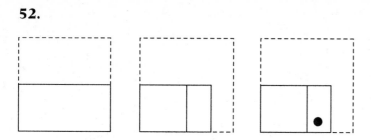

A.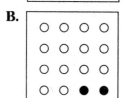

B.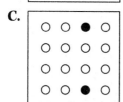

C.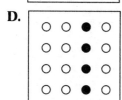

D.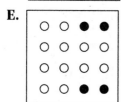

E.

53.

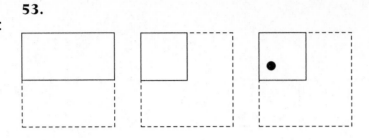

A.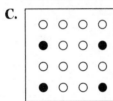

B.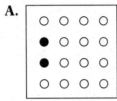

C.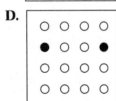

D.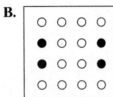

E.

54.

A.

B.

C.

D.

E.

55.

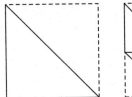
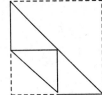
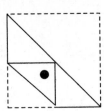

A.

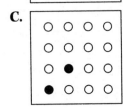

B.

C.

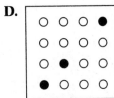

D.

E.

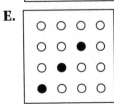

56.

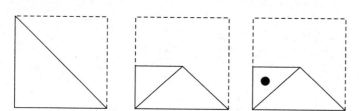

A.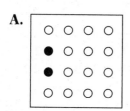

B.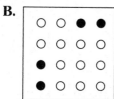

C.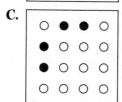

D.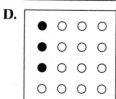

E.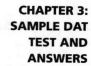

57.

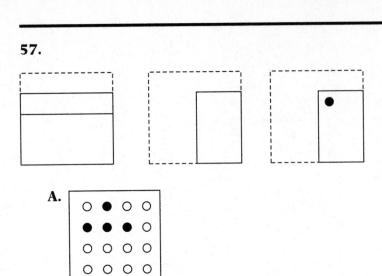

A.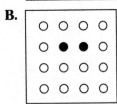

B.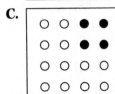

C.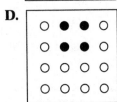

D.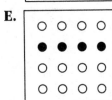

E.

58.

59.

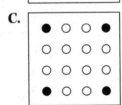

A.

B.

C.

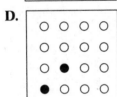

D.

E.

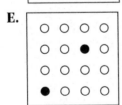

60.

A.

B.

C.

D.

E.

Part 5: Cube Stacking

Questions 61–75

In this section, you will see a figure that has been made by cementing a number of cubes of the same size together. After being cemented together, the figure is painted on all sides, except for the bottom, on which it is resting. The only hidden cubes are those needed to support other cubes. You will examine each figure to determine how many cubes in the figure have a given number of their sides painted: none, one, two, three, four, or five sides.

Example (Do not mark the answer to this example on the answer sheet)

Figure K

In Figure K, how many cubes have four of their exposed sides painted?
A. 1 cube
B. 2 cubes
C. 3 cubes
D. 4 cubes
E. 5 cubes

There are four cubes in Figure K: three that are visible and one that is invisible and is supporting the top cube. The invisible cube has only two sides painted. The top cube has five sides painted. The two side cubes each have four sides painted, so the answer is B.

Proceed to the questions. Select the answer that corresponds to the number of cubes that have the different numbers of sides painted. Remember, after being cemented together, each figure was PAINTED ON ALL EXPOSED SIDES EXCEPT THE BOTTOM.

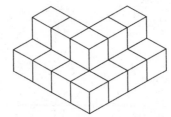

Figure A

61. In Figure A, how many cubes have one of their exposed sides painted?
A. 1 cube
B. 2 cubes
C. 3 cubes
D. 4 cubes
E. 5 cubes

62. In Figure A, how many cubes have two of their exposed sides painted?
    A. 3 cubes
    B. 4 cubes
    C. 5 cubes
    D. 6 cubes
    E. 7 cubes

63. In Figure A, how many cubes have three of their exposed sides painted?
    A. 3 cubes
    B. 4 cubes
    C. 5 cubes
    D. 6 cubes
    E. 7 cubes

64. In Figure A, how many cubes have four of their exposed sides painted?
    A. 1 cube
    B. 2 cubes
    C. 3 cubes
    D. 4 cubes
    E. 5 cubes

65. In Figure A, how many cubes have NO exposed sides painted?
    A. 1 cube
    B. 2 cubes
    C. 3 cubes
    D. 4 cubes
    E. 5 cubes

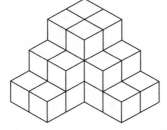

Figure B

66. In Figure B, how many cubes have NO exposed sides painted?
    A. 1 cube
    B. 2 cubes
    C. 3 cubes
    D. 4 cubes
    E. 5 cubes

67. In Figure B, how many cubes have one of their exposed sides painted?

    A. 4 cubes

    B. 5 cubes

    C. 6 cubes

    D. 7 cubes

    E. 8 cubes

68. In Figure B, how many cubes have two of their exposed sides painted?

    A. 1 cube

    B. 2 cubes

    C. 3 cubes

    D. 4 cubes

    E. 5 cubes

69. In Figure B, how many cubes have three of their exposed sides painted?

    A. 8 cubes

    B. 9 cubes

    C. 10 cubes

    D. 11 cubes

    E. 12 cubes

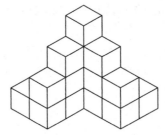

Figure C

70. In Figure C, how many cubes have NO exposed sides painted?

    A. 0 cubes

    B. 1 cube

    C. 2 cubes

    D. 3 cubes

    E. 4 cubes

71. In Figure C, how many cubes have only one of their exposed sides painted?

    A. 0 cubes

    B. 1 cube

    C. 2 cubes

    D. 3 cubes

    E. 4 cubes

72. In Figure C, how many cubes have only two of their exposed sides painted?
- **A.** 5 cubes
- **B.** 6 cubes
- **C.** 7 cubes
- **D.** 8 cubes
- **E.** 9 cubes

73. In Figure C, how many cubes have only three of their exposed sides painted?
- **A.** 0 cubes
- **B.** 1 cube
- **C.** 2 cubes
- **D.** 3 cubes
- **E.** 4 cubes

74. In Figure C, how many cubes have only four of their exposed sides painted?
- **A.** 3 cubes
- **B.** 4 cubes
- **C.** 5 cubes
- **D.** 6 cubes
- **E.** 7 cubes

75. In Figure C, how many cubes have five of their exposed sides painted?
- **A.** 1 cube
- **B.** 2 cubes
- **C.** 3 cubes
- **D.** 4 cubes
- **E.** 5 cubes

Part 6: Form Creation

Questions 76–90

In this section you will see a flat pattern that you will mentally fold into a three-dimensional figure. The original flat pattern is shown to the left in each question and is followed by four possible figures. Choose among these for the correct figure into which the flat pattern can be folded. There is only one correct answer.

Example (Do not mark the answer to this example on the answer sheet)

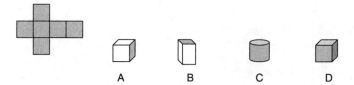

The flat figure is a design for a cube-shaped box. All sides are shaded. Choice D shows what the figure would look like in three dimensions. Choice A is also a cube, but not all sides are shaded.

76.

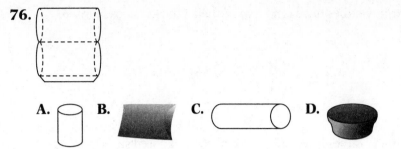

A.   B.   C.   D.

77.

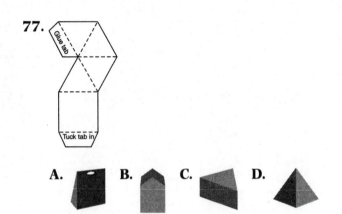

A.   B.   C.   D.

78.

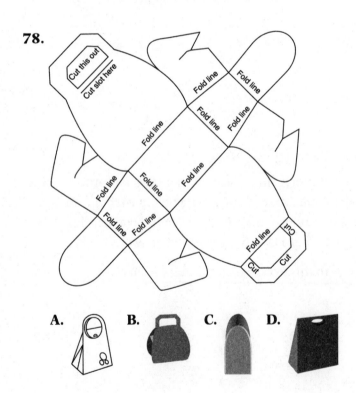

A.   B.   C.   D.

79.

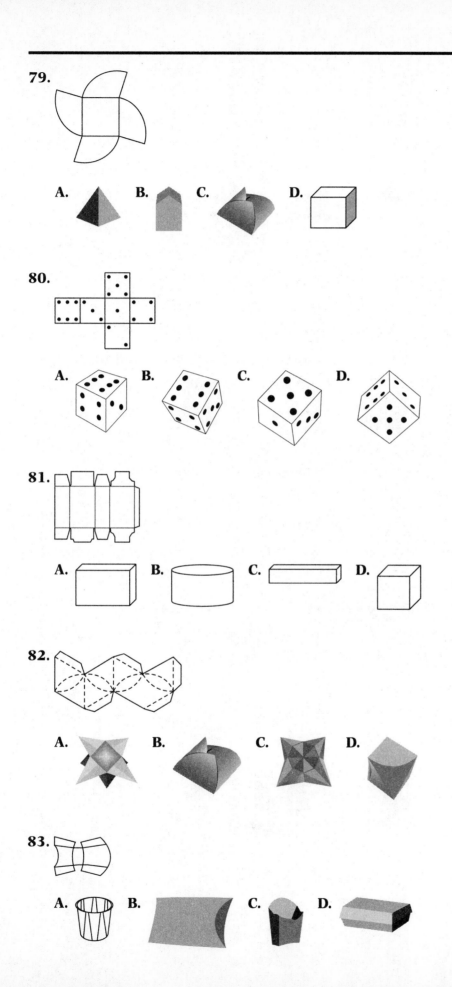

80.

81.

82.

83.

84.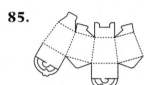

A.   B. 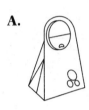   C.   D.

85.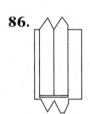

A. 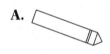   B. 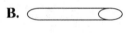   C.   D.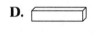

86.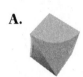

A.   B.   C.   D.

87.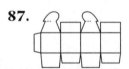

A.   B.   C.   D.

88.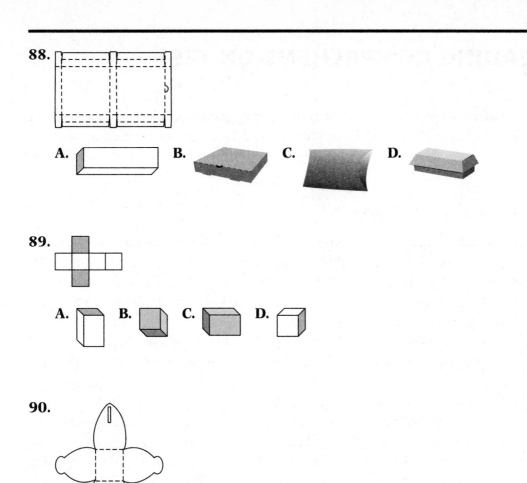

89.

    A.   B.   C.   D.

90.

    A.   B.   C.   D.

READING COMPREHENSION TEST

Directions: This section consists of three reading passages, followed by a series of questions or incomplete statements. Choose the correct answer for each question or incomplete statement. There are **50 items**, and you will have **60 minutes** to complete them.

Lip and Oral Cavity Cancer

1. The oral cavity extends from the skin-vermilion junctions of the anterior lips to the junction of the hard and soft palates above and to the line of circumvallate papillae below and is divided into the following specific areas: lip, anterior two-thirds of tongue, buccal mucosa, floor of mouth, lower gingival, retromolar trigone, upper gingival, and hard palate.

2. The main routes of lymph node drainage are into the first station nodes (i.e., buccinator, jugulodigastric, submandibular, and submental). Sites close to the midline often drain bilaterally. Second station nodes include the parotid, jugular, and the upper and lower posterior cervical nodes.

3. Early cancers (stage I and stage II) of the lip and oral cavity are highly curable by surgery or by radiation therapy, and the choice of treatment is dictated by the anticipated functional and cosmetic results of treatment and by the availability of the particular expertise required of the surgeon or radiation oncologist for the individual patient. The presence of a positive margin or a tumor depth of more than 5 mm significantly increases the risk of local recurrence and suggests that combined modality treatment may be beneficial.

4. Advanced cancers (stage III and stage IV) of the lip and oral cavity represent a wide spectrum of challenges for the surgeon and radiation oncologist. Except for patients with small T3 lesions and no regional lymph node and no distant metastases or who have no lymph nodes larger than 2 cm in diameter, for whom treatment by radiation therapy alone or surgery alone might be appropriate, most patients with stage III or stage IV tumors are candidates for treatment by a combination of surgery and radiation therapy. Furthermore, because local recurrence and/or distant metastases are common in this group of patients, they should be considered for clinical trials. Such trials evaluate the potential role of radiation modifiers or combination chemotherapy combined with surgery and/or radiation therapy.

5. Patients with head and neck cancers have an increased chance of developing a second primary tumor of the upper aerodigestive tract. A study has shown that daily treatment of these patients with moderate doses of isotretinoin (13-cis-retinoic acid) for one year can significantly reduce the incidence of second tumors. No survival advantage has yet been demonstrated, however, in part due to recurrence and death from the primary malignancy. An additional trial has shown no benefit of retinyl palmitate or retinyl palmitate plus beta-carotene when compared to retinoic acid alone.

6. The rate of curability of cancers of the lip and oral cavity varies depending on the stage and specific site. Most patients present with early cancers of the lip, which are highly curable by surgery or by radiation therapy with cure rates of 90 to 100 percent. Small cancers of the retromolar trigone, hard palate, and upper gingiva are highly curable by either radiation therapy or surgery with survival rates of as much as 100 percent. Local control rates of as much as 90 percent can be achieved with either radiation therapy or surgery in small cancers of the anterior tongue, the floor of the mouth, and buccal mucosa.

7. Moderately advanced and advanced cancers of the lip also can be controlled effectively by surgery or radiation therapy or a combination of these. The choice of treatment is generally dictated by the anticipated functional and cosmetic results of the treatment. Moderately advanced lesions of the retromolar trigone without evidence of spread to cervical lymph nodes are usually curable and have shown local control rates of as much as 90 percent; such lesions of the hard palate, upper gingiva, and buccal mucosa have a local control rate of as much as 80 percent. In the absence of clinical evidence of spread to cervical lymph nodes, moderately advanced lesions of the floor of the mouth and anterior tongue are generally curable with survival rates of as much as 70 percent and 65 percent, respectively.

8. Depending on the site and extent of the primary tumor and the status of the lymph nodes, some general considerations for the treatment of lip and oral cavity cancer include surgery alone, radiation therapy alone, or a combination of the two.

9. For lesions of the oral cavity, surgery must adequately encompass all of the gross as well as the presumed microscopic extent of the disease. If regional nodes are positive, cervical node dissection is usually done in continuity. With modern approaches, the surgeon can successfully ablate large posterior oral cavity tumors and with reconstructive methods can achieve satisfactory functional results. Prosthodontic rehabilitation is important, particularly in early stage cancers, to assure the best quality of life.

10. Radiation therapy for lip and oral cavity cancers can be administered by external-beam radiation therapy (EBRT) or interstitial implantation alone, but for many sites the use of both modalities produces better control and functional results. Small superficial cancers can be very successfully treated by local implantation using any one of several radioactive sources, by intraoral cone radiation therapy, or by electrons. Larger lesions are frequently managed using EBRT to include the primary site and regional lymph nodes, even if they are not clinically involved. Supplementation with interstitial radiation sources may be necessary to achieve adequate doses to large primary tumors and/or bulky nodal metastases. A review of published clinical results of radical radiation therapy for head and neck cancer suggests a significant loss of local control when the administration of radiation therapy was prolonged; therefore, lengthening of standard treatment schedules should be avoided whenever possible.

11. Early cancers (stage I and stage II) of the lip, floor of the mouth, and retromolar trigone are highly curable by surgery or radiation therapy. The choice of treatment is dictated by the anticipated functional and cosmetic results. Availability of the particular expertise required of the surgeon or radiation oncologist for the individual patient is also a factor in treatment choice.

12. Advanced cancers (stage III and stage IV) of the lip, floor of the mouth, and retromolar trigone represent a wide spectrum of challenges for the surgeon and radiation oncologists. Most patients with stage III or stage IV tumors are candidates for treatment by a combination of surgery and radiation therapy. Patients with small T3 lesions and no regional lymph nodes and no distant metastases, or patients who have no lymph nodes larger than 2 cm in diameter, for whom treatment by radiation therapy alone or surgery alone might be appropriate, are the exceptions. Because local recurrence and/or distant metastases are common in this group of patients, they should be considered for clinical trials that are evaluating the potential role of radiation modifiers to improve local control or decrease morbidity and the role of combinations of chemotherapy with surgery and/or radiation therapy both to improve local control and to decrease the frequency of distant metastases.

13. Early cancers of the buccal mucosa are equally curable by radiation therapy or by adequate excision. Patient factors and local expertise influence the choice of treatment. Larger cancers require composite resection with reconstruction of the defect by pedicle flaps.

14. Early lesions (T1 and T2) of the anterior tongue may be managed by surgery or by radiation therapy alone. Both modalities produce 70 to 85 percent cure rates in early lesions. Moderate excisions of tongue, even hemiglossectomy, can often result in little speech disability provided the wound closure is such that the tongue is not bound down. If, however, the resection is more extensive, problems may include aspiration of liquids and solids and difficulty in swallowing in addition to speech difficulties. Occasionally, patients with tumor of the tongue require almost total glossectomy. Large lesions generally require combined surgical and radiation treatment. The control rates for larger lesions are about 30 to 40 percent. According to clinical and radiological evidence of involvement, cancers of the lower gingiva that are exophytic and amenable to adequate local excision may be excised to include portions of bone. More advanced lesions require segmental bone resection, hemimandibulectomy, or maxillectomy, depending on the extent of the lesion and its location.

15. Early lesions of the upper gingiva or hard palate without bone involvement can be treated with equal effectiveness by surgery or by radiation therapy alone. Advanced infiltrative and ulcerating lesions should be treated by a combination of radiation therapy and surgery. Most primary cancers of the hard palate are of minor salivary gland origin. Primary squamous cell carcinoma of the hard palate is uncommon, and these tumors generally represent invasion of squamous cell carcinoma arising on the upper gingiva, which is much more common. Management of squamous cell carcinoma of the upper gingiva and hard palate are usually considered together. Surgical treatment of cancer of the hard palate usually

requires excision of underlying bone producing an opening into the antrum. This defect can be filled and covered with a dental prosthesis, which is a maneuver that restores satisfactory swallowing and speech.

16. Patients who smoke while on radiation therapy appear to have lower response rates and shorter survival durations than those who do not; therefore, patients should be counseled to stop smoking before beginning radiation therapy. Dental status evaluation should be performed prior to therapy to prevent late sequelae.

1. What is the likely treatment for a patient with stage III cancer of the retromolar trigone?
   A. Radiation therapy alone
   B. Surgery alone
   C. Chemotherapy alone
   D. A combination of surgery and radiation therapy
   E. There is no treatment option for stage III cancer of the retromolar trigone.

2. Which of the following is NOT a first station node for lymph node drainage?
   A. Submental
   B. Submandibular
   C. Parotid
   D. Jugulodigastric
   E. Buccinator

3. According to the passage, why should a dental evaluation be performed before a patient begins treatment for cancer of the lip or oral cavity?
   A. To assess the probability of success for a particular course of treatment
   B. To determine whether the patient requires a glossectomy
   C. To measure for dental prosthesis
   D. To prevent a pathological condition resulting from the disease
   E. To evaluate tumor depth

4. What is the cure rate for radiation therapy alone in a T2 lesion of the anterior tongue?
   A. 70 to 85 percent
   B. 30 to 40 percent
   C. 90 to 100 percent
   D. 65 percent
   E. 80 percent

5. What is the most likely origin of a primary cancer of the hard palate?
   A. The minor salivary gland
   B. The lower gingiva
   C. The primary squamous cell
   D. The buccal mucosa
   E. The lower posterior cervical nodes

6. Each of the following moderate lesion locations has a local control rate of higher than 75 percent, provided that there is no spread to the cervical lymph nodes, EXCEPT
   A. the retromolar trigone
   B. the buccal mucosa
   C. the upper gingiva
   D. the hard palate
   E. the anterior tongue

7. According to the passage, a patient with stage I cancer of the lip should consider which of the following in determining course of treatment?
   A. The cosmetic results of the treatment
   B. The convenience of the location for treatment
   C. The survival rate for the treatment
   D. The availability of home health care posttreatment
   E. The possible complications of the treatment

8. Cancer of the hard palate treated with surgery usually requires which of the following procedures?
   A. Glossectomy
   B. Excising bone to open the antrum
   C. Maxillectomy
   D. Segmental bone resection
   E. Hemimandibulectomy

9. Which of the following cancers has the lowest cure rate?
   A. Moderately advanced lesions of the retromolar trigone without evidence of spread to cervical lymph nodes
   B. Small cancers of the buccal mucosa
   C. Small cancers of the retromolar trigone
   D. Moderately advanced lesions of the floor of the mouth without evidence of spread to cervical lymph nodes
   E. Early cancers of the lip

10. A stage IV oral cavity patient might be considered for a clinical trial because
    A. it is the best option for survival
    B. it offers treatments that are not normally available and may have better results
    C. recurrence of cancer has a higher probability in these patients
    D. this type of cancer is the most challenging to treat successfully
    E. researchers can learn more from the difficulties presented by treating stage IV cancers

11. Patients undergoing radiation therapy are advised to stop smoking prior to beginning treatment because smoking
    A. increases the probability of the patient needing dental prosthesis posttreatment
    B. increases the probability of later recurrences of cancer

    C. increases the probability of metastasis

    D. can cause dangerous side effects when combined with radiation therapy

    E. may lower long-term survival rates

12. The author would most likely agree that patients with neck cancers should

    A. undergo both surgical and radiation therapy

    B. be treated with retinyl palmitate

    C. be placed in clinical trials due to the low survival rate of this type of cancer

    D. be treated with retinyl palmitate plus beta-carotene

    E. be treated with isotretinoin for a period of one year

13. Which of the following is a proper treatment for a small superficial tumor of the lip?

    A. External-beam radiation therapy of the primary site and regional lymph nodes

    B. Local implantation by intraoral cone radiation therapy

    C. Chemotherapy, followed by interstitial radiation

    D. Surgical removal of the tumor mass, followed by EBRT

    E. Tumor excision, followed by chemotherapy

14. A hemiglossectomy is a(n)

    A. removal of the anterior surface of the tongue

    B. surgery to remove a tumor on the lower gingiva

    C. excision of one side of the tongue

    D. excision of underlying bone producing an opening into the antrum

    E. reconstruction by pedicle flaps

15. An extensive resection of the tongue might cause

    A. problems with swallowing

    B. a loss of function in the lower gingiva

    C. difficulty with managing secretions

    D. excess production of saliva

    E. external cosmetic abnormalities

16. A hemimandibulectomy is used to treat which of the following?

    A. A squamous cell carcinoma arising on the upper gingiva

    B. A cancer of the hard palate

    C. A T1 lesion of the anterior tongue

    D. An advanced cancer of the lower gingiva

    E. An early cancer of the buccal mucosa

Infection Control

1. In the United States, an estimated 9 million persons work in healthcare professions, including approximately 168,000 dentists, 112,000 registered dental hygienists, 218,000 dental assistants, and 53,000 dental laboratory technicians. In this report, dental healthcare personnel (DHCP) refers to all paid and unpaid personnel in the dental healthcare setting who might be occupationally exposed to infectious materials, including body substances and contaminated supplies, equipment, environmental surfaces, water, or air. DHCP include dentists, dental hygienists, dental assistants, dental laboratory technicians (in-office and commercial), students and trainees, contractual personnel, and other persons not directly involved in patient care but potentially exposed to infectious agents (e.g., administrative, clerical, housekeeping, maintenance, or volunteer personnel). Recommendations in this report are designed to prevent or reduce potential for disease transmission from patient to DHCP, from DHCP to patient, and from patient to patient. Although these guidelines focus mainly on outpatient, ambulatory dental healthcare settings, the recommended infection-control practices are applicable to all settings in which dental treatment is provided.

2. Dental patients and DHCP can be exposed to pathogenic microorganisms including cytomegalovirus (CMV), HBV, HCV, herpes simplex virus types 1 and 2, HIV, *Mycobacterium tuberculosis*, staphylococci, streptococci, and other viruses and bacteria that colonize or infect the oral cavity and respiratory tract. These organisms can be transmitted in dental settings through direct contact with blood, oral fluids, or other patient materials; indirect contact with contaminated objects (e.g., instruments, equipment, or environmental surfaces); contact of conjunctival, nasal, or oral mucosa with droplets (e.g., spatter) containing microorganisms generated from an infected person and propelled a short distance (e.g., by coughing, sneezing, or talking); and inhalation of airborne microorganisms that can remain suspended in the air for long periods.

3. Infection through any of these routes requires that all of the following conditions be present: a pathogenic organism of sufficient virulence and in adequate numbers to cause disease; a reservoir or source that allows the pathogen to survive and multiply (e.g., blood); a mode of transmission from the source to the host; a portal of entry through which the pathogen can enter the host; and a susceptible host (i.e., one who is not immune). Occurrence of these events provides the chain of infection. Effective infection-control strategies prevent disease transmission by interrupting one or more links in the chain.

4. Previous CDC recommendations regarding infection control for dentistry focused primarily on the risk of transmission of blood-borne pathogens among DHCP and patients and use of universal precautions to reduce that risk. Universal precautions were based on the concept that all blood and body fluids that might be contaminated with blood should be treated as infectious because patients with blood-borne infections can be asymptomatic or unaware they are infected. Preventive practices used to reduce blood exposures, particularly percutaneous exposures, include careful handling of sharp instruments, use of rubber dams to minimize blood spattering, hand washing, and use of protective barriers (e.g., gloves, masks, protective eyewear, and gowns).

5. The relevance of universal precautions to other aspects of disease transmission was recognized, and in 1996, CDC expanded the concept and changed the term to *standard precautions*. Standard precautions integrate and expand the elements of

universal precautions into a standard of care designed to protect HCP and patients from pathogens that can be spread by blood or any other body fluid, excretion, or secretion. Standard precautions apply to contact with blood; all body fluids, secretions, and excretions (except sweat), regardless of whether they contain blood; nonintact skin; and mucous membranes. Saliva has always been considered a potentially infectious material in dental infection control; thus, no operational difference exists in clinical dental practice between universal precautions and standard precautions.

6. In addition to standard precautions, other measures (e.g., expanded or transmission-based precautions) might be necessary to prevent potential spread of certain diseases (e.g., TB, influenza, and varicella) that are transmitted through airborne, droplet, or contact transmission (e.g., sneezing, coughing, and contact with skin). When acutely ill with these diseases, patients do not usually seek routine dental outpatient care. Nonetheless, a general understanding of precautions for diseases transmitted by all routes is critical because some DHCP are hospital-based or work part-time in hospital settings, patients infected with these diseases might seek urgent treatment at outpatient dental offices, and DHCP might become infected with these diseases. Necessary transmission-based precautions might include patient placement (e.g., isolation), adequate room ventilation, respiratory protection (e.g., N-95 masks) for DHCP, or postponement of nonemergency dental procedures.

7. DHCP should also be familiar with the hierarchy of controls that categorizes and prioritizes prevention strategies. For blood-borne pathogens, engineering controls that eliminate or isolate the hazard (e.g., puncture-resistant sharps containers or needle-retraction devices) are the primary strategies for protecting DHCP and patients. Where engineering controls are not available or appropriate, work-practice controls that result in safer behaviors (e.g., one-hand needle recapping or not using fingers for cheek retraction while using sharp instruments or suturing) and use of personal protective equipment (PPE) (e.g., protective eyewear, gloves, and mask) can prevent exposure. In addition, administrative controls (e.g., policies, procedures, and enforcement measures targeted at reducing the risk of exposure to infectious persons) are a priority for certain pathogens (e.g., *M. tuberculosis*), particularly those spread by airborne or droplet routes.

8. DHCP are at risk for exposure to, and possible infection with, infectious organisms. Immunizations substantially reduce both the number of DHCP susceptible to these diseases and the potential for disease transmission to other DHCP and patients. Thus, immunizations are an essential part of prevention and infection-control programs for DHCP, and a comprehensive immunization policy should be implemented for all dental healthcare facilities. The Advisory Committee on Immunization Practices (ACIP) provides national guidelines for immunization of HCP, which includes DHCP. Dental practice immunization policies should incorporate current state and federal regulations as well as recommendations from the U.S. Public Health Service and professional organizations.

9. On the basis of documented healthcare-associated transmission, HCP are considered to be at substantial risk for acquiring or transmitting hepatitis B, influenza, measles, mumps, rubella, and varicella. All of these diseases are vaccine-preventable. ACIP recommends that all HCP be vaccinated or have documented immunity to these diseases. ACIP does not recommend routine immunization of HCP against TB (i.e., inoculation with bacillus Calmette-Guérin vaccine) or hepatitis A. No vaccine exists for HCV. ACIP guidelines also provide recommendations regarding immunization of HCP with special conditions (e.g., pregnancy, HIV infection, or diabetes).

10. Immunization of DHCP before they are placed at risk for exposure remains the most efficient and effective use of vaccines in healthcare settings. Some educational institutions and infection-control programs provide immunization schedules for students and DHCP. OSHA requires that employers make hepatitis B vaccination available to all employees who have potential contact with blood or other potentially infectious materials (OPIM). Employers are also required to follow CDC recommendations for vaccinations, evaluation, and follow-up procedures. Non-patient-care staff (e.g., administrative or housekeeping) might be included, depending on their potential risk of coming into contact with blood or OPIM. Employers are also required to ensure that employees who decline to accept hepatitis B vaccination sign an appropriate declination statement. DHCP unable or unwilling to be vaccinated as required or recommended should be educated regarding their exposure risks, infection-control policies and procedures for the facility, and the management of work-related illness and work restrictions (if appropriate) for exposed or infected DHCP.

11. Avoiding exposure to blood and OPIM, as well as protection by immunization, remain primary strategies for reducing occupationally acquired infections, but occupational exposures can still occur. A combination of standard precautions, engineering, work practice, and administrative controls is the best means to minimize occupational exposures.

12. Dental practices should develop a written infection-control program to prevent or reduce the risk of disease transmission. Such a program should include establishment and implementation of policies, procedures, and practices (in conjunction with selection and use of technologies and products) to prevent work-related injuries and illnesses among DHCP as well as healthcare-associated infections among patients. The program should embody principles of infection control and occupational health, reflect current science, and adhere to relevant federal, state, and local regulations and statutes. An infection-control coordinator (e.g., dentist or other DHCP) knowledgeable or willing to be trained should be assigned responsibility for coordinating the program. The effectiveness of the infection-control program should be evaluated on a day-to-day basis and over time to help ensure that policies, procedures, and practices are useful, efficient, and successful.

13. Although the infection-control coordinator remains responsible for overall management of the program, creating and maintaining a safe work environment ultimately requires the commitment and accountability of all DHCP. This report is

designed to provide guidance to DHCP for preventing disease transmission in dental healthcare settings, for promoting a safe working environment, and for assisting dental practices in developing and implementing infection-control programs. These programs should be followed in addition to practices and procedures for worker protection required by the Occupational Safety and Health Administration's (OSHA) standards for occupational exposure to blood-borne pathogens, including instituting controls to protect employees from exposure to blood or OPIM and requiring implementation of a written exposure-control plan, annual employee training, HBV vaccinations, and postexposure follow-up. Interpretations and enforcement procedures are available to help DHCP apply this OSHA standard in practice. Also, manufacturer's Material Safety Data Sheets (MSDS) should be consulted regarding correct procedures for handling or working with hazardous chemicals.

17. According to the passage, who is responsible for creating a safe work environment?
   A. All DHCP
   B. OSHA
   C. Employers of HCP
   D. Federal and local authorities
   E. ACIP

18. An administrative control is a
   A. policy, the purpose of which is to reduce the risk of infection
   B. procedure, the purpose of which is to prevent the spread of airborne infection
   C. training program to educate DHCP about tuberculosis
   D. behavior, such as wearing PPE, to prevent infection
   E. hierarchy of controls to categorize and prioritize prevention strategies

19. According to the passage, when is the best time to vaccinate DHCP?
   A. Immediately following a potential exposure
   B. On a regular schedule
   C. Vaccinations are optional and may be done at any time
   D. Before placing DHCP at risk of exposure
   E. When required by OSHA

20. Which of the following is NOT a precaution against transmission of varicella?
   A. Putting the patient in a properly ventilated room
   B. Allowing only DHCP who have had varicella to treat the patient
   C. Having DHCP wear N-95 masks
   D. Deferring any nonessential procedures
   E. Isolating the patient

21. Herpes simplex virus type 2 may be transmitted by any of the following EXCEPT
   A. inhalation of airborne microorganisms
   B. direct contact with oral fluids
   C. nasal contact with spatter
   D. indirect contact with contaminated equipment
   E. touching unbroken skin without gloves

22. The purpose of preventive practices is to
  A. reduce the risk of exposure to blood that might contain pathogens
  B. encourage safe handling of sharp instruments
  C. minimize blood spattering
  D. train DHCP to use protective barriers
  E. prevent inhalation of airborne microorganisms

23. One type of engineering control is
  A. a training program
  B. using non-latex gloves
  C. a container for needles that cannot be punctured
  D. to recap needles with one hand
  E. adequate room ventilation

24. To which of the following microorganisms are DCHP at risk of exposure?
  A. Herpes simplex virus type 1
  B. Cytomegalovirus
  C. HIV
  D. Streptococci
  E. All of the above

25. Which of the following is NOT preventable by vaccine?
  A. Rubella
  B. Varicella
  C. Hepatitis B
  D. HCV
  E. Measles

26. The CDC changed from universal to standard precautions because
  A. the previous term was too broadly defined
  B. it realized that universal precautions could apply to other aspects of disease transmission
  C. the latter term was more specific to preventing blood-borne illnesses
  D. the previous term did not adequately cover the risks to which DHCP are exposed
  E. universal precautions did not include transmission through saliva

27. Which of the following is NOT in the chain of infection?
  A. Entry portal to the host
  B. Adequate time for the host to infect others
  C. A host who is vulnerable to the infection
  D. Mode of transmission to the host
  E. Source that allows the pathogen to grow

28. A work-practice control is a
  A. policy, the purpose of which is to reduce the risk of infection
  B. procedure, the purpose of which is to prevent the spread of airborne infection
  C. training program to educate DHCP about tuberculosis

    D. behavior, such as wearing PPE, to prevent infection

    E. hierarchy of controls to categorize and prioritize prevention strategies

29. What organization provides national immunization guidelines for DHCP?

    A. ACIP

    B. NIH

    C. The Dental Association of America

    D. U.S. Public Health Service

    E. CDC

30. DCHP includes each of the following EXCEPT

    A. dental hygienists

    B. dental laboratory technicians

    C. a person who volunteers in a dental office

    D. dentists

    E. dental supply manufacturers

31. An infection-control program should be evaluated

    A. yearly

    B. monthly

    C. daily

    D. whenever an exposure incident occurs

    E. weekly

32. Standard precautions apply to

    A. sweat

    B. saliva

    C. toothpaste

    D. disinfectants

    E. room ventilation

33. Which of the following agencies provides practices for worker safety?

    A. HCV

    B. MSDS

    C. DHCP

    D. OPIM

    E. OSHA

Practical Oral Care for People with Autism

    1. Autism is a complex developmental disability that impairs communication and social, behavioral, and intellectual functioning. Some people with the disorder appear distant, aloof, or detached from other people or from their surroundings. Others do not react appropriately to common verbal and social cues, such as a parent's tone of voice or smile. Obsessive routines, repetitive behaviors, unpredictable body movements, and self-injurious behavior may all be symptoms that complicate dental care. Autism varies widely in symptoms and severity, and some people have coexisting conditions such as intellectual disability or epilepsy. They can be among the most challenging of patients, but providing oral care to people with autism merely requires adaptation of the skills you use every day. In fact, most people with mild or moderate forms of autism can be treated successfully in the general practice setting. Making a difference in the oral health of a person with autism may go slowly at first, but determination can bring positive results and invaluable rewards.

2. Communication and mental capabilities are central concerns when treating people with autism. Before the appointment, obtain and review the patient's medical history. Consultation with physicians, family, and caregivers is essential to assembling an accurate medical history. Also, determine who can legally provide informed consent for treatment. Talk with the parent or caregiver to determine your patient's intellectual and functional abilities, and then communicate with the patient at a level he or she can understand. Use a "tell-show-do" approach to providing care. Start by explaining each procedure before it occurs. Take the time to show what you have explained, such as the instruments you will use and how they work. Demonstrations can encourage some patients to be more cooperative.

3. Behavior problems, which may include hyperactivity and quick frustration, can complicate oral health care for patients with autism. The invasive nature of oral care may trigger violent and self-injurious behavior such as temper tantrums or head banging. Plan a desensitization appointment to help the patient become familiar with the office, staff, and equipment through a step-by-step process. These steps may take several visits to accomplish.

4. Have the patient sit alone in the dental chair to become familiar with the treatment setting. Some patients may refuse to sit in the chair and choose instead to sit on the operator's stool. Once your patient is seated, begin a cursory examination using your fingers. Next, use a toothbrush to brush the teeth and gain additional access to the patient's mouth. The familiarity of a toothbrush will help your patient feel comfortable and provide you with an opportunity to further examine the mouth. When the patient is prepared for treatment, make the appointment short and positive.

5. Pay special attention to the treatment setting. Keep dental instruments out of sight and light out of your patient's eyes. Praise and reinforce good behavior after each step of a procedure. Ignore inappropriate behavior as much as you can. Try to gain cooperation in the least restrictive manner. Some patients' behavior may improve if they bring comfort items such as a stuffed animal or a blanket. Asking the caregiver to sit nearby or hold the patient's hand may be helpful as well.

6. Use immobilization techniques only when absolutely necessary to protect the patient and staff during dental treatment—not as a convenience. There are no universal guidelines on immobilization that apply to all treatment settings. Before employing any kind of immobilization, it may help to consult available guidelines on federally funded care, your state department of mental health/disabilities, and your state Dental Practice Act. Guidelines on behavior management are published by the American Academy of Pediatric Dentistry and may also be useful. Obtain consent from your patient's legal guardian and choose the least restrictive technique that will allow you to provide care safely. Immobilization should not cause physical injury or undue discomfort.

7. If all other strategies fail, pharmacological options are useful in managing some patients. Others need to be treated under general anesthesia. However, caution is necessary because some patients with developmental disabilities can have unpredictable reactions to medications.

8. People with autism often engage in perseveration, a continuous, meaningless repetition of words, phrases, or movements. Your patient may mimic the sound of the suction, for example, or repeat an instruction over and again. Avoid demonstrating dental equipment if it triggers perseveration, and note this in the patient's record.

9. Unusual responses to stimuli can create distractions and interrupt treatment. People with autism need consistency and can be especially sensitive to changes in their environment. They may exhibit unusual sensitivity to sensory stimuli such as sound, bright colors, and touch. Reactions vary: some people with autism may overreact to noise and touch, while exposure to pain and heat may not provoke much reaction at all. Use the same staff, dental operatory, and appointment time to sustain familiarity. These details can help make dental treatment seem less threatening. Minimize the number of distractions. Try to reduce unnecessary sights, sounds, odors, or other stimuli that might be disruptive. Use an operatory that is somewhat secluded instead of one in the middle of a busy office. Also, consider lowering ambient light and asking the patient's caregiver whether soft music would help. Allow time for your patient to adjust and become desensitized to the noise of a dental setting. Some patients may be hypersensitive to the sound of dental instruments. Talk to the caregiver to get a sense of the patient's level of tolerance. People with autism differ in how they accept physical contact. Some are defensive and refuse any contact in or around the mouth, or cradling of the head or face. Others find such cradling comforting. Note your findings and experiences in the patient's chart.

10. Unusual and unpredictable body movements are sometimes observed in people with autism. These movements can jeopardize safety as well as your ability to deliver oral health care.

11. Make sure the path from the reception area to the dental chair is clear. Observe the patient's movements and look for patterns. Try to anticipate the movements, either blending your movements with those of your patient or working around them.

12. Seizures may accompany autism but can usually be controlled with anticonvulsant medications. The mouth is always at risk during a seizure: patients may chip teeth or bite the tongue or cheeks. People with controlled seizure disorders can easily be treated in the general dental office. Consult your patient's physician. Record information in the chart about the frequency of seizures and the medications used to control them. Determine before the appointment whether medications have been taken as directed. Know and avoid any factors that trigger your patient's seizures. Be prepared to manage a seizure. If one occurs during oral care, remove any instruments from the mouth and clear the area around the dental chair. Attaching dental floss to rubber dam clamps and mouth props when treatment begins can help you remove them quickly. Do not attempt to insert any objects between the teeth during a seizure.

13. Stay with your patient, turn him or her to one side, and monitor the airway to reduce the risk of aspiration.

14. Record in the patient's chart strategies that were successful in providing care. Note your patient's preferences and other unique details that will facilitate treatment, such as music, comfort items, and flavor choices.

15. People with autism experience few unusual oral health conditions. Although commonly used medications and damaging oral habits can cause problems, the rates of caries and periodontal disease in people with autism are comparable to those in the general population. Communication and behavioral problems pose the most significant challenges in providing oral care.

16. Damaging oral habits are common and include bruxism; tongue thrusting; self-injurious behavior such as picking at the gingiva or biting the lips; and pica—eating objects and substances such as gravel, cigarette butts, or pens. If a mouth guard can be tolerated, prescribe one for patients who have problems with self-injurious behavior or bruxism.

17. Dental caries risk increases in patients who have a preference for soft, sticky, or sweet foods; damaging oral habits; and difficulty brushing and flossing. Recommend preventive measures such as fluorides and sealants. Caution patients or their caregivers about medicines that reduce saliva or contain sugar. Suggest that patients drink water often, take sugar-free medicines when available, and rinse with water after taking any medicine. Advise caregivers to offer alternatives to cariogenic foods and beverages as incentives or rewards.

18. Encourage independence in daily oral hygiene. Ask patients to show you how they brush, and follow up with specific recommendations. Perform hands-on demonstrations to show patients the best way to clean their teeth. If appropriate, show patients and caregivers how a modified toothbrush or floss holder might make oral hygiene easier. Some patients cannot brush and floss independently. Talk to caregivers about daily oral hygiene and do not assume that they know the basics. Use your experiences with each patient to demonstrate oral hygiene techniques and sitting or standing positions for the caregiver. Emphasize that a consistent approach to oral hygiene is important—caregivers should try to use the same location, timing, and positioning.

19. Periodontal disease occurs in people with autism in much the same way it does in persons without developmental disabilities. Some patients benefit from the daily use of an antimicrobial agent such as chlorhexidine. Stress the importance of conscientious oral hygiene and frequent prophylaxis.

20. Tooth eruption may be delayed due to phenytoin-induced gingival hyperplasia. Phenytoin is commonly prescribed for people with autism.

21. Trauma and injury to the mouth from falls or accidents occur in people with seizure disorders. Suggest a tooth saving kit for group homes. Emphasize to caregivers that traumas require immediate professional attention and explain the procedures to follow if a permanent tooth is knocked out. Also, instruct caregivers to locate any missing pieces of a fractured tooth, and explain that radiographs of the patient's chest may be necessary to determine whether any fragments have been aspirated.

34. According to the passage, what might trigger head banging?
A. Bright lights
B. Sudden noises
C. Hyperactivity
D. The intrusive nature of a dental exam
E. Insensitive behavior by the provider

35. Tooth eruption in a patient with autism may be delayed due to
A. a phenytoin deficiency
B. obstruction due to mucosal barrier
C. phenytoin-induced gingival hyperplasia
D. global developmental delays
E. the presence of supernumerary teeth

36. Seizures can be a problem because the patient may
A. hit his or her head
B. chip teeth
C. choke on his or her tongue
D. injure staff
E. incur brain injury

37. Which of the following types of functions is NOT affected by autism?
A. Physical
B. Communication
C. Behavioral
D. Social
E. Intellectual

38. The best way to determine how best to make a patient with autism comfortable is to
A. ask the patient
B. consult the patient's physician
C. talk to the caregiver
D. read up on the condition in medical journals
E. do a thorough medical history

39. According to the passage, what approach to care should a dentist use with a patient who has autism?
A. Demonstrative
B. Explain-perform
C. Desensitization
D. Tell-show-do
E. Cooperative

40. Each of the following is a damaging oral habit that a patient with autism may exhibit EXCEPT
A. tongue-thrusting
B. pica

C. making repetitive sounds

D. bruxism

E. lip biting

41. What should be done prior to the first appointment with a patient who has autism?

    A. A consultation with the patient

    B. Determination of legal responsibility

    C. Intelligence testing

    D. Dental x-rays

    E. Functional testing

42. The passage mentions each of the following types of stimuli that might be distracting to a patient who has autism EXCEPT

    A. noise

    B. odor

    C. touch

    D. light

    E. taste

43. Which of the following is often a coexisting condition of autism?

    A. Epilepsy

    B. Respiratory diseases

    C. Halitosis

    D. Periodontal disease

    E. Diabetes

44. All of the following should be done to protect a patient during a seizure EXCEPT

    A. remove dental instruments from the mouth

    B. clear a space around the patient

    C. turn the patient on his or her side

    D. monitor the patient's airway

    E. help the patient bite down on a hard object

45. Which of the following may complicate the dental care of a person with autism?

    A. The presence of a caregiver

    B. A patient's tendency to get frustrated quickly

    C. Impaired intellectual function

    D. Self-injurious behavior

    E. Detachment from surroundings

46. What is perseveration?

    A. A drawing in of limbs

    B. Verbal or physical repetition

    C. Determination to succeed

    D. Sensitivity to loud noises

    E. An aversion to touch

47. The rate of caries in people with autism is
  A. lower than in the general population
  B. slightly higher than in the general population
  C. the same as in the general population
  D. noticeably higher than in the general population
  E. not something that has been studied adequately

48. What is the purpose of a desensitization appointment?
  A. To acclimate the patient to the office, staff, and equipment
  B. To get the patient used to having his or her mouth touched
  C. To help the patient become familiar with medical personnel
  D. To decrease the patient's sensitivity to loud noises
  E. To answer questions that the patient may have

49. When should a dentist use immobilization techniques?
  A. When the patient is unable to control involuntary movements
  B. When necessary to protect the patient and staff
  C. To prevent a patient from engaging in perseveration
  D. If a patient refuses to sit in the dental chair
  E. When it helps make the exam more convenient

50. The risk of caries increases in people who
  A. have obsessive oral behaviors
  B. take phenytoin
  C. cannot perform dental hygiene tasks independently
  D. have been diagnosed with autism
  E. have difficulty brushing and flossing

QUANTITATIVE REASONING

Directions: This section consists of **40 mathematics questions**. You will have **45 minutes** to complete them.

1. The end of a dog's leash is attached to the top of a 5-foot-tall fence post. The dog is 7 feet away from the base of the fence post. What is the length of the leash in feet?

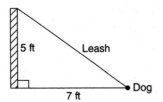

   A. 4.9
   B. 8.6
   C. 6.0
   D. 9.0
   E. 12.0

2. What is the slope of the line passing through the two points shown?

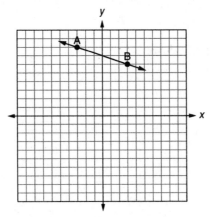

   A. −3
   B. $-\dfrac{1}{3}$
   C. 0
   D. 3
   E. $\dfrac{1}{3}$

3. In a recent town election, 1,860 people voted for either candidate A or candidate B. If candidate A received 55% of the votes, how many votes did candidate B receive?
   A. 186
   B. 837

C. 45

D. 1,023

E. 1,805

4. Which expression is equivalent to $121 - x^2$?

 A. $(x - 11)(x - 11)$

 B. $(x + 11)(x - 11)$

 C. $(11 - x)(11 + x)$

 D. $(11 - x)(11 - x)$

 E. $11(11 - x)$

5. Which value of x is the solution of

$$\frac{2x - 3}{x - 4} = \frac{2}{3}$$

 A. $-\dfrac{1}{4}$

 B. $\dfrac{3}{2}$

 C. -4

 D. $\dfrac{1}{4}$

 E. 4

6. What is the perimeter of a regular pentagon with a side whose length is $x + 4$?

 A. $x^2 + 16$

 B. $4x + 16$

 C. $5x + 4$

 D. $x^5 + 20$

 E. $5x + 20$

7. Which point lies on the line whose equation is $2x - 3y = 9$?

 A. $(-1, -3)$

 B. $(-1, 3)$

 C. $(9, 0)$

 D. $(0, 3)$

 E. $(0, -3)$

8. The probability that it will snow on Sunday is $\dfrac{3}{5}$. The probability that it will snow on both Sunday and Monday is $\dfrac{3}{10}$. What is the probability that it will snow on Monday, if it snowed on Sunday?

 A. $\dfrac{1}{2}$

 B. $\dfrac{9}{50}$

C. 2

D. $\dfrac{9}{10}$

E. $\dfrac{7}{10}$

9. Which graph represents an exponential equation?

A.

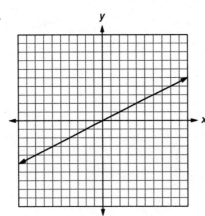

C.

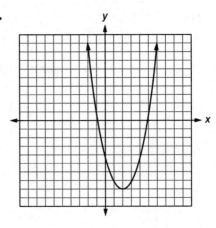

B.

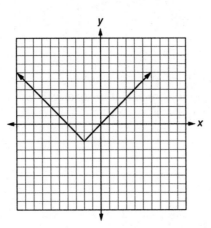

D.

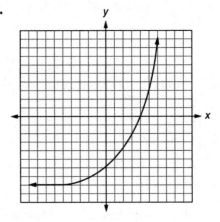

E. None of the above

10. The value of the tangent of angle B is

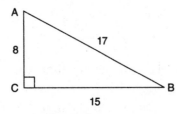

A. 0.4706
B. 0.5333
C. 0.8824
D. 1.8750
E. 1.2890

11. Expressed in simplest form, what is the value of the problem below?

$$\frac{2+x}{5x} - \frac{x-2}{5}$$

  A. 0

  B. $\dfrac{5}{2}$

  C. $\dfrac{4}{5x}$

  D. $\dfrac{2}{5}$

  E. $\dfrac{2x+4}{5x}$

12. How many different four-letter arrangements are possible with the letters *G*, *A*, *R*, *D*, *E*, *N* if each letter may be used only once?

  A. 15
  B. 24
  C. 180
  D. 360
  E. 720

13. Expressed in simplest radical form, $-3\sqrt{48}$ is

  A. $-3(2)\sqrt{12}$
  B. $-6\sqrt{24}$
  C. $-3\sqrt{12}$
  D. $-3\sqrt{2}\sqrt{12}$
  E. $-12\sqrt{3}$

14. Given the rectangular prism shown

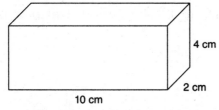

  A. The volume is 80 cm³ only.
  B. The surface area is 136 cm² only.
  C. The length of all of the edges is 64 cm only.
  D. The surface area is 136 cm² and the length of all of the edges is 64 cm only.
  E. The volume is 80 cm³, the surface area is 136 cm², and the length of all of the edges is 64 cm.

15. The height of the hot-air balloon above the ground in the following picture is approximately

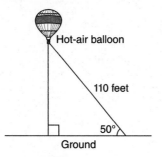

A. 84 feet
B. 110 feet
C. 48 feet
D. 168 feet
E. 100 feet

16. The equation of a circle is $x^2 + (y - 7)^2 = 16$. What are the center and radius of the circle?
A. center = (7, 0); radius = 4
B. center = (0, 7); radius = 4
C. center = (0, 7); radius = 16
D. center = (0, −7); radius = 4
E. center = (0, −7); radius = 16

17. What is the length of the line segment with endpoints A (−6, 4) and B (2, −5)?
A. $\sqrt{13}$
B. $\sqrt{17}$
C. $\sqrt{72}$
D. $\sqrt{145}$
E. $\sqrt{155}$

18. What is the slope of a line perpendicular to the line whose equation is $2y = -6x + 8$?
A. −3
B. $\dfrac{1}{6}$
C. $\dfrac{1}{3}$
D. −6
E. $-\dfrac{1}{6}$

19. The following diagram shows isosceles trapezoid ABCD with line AB parallel to line DC and line AD the same length as line BC. The measure of angle BAD is $2x$ and the measure of angle BCD is $3x + 5$.

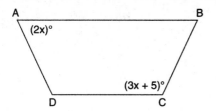

Angle ABC has a value of

A. $3x + 5$

B. $4x$

C. $180°$

D. $6x^2 + 10x$

E. $70°$

20. The value of angle BCD is

A. $35°$

B. $70°$

C. $75°$

D. $110°$

E. $180°$

21. The total number of degrees in the trapezoid is

A. 180

B. $10x + 10$

C. x

D. 90

E. 240

Questions 22 through 24 refer to the following:

In the diagram of $\triangle HQP$, side $\overline{HP}$ is extended through P to T, $m \angle QPT = 6x + 20$, $m \angle HQP = x + 40$, and $m \angle PHQ = 4x - 5$.

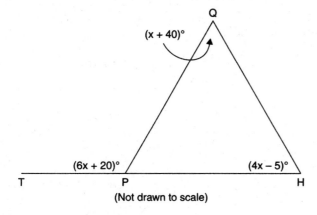

(Not drawn to scale)

22. The value of angle QPH is

A. $6x + 20 - 180$

B. $180 - 6x + 20$

C. $180 - 6x - 20$

D. $6x + 20 + 180$

E. $180 + 6x + 20$

23. The value of x is

    A. 5

    B. 10

    C. 15

    D. 20

    E. 25

24. Triangle HQP can best be described as being

    A. isosceles

    B. right

    C. obtuse

    D. acute

    E. equilateral

Questions 25 through 27 refer to the following:

In the diagram of quadrilateral ABCD with diagonal $\overline{BD}$, m $\angle A = 93$, m $\angle ADB = 43$, m $\angle C = 3x + 5$, m $\angle BDC = x + 19$, and m $\angle DBC = 2x + 6$.

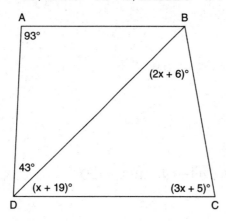

25. The total number of degrees in triangle BCD is

    A. 90

    B. 360

    C. 25

    D. $6x + 30$

    E. None of the above

26. The value of x is

    A. 5

    B. 10

    C. 15

    D. 20

    E. 25

27. Line segments AB and CD can best be described as being
   A. perpendicular
   B. parallel
   C. intersecting
   D. equivalent
   E. congruent

28. If $f(x) = x^2 - 9$ and $g(x) = 2x + 1$, what is $f(g(x))$?
   A. $4x^2 + 4x - 8$
   B. $2x^2 - 17$
   C. $x^2 + 4x + 8$
   D. $(x + 3)(x - 3)(2x + 1)$
   E. $2x^2 - 8$

29. Which equation is sketched in the following diagram?

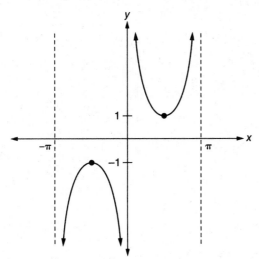

   A. $y = \sin x$
   B. $y = \cot x$
   C. $y = \csc x$
   D. $y = \tan x$
   E. $y = \cos x$

30. $\dfrac{3}{8}$ multiplied by $\dfrac{1}{2}$ is

   A. $\dfrac{6}{8}$

   B. $\dfrac{1}{3}$

   C. $\dfrac{3}{4}$

   D. $\dfrac{2}{5}$

   E. $\dfrac{3}{16}$

31. $\frac{5}{6}$ minus $\frac{1}{4}$ is

    A. $\frac{7}{12}$

    B. 2

    C. $\frac{1}{2}$

    D. $\frac{15}{12}$

    E. $\frac{2}{3}$

32. If $\frac{1}{x-2} = \frac{7}{x}$, what is the value of x?

    A. $\frac{1}{14}$

    B. $\frac{3x}{7}$

    C. $\frac{3}{7}$

    D. $\frac{7}{3}$

    E. $-\frac{3}{7}$

33. How many seconds are there in one week?

    A. 168

    B. 3600

    C. 10,080

    D. 604,800

    E. 3.63×10^7

34. Assuming a standard deck of playing cards, what is the probability of picking a card with a heart on it?

    A. $\frac{1}{26}$

    B. $\frac{1}{4}$

    C. $\frac{1}{52}$

    D. $\frac{1}{2}$

    E. $\frac{2}{13}$

Questions 35 and 36 refer to the following set of numbers:

$\{56, 65, 45, 97, 78, 60, 81\}$

35. Which of the following is true?

    I. The mean is 68.9.

    II. The median is 65.

    III. The mode is 62.5.

  A. I only

  B. II only

  C. I and II only

  D. II and III only

  E. III only

36. The range for the set of numbers is

  A. 97

  B. 52

  C. 45

  D. 142

  E. 65

Questions 37 through 39 refer to the following choices:

  A. $A = \dfrac{1}{2}(a + b)h$

  B. $\dfrac{(x_2 + x_1, y_2 + y_1)}{2}$

  C. $\dfrac{1}{2}bh$

  D. $A = s^2$

  E. $ax^2 + bx + c$

37. Will require the quadratic equation to find the roots.

38. Will find the midpoint of two points.

39. Will find the area of a trapezoid.

40. Which of the following is true regarding a circle with a radius of 3.8 meters?

    I. The diameter is 1.9 meters.

    II. The circumference of the circle is 23.86 meters.

    III. The area of the circle is 45.34 meters.

    IV. The number of degrees in the circle is 360.

  A. I and III only

  B. II, III, and IV only

  C. II and IV only

  D. II and III only

  E. I, II, III, and IV

DIAGNOSTICS TEST ANSWER KEY

Natural Sciences

1. C	35. B	68. B
2. C	36. D	69. C
3. B	37. A	70. D
4. D	38. B	71. E
5. A	39. B	72. B
6. E	40. B	73. C
7. A	41. D	74. A
8. E	42. D	75. E
9. B	43. A	76. C
10. D	44. E	77. D
11. D	45. A	78. E
12. C	46. B	79. B
13. E	47. C	80. C
14. B	48. E	81. D
15. A	49. D	82. A
16. E	50. A	83. D
17. E	51. C	84. B
18. D	52. E	85. C
19. D	53. C	86. E
20. E	54. B	87. D
21. B	55. B	88. B
22. A	56. E	89. D
23. B	57. C	90. A
24. E	58. A	91. E
25. C	59. D	92. C
26. E	60. A	93. C
27. E	61. C	94. A
28. D	62. C	95. B
29. B	63. E	96. E
30. C	64. B	97. D
31. A	65. E	98. D
32. A	66. D	99. B
33. E	67. A	100. C
34. A		

Perceptual Ability

1. B	**31.** C	**61.** B
2. D	**32.** B	**62.** D
3. C	**33.** A	**63.** D
4. A	**34.** D	**64.** B
5. E	**35.** C	**65.** A
6. E	**36.** B	**66.** B
7. B	**37.** A	**67.** E
8. D	**38.** C	**68.** B
9. C	**39.** D	**69.** E
10. D	**40.** C	**70.** A
11. B	**41.** B	**71.** A
12. E	**42.** C	**72.** E
13. A	**43.** D	**73.** A
14. C	**44.** A	**74.** D
15. D	**45.** A	**75.** A
16. A	**46.** E	**76.** B
17. C	**47.** A	**77.** D
18. A	**48.** B	**78.** B
19. D	**49.** C	**79.** C
20. B	**50.** D	**80.** A
21. D	**51.** E	**81.** A
22. A	**52.** E	**82.** D
23. C	**53.** B	**83.** C
24. C	**54.** C	**84.** B
25. D	**55.** A	**85.** B
26. B	**56.** C	**86.** A
27. B	**57.** D	**87.** C
28. D	**58.** A	**88.** B
29. A	**59.** B	**89.** D
30. C	**60.** A	**90.** B

Reading Comprehension

1. D	18. A	35. C
2. C	19. D	36. B
3. D	20. B	37. A
4. A	21. E	38. C
5. A	22. A	39. D
6. E	23. C	40. C
7. A	24. E	41. B
8. B	25. D	42. E
9. D	26. B	43. A
10. C	27. B	44. E
11. E	28. D	45. D
12. E	29. A	46. B
13. B	30. E	47. C
14. C	31. C	48. A
15. A	32. B	49. B
16. D	33. E	50. E
17. A	34. D	

Quantitative Reasoning

1. B	15. A	28. A
2. B	16. B	29. C
3. B	17. D	30. E
4. C	18. C	31. A
5. D	19. E	32. D
6. E	20. D	33. D
7. E	21. B	34. B
8. A	22. C	35. C
9. D	23. C	36. B
10. B	24. A	37. E
11. C	25. D	38. B
12. D	26. E	39. A
13. E	27. B	40. C
14. E		

EXPLANATIONS

Natural Sciences

1. **C** A prokaryotic cell is going to have a single loop of DNA. The other choices describe eukaryotes.

2. **C** The mitochondria will take on the reactions that produce ATP, the molecule that supplies energy to our cells. This is why some people refer to the mitochondria as the "mighty-chondria" or the "powerhouse of the cell."

3. **B** The cell membrane is selectively permeable, allowing it to control what goes in and out of the cell.

4. **D** The lysosomes contain digestive enzymes in the cell.

5. **A** The Golgi apparatus is responsible for "processing, packing, and shipping" materials throughout the cell.

6. **E** Centrioles are composed of microtubules. Most of the time, the microtubules are found in bundles of three, depending upon the organism.

7. **A** Catalysts are not consumed during a reaction. Instead, they do their work of speeding up reactions without any (major) deformation or denaturation to their structures. This allows them to continue to function and catalyze reactions.

8. **E** Choices A through D are serious types of damage that can occur to chromosomes during meiosis. These damages can have terrible or fatal consequences to the offspring.

9. **B** Rubisco is an enzyme found in plants, not in humans. The other choices are all part of the electron transport chain.

10. **D** Mitochondria are not found in chloroplasts, while the other four choices are.

11. **D** This question can be a little tricky because one would expect the answer to read prophase, prometaphase, metaphase, anaphase, telophase, and so on. Instead, it sequences from the end of meiosis I into the beginning of meiosis II.

12. **C** Archaea lack a nucleus. Choice A is wrong because eukaryotes can be multi- or unicellular. Choices B and D are wrong because bacteria and viruses are not eukaryotic or nucleus-containing organisms.

13. **E** Depending upon the species of fungus and the current environmental conditions, reproduction for fungi can vary. Yeasts are unicellular fungi, while molds and mushrooms are multicellular. Finally, the mycelium helps the fungi obtain nutrition.

14. **B** Bacteria can multiply very quickly, but because of this tremendous rate of growth, they reach their carrying capacity quickly. This makes resources scarce and forces the population to decline.

15. **A** Choices B through E are the reproductive portions of flowering plants. Hyphae are located in fungi and make up the mycelium.

16. **E** Choices A through D are all parts of the nerve cell, while stomata control transpiration and the exchange of gases within a plant.

17. **E** The cerebellum is responsible for the actions described in the question, such as balance and complex movements. This is not to be confused with the cerebrum, which is divided into two hemispheres that regulate intelligence, learning, memory, the senses, and other functions.

18. **D** The sacrum is a large, triangular bone located at the base of the spine. The other four choices are related to the head: The mandible is the lower jawbone, and the skull is composed of the cranium and the mandible. The maxilla is a bone that forms part of the upper jaw.

19. **D** Hormones are chemical signals that are produced to communicate with the cells of the body. Choices A, B, C, and E are incorrectly paired, and only D is correct since the small intestine releases cholecystokinin (CCK) to stimulate the pancreas and gallbladder to release insulin and bile, respectively. These accessory organs aid with chemical digestion.

20. **E** The valves in veins prevent blood backflow so that blood can only flow in one direction. Arterioles and venules are smaller versions of arteries and veins, respectively, and are connected by the one-cell-wide capillaries. In general, veins have thinner walls than arteries.

21. **B** Air enters the body through the nose or mouth and makes its way through several passageways until it finally reaches the bronchioles and alveoli. While the diaphragm is important for helping air to get to the lungs, it is not a passageway along the respiratory system. Choices A, C, and E are out of order, leaving B as the answer.

22. **A** Chemical digestion is facilitated by enzymes and digestive juices. Choices B, C, and D are all related to mechanical digestion. Choice E is the contraction of the muscle in the digestive system to move materials along the digestive tract.

23. **B** The nephron contains the Bowman's capsule. The other four choices name parts of the urinary system.

24. **E** Primary defenses aim to keep pathogens out of the body (skin, tears, etc.). A secondary line of defense fights infection once it is in the body (white blood cells). A tertiary line of defense remembers what the invaders "looked like" so that, should they invade again, the response against them is quicker.

25. **C** The different hormones will have various levels depending upon what part of the menstrual cycle is in question. This allows processes to occur at certain times during the cycle so that they are in the right sequence and play a proper role.

26. **E** All the mentioned structures are part of the human male reproductive system. The vas deferens will transport sperm from the epididymis during ejaculation. The seminal vesicles secrete the fluid that makes up a major part of semen.

27. **E** During the gastrula stage there is the formation of the ectoderm (which will become the skin and nervous system), mesoderm (which becomes the muscles, bones, and internal organs), and endoderm (which becomes a number of internal linings).

28. **D** The placenta will develop from the chorion and allow materials to be exchanged between fetus and mother via the umbilical cord. The yolk sac is a source of nutrients. The allantois is a membrane that aids with waste collection and gas exchange. The amnion is the fluid-filled sac that serves as protection and cushioning.

29. **B** The posterior pituitary gland produces oxytocin, which will commence contractions. Choices A, C, and D are important in the maintenance of pregnancy, but they do not trigger labor.

30. **C** rRNA stands for ribosomal RNA, which is a component of ribosomes.

31. **A** The *D* in DNA stands for *deoxyribose*, indicating the lack of an oxygen atom.

32. **A** The nitrogen bases for DNA are adenine, thymine, guanine, and cytosine. In RNA the thymine is replaced by uracil.

33. **E** tRNA is transfer RNA, which moves amino acids to the ribosome during translation.

34. **A** The work of Watson, Crick, and Franklin led to the discovery of the double helix of DNA. This was accomplished with the painstaking work of using x-ray crystallography and months of calculations.

35. **B** Choice B is correct because a recessive trait will never be expressed with just one recessive allele: the individual must be homozygous recessive in order to express the recessive trait. This is true regardless of the sex of the person, as long as the gene is on an autosomal chromosome and not a sex chromosome.

36. **D** Differentiation is important because only the genes necessary for a cell to perform its function need to be expressed. This allows the cell to do its job and its job only.

37. **A** Autotrophs (producers) are the lowest tier of the food pyramid but are the level that contains the most energy.

38. **B** Herbivores maintain a diet that relies on plants and vegetation. These animals are hunted for their meat by carnivores.

39. **B** Paleontologists examine the fossil record in an effort to understand the organisms that have lived on earth. This, however, is not the only means for understanding evolution. Now that DNA can be manipulated in the laboratory like any other chemical, the use of DNA sequencing has showed a tremendous amount of insight to ancestry.

40. **B** Altruism is when the organisms that are closely related to each other function together for their own good. A family of baboons will sound an alarm when a predator has been spotted. Doing so alerts the family and offspring about the incoming danger. While the alarm is meant for the baboons, other species of organisms (like gazelles) can also identify this warning and be on high alert as well. Choices E and A are not winning situations for an injured wildebeest being hunted by a lion or for a dog that has intestinal worms. With competition, one organism is more likely to thrive than another. Extinction shows that the species could not adapt and maintain a successful gene pool.

41. **D** The mass of sulfuric acid is 98 g/mol ($H \times 2 = 2$, $S \times 1 = 32$, $O \times 4 = 64$). It is a diprotic acid with two hydronium ions to yield. However, red litmus paper will turn blue in a basic solution. Remember the mnemonic device *Litmus* BRA, meaning "Blue → Red = Acid."

42. **D** First, start with a balanced equation: $CH_4 + 2O_2 \rightarrow CO_2 + 2H_2O$. 32 grams of methane is two moles of methane. So now we can modify the coefficients to show that two moles are reacting: $2CH_4 + 4O_2 \rightarrow 2CO_2 + 4H_2O$. There will be 2×22.4 L of carbon dioxide formed, or 44.8L because one mole of a gas at STP will occupy 22.4 L.

43. **A** Regarding glucose, the oxygen makes up the largest percentage of the mass. The molecule is polar and dissolves in water. The molecule is used during cellular respiration, and finally, with solids, more can dissolve with an increase in temperature of the solvent. Because the empirical formula $C_3H_6O_3$ has the same ratio as the molecular formula, $C_6H_{12}O_6$, the percent composition for each element is the same.

44. **E** The lowest density of the noble gases goes to helium, the element with the greater root mean square velocity. Because more helium will escape the container, it will have the lowest partial pressure remaining.

45. **A** Gas molecules having an attraction for each other is not part of the Kinetic Molecular Theory. As a refresher remember that:

   ➤ Particles of gases are separated from one another by large distances when compared to the size of the particles.
   ➤ Particles of a gas are in constant and random motion.
   ➤ When the particles of a gas collide with other particles or the sides of the container, no energy is lost, that is, the collisions are elastic.
   ➤ The particles exert neither repulsive nor attractive forces on one another.
   ➤ The average kinetic energy of gas particles is directly proportional to the absolute temperature in Kelvin.

46. **B** Going back to the equation for the ideal gas law, $PV = nRT$, we need to solve for R, so $\dfrac{PV}{nT} = R$. The units will be $\dfrac{L \cdot atm}{mol \cdot K}$.

47. **C** Methane is nonpolar and will exhibit dispersion forces. HBr is a polar molecule and will show dipole forces between the molecules. NaCl is ionic as it is a salt made from a metal and nonmetal. In the case of carbon dioxide, even though the bonds are polar, the molecule is nonpolar because of the linear shape and will exhibit dispersion forces. HF shows hydrogen bonding. Hydrogen bonds are formed when H is bonded to F, O, or N. This can be remembered by the mnemonic device, "I heard about hydrogen bonding on the FON."

48. **E** Ethanol, acetone, and butane are organic compounds and will have low boiling points. In fact, ethanol boils at 78 °C. Acetone and butane boil at even lower temperatures because of their weak intermolecular forces. Water is polar and boils at 100 °C, but that colligative property will change and the boiling point become higher when a solute is dissolved in the water.

49. **D** At a certain temperature and pressure, a substance can exist in all three phases at once. This is called the triple point.

50. **A** 58.5 grams of NaCl dissolved to make 2 liters of solution is $\dfrac{1 \text{ mol NaCl}}{2\text{L}} = 0.5 \text{ M}$ NaCl. The freezing point will be depressed because of the ions in solution and their effect on the freezing point. The salt is a neutral salt because it was made from a strong base (NaOH) and a strong acid (HCl).

51. **C** Remember that:

   ➤ All salts of Group 1 cations, Li^+, Na^+, and K^+, and the ammonium ion, $NH_4{}^+$, are soluble.
   ➤ All nitrates, $NO_3{}^-$, and acetates, CH_3COO^-, are soluble.
   ➤ All chlorides, Cl^-, bromides, Br^-, and iodides, I^-, are soluble except when combined with Ag^+, Pb^{2+}, or $Hg_2{}^{2+}$.
   ➤ Carbonates are insoluble except when combined with group 1 metals or ammonium ion.

   The precipitates will be (A.) Silver chloride, (B.) Lead chloride, (D.) Silver iodide, (E.) Calcium carbonate (marble).

52. **E** 50 grams of LiCl (GFM = 42.4 g/mol) is 0.848 mol LiCl. Dissolved in 750 mL of solution, the molarity of the solution is 1.13 M. Dissolved to make 1 liter of solution, the molarity is 0.848 M. A is correct as per question 48. B is correct as per the calculation shown. Finally, C is correct because as the solvent evaporates, the volume of solution decreases, increasing the concentration.

53. **C** The equilibrium constant K_a is equal to $\dfrac{[H+][A-]}{[HA]}$. Substituting, we get $1.5 \times 10^{-5}[0.2] = x^2$. Next we find that $x^2 = 3.0 \times 10^{-6}$. The square root of this is equal to the concentration of hydronium ions $= 1.73 \times 10^{-3}$. Taking the $-\log[H^+]$ we get the pH to be about 2.76.

54. **B** NaCl is a neutral salt as is LiCl. H_2SO_4 is an acid, and NH_4Cl is an acid salt. Examining the parent base and acid for sodium acetate ($NaC_2H_3O_2$), we find them to be NaOH and $HC_2H_3O_2$. This is a strong base and a weak acid that yielded a basic salt.

55. **B** Be careful of too many unnecessary calculations! 0.0284 L × 0.18 M NaOH gives 0.005 mol NaOH to be titrated no matter how much the solution is diluted. Using the equation $M_aV_a = M_bV_b$ we get (X)(0.0249 L) = (0.18 M)(0.0284 L). Looking at the numbers, we see that more base was used, meaning that it was lower in concentration than the acid. Completing the calculation, we find that the molarity of the HCl is 0.205 M.

56. **E** If A is removed the reaction shifts left to replace the loss. If D is added, the reaction shifts left to use up the excess. If the temperature is decreased, it has the same effect as removing a reactant, causing a shift to the left. A decrease in pressure means a greater volume, which is on the left side of the equation. If C is removed, there is missing product. The reaction will shift to the right to make up for the loss of product.

57. **C** Because the hydrogen gas is being used up, the sign must be negative. Because the coefficient is 3, the 3 must appear in the denominator.

58. **A** Examining the data in experiments 1 and 2, doubling the concentration of B doubled the rate. This means that y = 1. Examining experiments 2 and 4, doubling the concentration of A quadrupled the rate. This means that x = 2.

59. **D** A negative value for the change in entropy means less chaos and less randomness. The raking up of leaves and the collection of hockey pucks makes the garden and rink more organized. The same cannot be said for the kids who had the eggs thrown at them.

60. **A** ΔH is the heat of reaction and is the potential energy of the reactants minus the potential energy of the products.

61. **C** The activation energy can be calculated by subtracting the $PE_{reactants}$ from the $PE_{activated\ complex}$.

62. **C** The energy needed to start the reaction is the activation energy.

63. **E** Oxygen can have a wide range of oxidation states, depending upon the elements that it is bonded to. Choices B and C are explained by O_2 and H_2O respectively. The oxygen atom could be +2 in the compound OF_2. Finally, not listed, oxygen can be −1 as it is in a peroxide, such as H_2O_2 or Na_2O_2.

64. **B** Redox and electrochemistry are loaded with mnemonic devices. The first is "LEO says GER" and stands for "lose electrons oxidation, gain electrons reduction." Also, there is "An Ox and Red Cat," which stands for "anode is oxidation, cathode is reduction." Oxidation takes place at the anode, making A incorrect. C is incorrect

because the whole idea behind reduction is the reduction of the oxidation number—it gets lower in value during reduction. B is the redox definition of oxidation: the loss of electrons.

65. **E** $1s^2 2s^2 2p^6 3s^2 3p^6$ demonstrates a noble gas configuration. This is the configuration for Ar. A potassium ion has one less electron than the potassium atom (19 electrons). Chlorine has 17 electrons and has a configuration of $1s^2 2s^2 2p^6 3s^2 3p^5$.

66. **D** m_s is the spin quantum number for an electron. It can be $+\dfrac{1}{2}$ or $-\dfrac{1}{2}$.

67. **A** The molecular geometries are, respectively, trigonal bipyramidal, tetrahedral, bent, linear, and octahedral. Three of the chlorine atoms will be in the equatorial position and two will be in the axial position.

68. **B** The halogens (salt formers) are known for their terrible odors. Their colors are F: pale yellow, Cl: green, Br: orange-brown, and I: purple. Respectively, their phases at room temperature are gas, gas, liquid, and solid. Being a solid, iodine can sublime and enter the gas phase with no apparent liquid phase in between. This is not to be confused with $KMnO_4$, which is a purple-colored salt.

69. **C** Ca and Sr are in the same family. The same concept from biology, that people in the same family look alike, can be applied to chemistry as well because both elements have the same number of valence electrons and will form ions with a +2 charge.

70. **D** Beta particles are the same size as an electron, approximately 1/1836 AMU. An alpha particle is a helium nucleus (not a helium ion!). It has a mass of 4 AMU, hence the symbol: $^4_2 He$.

71. **E** The modifier *oxo* is used when a C=O group of an aldehyde or ketone is located in the molecule but the molecule has a functional group of higher priority present. An example could be $HOOC\text{-}CH_2\text{-}CHO$, 3-oxo-propanoic acid.

72. **B** R and S refer to the configurations about a chiral center, which is missing from this molecule in question. Given that the configuration is trans, the E can be used in the name. If it were cis, then the Z could be used. A terrific mnemonic device to use is: *E-pposite* (opposite) side and *Z-ame* (same) side.

73. **C** A shoe will not superimpose upon its mirror image, while all of the other items or molecules will.

74. **A** Bimolecular nucleophilic substitution takes place via a backside attack leaving 100% inversion of configuration. This is opposed to unimolecular nucleophilic substitution, which has a trigonal planar intermediate that then yields a 50/50 mixture of racemates.

75. **E** Zaitsef's rule points out that reactions will take place to form double bonds, but the double bond formation will be stabilized by more R groups resulting on the C=C.

76. **C** This is the classic definition of Markovnikov's rule: the addition of HX adds the H atoms to the carbon atom of the double bond that already has a greater number of H atoms.

77. **D** This hyboration reaction proceeds in an anti-Markovnikov fashion. In this case, the OH group went to the carbon atom, which had more H atoms.

78. **E** The degradation of the C=O in the amide to yield an amine is textbook Hofmann rearrangement.

79. **B** The sodium borohydride is rich in H atoms, meaning that it is likely a reducing agent. Keep in mind that the definitions of oxidation and reduction change in organic chemistry. The addition of oxygen or the removal of hydrogen is considered to be oxidation. The addition of hydrogen or the removal of oxygen is considered to be reduction.

80. **C** This is a classic organometallic reaction via the use of a Grignard reagent.

81. **D** The use of ozone should give away the answer here. However, keep in mind the importance of this reaction as it can be used to make derivatives of an alkene or help to determine the structure of an alkene.

82. **A** Nitration will yield $C_6H_5NO_2$. The reduction of the nitrobenzene will yield $C_6H_5NH_2$.

83. **D** A Friedel-Crafts alkylation will place an R group on the benzene. Reaction with the oxidation power of potassium permanganate will produce benzoic acid after acidification.

84. **B** The sulfonation or halogenation of benzene followed up with a reaction with molten NaOH will produce a phenol.

85. **C** Both choices C and D will place ortho, para directors on the benzene. However, it is the halogens that are deactivating. Choices A, B, and E are all meta directors.

86. **E** Conjugated systems will have a λ_{max} of over 200 nm in the UV region. This is opposed to simple alkenes, which have a λ_{max} of approximately 171 nm, and alkynes, which have a λ_{max} of approximately 185 nm. Both the benzene ring and the conjugated diene will have λ_{max} greater than 200 nm.

87. **D** The mass of benzyl chloride will have a base ion peak at 91 m/z showing the stability of the fragmentation when the chlorine is lost. 91 + 35 and 91 + 37 explain the peaks at 126 and 128 m/z. The M+2 peak being one-third the relative abundance of the M+ peak is consistent with the isotopic relative abundances for Cl-35 and Cl-37 being 75% and 25%, respectively. There will not be a peak at 77 m/z even though a benzene ring is present. This is because of the resonance stabilization of the benzyl fragment.

88. **B** There will not be any peaks with a chemical shift of 7.2 in the HNMR as peaks in this area indicate hydrogen atoms on a benzene ring. The peak at 1720 cm^{-1} indicates C=O in the IR. Despite there being seven carbon atoms in the molecule, only four of them will show because of the symmetry of the molecule creating equivalent carbon atoms.

89. **D** The para isomer, III, will show just three different hydrogen atom environments. I and II will show five different environments each because of the NH_2 and the four hydrogen atoms on the benzene ring not being equivalent in nature.

90. **A** This reaction needs a little time and drawing, but once completed, it is easy to spot the diene and dienophile forming the adduct. If that is hard to see, then just look at the other answers: there is no ketone present (B), there is no ester present (C), there is no aldehyde group present (D), and there is no proton bonding to an OH group to remove a water molecule (E). Instead, what we have here is a cycloaddition.

91. **E** The monochlorination of methane involves initiation, propagation, and termination. Choice A is endothermic and serves as the initiation step. Choices C and D are part of the propagation steps. Choice B is a possible termination step. However, choice E is not part of the reaction and is not likely to occur because of the formation of the chlorine and methyl radicals instead of a hydrogen radical.

92. **C** Choices A and E demonstrate the crowding of the substituents on the cyclohexane. Having axial substituents is not going to contribute to the stability of the molecule. Instead, any substituents placed on the molecule will cause ring inversion as to alleviate the strain by arranging the substituents into the equatorial position. Choices B and D are also true, as it takes much energy to overcome the half-chair conformation to reach the skew boat conformation.

93. **C** The number of stereoisomers is defined by 2^n, where n is the number of chiral carbon atoms present. $2^4 = 16$.

94. **A** A terminal alkyne like propyne is pretty acidic against other hydrocarbons, relatively speaking, but does not even come close to the other compounds listed. Aldehydes and alcohols have about the same acidity, pka values of 16 to 17. The chlorinated alcohol will be more acidic than the alcohol because of inductive effects. Choice C speaks for itself.

95. **B** The monobromination of propane demonstrates the relationship between reactivity and selectivity. Because the bromine is less reactive, the products will reflect only the most stable intermediates, showing that bromine is more selective. Because an aromatic (Ar) intermediate is more stable than a tertiary intermediate, which is more stable than a secondary intermediate (and so on), the bromine will react with the secondary carbon even though there are twice as many primary carbon atoms to react with. A trace of the 1-bromo product will appear, but it has no significance. The bromonium ion forms when bromine is added to an alkene via an anti-addition.

96. **E** This reaction shows an S_N1 mechanism. There will be racemization of the products in a 50/50 mixture. The rate law indicates that the reaction's rate depends upon the concentration of one substance. The intermediate will be a trigonal planar carbocation.

97. **D** Br outranks OH because of the greater atomic number of Br than O. The trend continues where OH > ethyl > methyl > H.

98. **D** Choice D refers to the strong, broad O-H stretch peak of alcohols. A describes aromatic overtones, B a monosubstituted benzene ring, C a carbonyl group, and E a peak that arises with nitriles.

99. **B** This compound is a bicyclic alkane called Bicyclo[2.2.1]heptane. The molecular formula is C_7H_{12}, four hydrogen atoms short of the alkane formula for heptane, C_7H_{16}. For each two hydrogen atoms short from the straight chain alkane, one degree of unsaturation exists.

100. **C** Tollen's test includes the reaction of an aldehyde to produce Ag(s), the silver mirror.

Perceptual Ability

1. **B** The object will fit through this aperture if introduced top or bottom first.

2. **D** If the letter A facing you is considered the front, then the object will fit through this aperture when introduced front or back. Choice A is very close, but the cutout in the A is not triangular.

3. **C** If the large rectangular base is considered the front, then the object will fit through this aperture if introduced side first.

4. **A** The object will fit through this aperture if introduced front or back first.

5. **E** The object will fit through this aperture if introduced front or back first. Note that the protrusion on the middle right extends beyond the edge of the cube. Choice B is close, but the protrusion is too large and not centered.

6. **E** The object will fit through this aperture if introduced top or bottom first.

7. **B** Since the object is symmetrical, it will fit through this aperture if introduced side, front, or back first.

8. **D** The object will fit through this aperture if introduced front or back first.

9. **C** The object will fit through this aperture if introduced side first.

10. **D** The object will fit through this aperture if introduced side first.

11. **B** The object will fit through this aperture if introduced front or back first.

12. **E** The object will fit through this aperture if flipped upside down and then introduced side first.

13. **A** The object will fit through this aperture if introduced top or bottom first.

14. **C** The object will fit through this aperture if introduced side first. Choice E is close, but note the tiny hooks on the top of the birdhouse. The aperture must leave room for those.

15. **D** The object will fit through this aperture if introduced front or back first.

16. **A** The top view shows two symmetrical corners at left and the front view shows a diamond shape to the corner, so the end view will show two diamond-shaped corners.

17. **C** The front view shows an overhang and the end view shows staggered levels, so the top view will show a stairway-like pattern.

18. **A** The top view shows that the figure is circular, with two irregularities on opposite sides. The end view shows that it is bell-shaped, with angled sides. Since it is a circular bell, the front view will be similar to the end view but will show the angled sides. Choices B and C also show a bell shape, but the bells are wider than the end view of the original figure.

19. **D** The front view shows that the top has three spikes.

20. **B** The top view shows a five-point cutout completely within a square base. The end view shows that the figure is a cube, so the front view will be the same as the end view since the cutout has five hidden points no matter what direction is facing the viewer.

21. **D** The top view shows an octagon with two blocks forming a cross through the center and a center vertical post. The front view shows that the figure narrows at the top and bottom.

22. **A** The end view shows that the figure has four sections at different heights. However, the left and right sections are the same height, so from the front view, the figure will appear as a square with three hidden lines.

23. **C** The end view will be similar to the front view, but flipped horizontally with the triangular shapes on the right side of the cube.

24. **C** The front view shows two cylinders inserted into opposite sides of a prism. The end view will be the rectangular side of the prism with one cylinder shown and one hidden.

25. **D** The top view shows that the figure is not symmetrical, so the end view will show the left side larger than the right. The front view shows that the circular part is on the top.

26. **B** Looking at the top view, there will be four points that show on the front view and one hidden point on the left side. Choice D also has four points with one hidden, but the narrow arm and the hidden point are on the wrong side in that choice.

27. **B** The top and front views show an inverted pyramid. The end view will appear triangular with the left side longer than the right.

28. **D** The top view shows two walls in a V-shape with a third wall intersecting them. The end view will show the intersecting wall on the left and the hidden side of the V on the right.

29. **A** The top and end views show that the figure is a sort of wall with a cylinder through it and another parallel cylinder on top.

30. **C** Looking at the top view, the front view will have four points shown, with a wide section on the left.

31. **C** The correct ranking is 2-4-3-1.

32. **B** The correct ranking is 4-1-2-3.

33. **A** The correct ranking is 2-1-4-3.

34. **D** The correct ranking is 3-1-2-4.

35. **C** The correct ranking is 4-3-1-2.

36. **B** The correct ranking is 3-4-2-1.

37. **A** The correct ranking is 3-1-2-4.

38. **C** The correct ranking is 1-2-4-3.

39. **D** The correct ranking is 3-1-4-2.

40. **C** The correct ranking is 4-1-3-2.

41. **B** The correct ranking is 4-1-2-3.

42. **C** The correct ranking is 2-1-3-4.

43. **D** The correct ranking is 3-2-4-1.

44. **A** The correct ranking is 4-3-2-1.

45. **A** The correct ranking is 2-1-3-4.

46. **E** The square is folded on the diagonal and the hole is punched in the upper left corner. When the paper is unfolded, there will be two holes, both in the upper left corner.

47. **A** The square is folded twice down from the top to the center and the hole is punched in the upper right corner. When the paper is unfolded, there will be three holes, all along the upper right side.

48. **B** The square is folded once from the bottom left corner toward the center and the hole is punched in the center of the folded triangle. When the paper is unfolded, there will be two holes: one in the lower left center and one in the lower left corner.

49. **C** The square is folded twice and the hole is punched in the lower right corner. When the paper is unfolded, there will be four holes in the center of the square.

50. **D** The lower left corner of the square is folded in toward the center and then the top half of the square is folded down over the bottom and the hole is punched along the upper left center of the folded paper. When the paper is unfolded, there will be three holes: one in the bottom left corner, one in the lower left center, and one in the upper left center.

51. **E** The square is folded once on the diagonal and then again on the diagonal. The hole is punched in the lower left side. When the paper is unfolded, there will be four holes: one in the lower left side, one in the bottom left side, one in the upper right side, and one in the top right side.

52. **E** The square is folded once down from the top and then the right end is folded in toward the center. The hole is punched in the bottom right corner of the folded paper. When the paper is unfolded, there will be four holes, two on the bottom right and two on the top right.

53. **B** The square is folded twice and the hole is punched along the left corner, just above the center. When the paper is unfolded, there will be four holes: two along the left center and two along the right center.

54. **C** The square is folded once down from the top to the center, and the hole is punched in the left center. When the paper is unfolded, there will be two holes: one in the left center and one in the upper left center.

55. **A** The square is folded down from the right corner on the diagonal and then the left corner is folded up toward the center. The hole is punched in the center of the folded triangle. When the paper is unfolded, there will be four holes along the diagonal from lower left corner to upper right corner.

56. **C** The square is folded down from the right corner on the diagonal and then the left corner is folded down toward the bottom. The hole is punched in the center of the folded triangle. When the paper is unfolded, there will be four holes: two in the middle of the left side and two in the middle of the top side.

57. **D** The top quarter of the square is folded once toward the center and then the paper is folded in half from left to right. The hole is punched in the top left corner of the folded part. When the paper is unfolded, there will be four holes: two each in the middle of the top two rows.

58. **A** The top quarter of the square is folded down to the center and the bottom quarter is folded up to the center. The hole is punched in the right side of the bottom folded part. When the paper is unfolded, there will be two holes on the bottom right side of the paper.

59. **B** The square is folded on the diagonal and the hole is punched in the lower left corner. When the paper is unfolded, there will be two holes: one in the lower left corner and one in the upper right corner.

60. **A** The square is folded in half from the bottom up and the hole is punched in the right center. When the paper is unfolded, there will be two holes in the right center.

61. **B** The figure is made up of 17 cubes total: 7 on the front bottom row, 5 on the top row, and 5 invisible cubes supporting the top row. The two cubes in the middle of the bottom invisible row have only one side painted.

62. **D** The figure is made up of 17 cubes total: 7 on the front bottom row, 5 on the top row, and 5 invisible cubes supporting the top row. The 2 cubes in the middle left of the front bottom row have only two sides painted, the 2 cubes in the middle right of the front bottom row have only two sides painted, and the 2 cubes on the ends of the invisible bottom row have only two sides painted. The correct answer is D, 6 cubes.

63. **D** The figure is made up of 17 cubes total: 7 on the front bottom row, 5 on the top row, and 5 invisible cubes supporting the top row. The 2 cubes on the ends of the front bottom row have three sides painted, the center cube in the front bottom row has three sides painted, and the 3 cubes in the center of the top row have three sides painted. The correct answer is D, 6 cubes.

64. **B** The figure is made up of 17 cubes total: 7 on the front bottom row, 5 on the top row, and 5 invisible cubes supporting the top row. The two cubes on the ends of the top row have four sides painted.

65. **A** The figure is made up of 17 cubes total: 7 on the front bottom row, 5 on the top row, and 5 invisible cubes supporting the top row. The center invisible cube has no sides painted.

66. **B** The figure is made up of 24 cubes total: 12 on the bottom level, 8 on the middle level, and 4 on the top level. There are a total of 10 invisible cubes supporting the levels (4 in the middle level and 6 in the bottom level). The central front invisible cubes on the middle level and the bottom level have no sides painted.

67. **E** The figure is made up of 24 cubes total: 12 on the bottom level, 8 on the middle level, and 4 on the top level. There are a total of 10 invisible cubes supporting the levels (4 in the middle level and 6 in the bottom level). On the bottom level, 4 of the invisible cubes plus the 2 center front visible ones have only one side painted. On the middle level, the invisible cubes on the left and right have only one side painted. There are 8 cubes total with only one side painted, so the correct answer is E.

68. **B** The figure is made up of 24 cubes total: 12 on the bottom level, 8 on the middle level, and 4 on the top level. There are a total of 10 invisible cubes supporting the levels (4 in the middle level and 6 in the bottom level). On the middle and bottom levels, the cube at the far back has only two sides painted. These are the only two cubes with two sides painted.

69. **E** The figure is made up of 24 cubes total: 12 on the bottom level, 8 on the middle level, and 4 on the top level. There are a total of 10 invisible cubes supporting the levels (4 in the middle level and 6 in the bottom level). All 4 cubes on the top level

have three sides painted. On both the middle and bottom levels, the 2 visible cubes on the left and the 2 visible cubes on the right each have three sides painted. There are 12 cubes total with three sides painted, so the correct answer is E.

70. **A** The figure is made up of 16 cubes total: 7 on the bottom level, 5 on the second level, 3 on the third level, and 1 on top. None of the cubes have no sides painted.

71. **A** The figure is made up of 16 cubes total: 7 on the bottom level, 5 on the second level, 3 on the third level, and 1 on top. None of the cubes have only one side painted.

72. **E** The figure is made up of 16 cubes total: 7 on the bottom level, 5 on the second level, 3 on the third level, and 1 on top. The following cubes have only two sides painted: a total of 5 cubes on the bottom level—the front left and right cubes and the center invisible cube in back, plus the two center visible cubes (fronts and backs are painted); on the second level, the 3 cubes in the center, including the invisible one; on the third level, the back center invisible cube. There are a total of 9 cubes with only two sides painted, so the answer is E.

73. **A** The figure is made up of 16 cubes total: 7 on the bottom level, 5 on the second level, 3 on the third level, and 1 on top. There are no cubes with three sides painted.

74. **D** The figure is made up of 16 cubes total: 7 on the bottom level, 5 on the second level, 3 on the third level, and 1 on top. The following cubes have only four sides painted: the far left and far right cubes on the back of the bottom level and the far left and far right cubes on the second and third levels. There are a total of 6 cubes with four sides painted, so the answer is D.

75. **A** The figure is made up of 16 cubes total: 7 on the bottom level, 5 on the second level, 3 on the third level, and 1 on top. Only the top cube has five sides painted.

76. **B** The design shows a rectangular pillow-shaped box with no sides and concave ends.

77. **D** This design shows a square base with triangular sides. When shown in three dimensions, this will make a pyramid.

78. **B** This design is of a handbag with a handle cutout. The sides of the handbag are slightly curved.

79. **C** This design shows a square base with sides that resemble waves and will overlap each other.

80. **A** This design is of a single die. You must pay careful attention to the placement of the dots on each side of the die. Only choice A has an arrangement that would be possible from the original design.

81. **A** This design is for a rectangular box. The end pieces that will be folded inward have odd shapes, but they will not show on the outside of the three-dimensional box. Choice C also shows a rectangular box, but it is too narrow and too long.

82. **D** This design is for a diamond-shaped box.

83. **C** The design is of a container with an open top with one side higher than the other, similar to a fast-food french fry container.

84. **B** This design is for a box that is shaped like a star.

85. **B** This design is for a take-out container with a handle on top that has a bow.

86. **A** This design shows a long box with triangular ends.

87. **C** The design is of a cube-shaped box with slits to join the top into a heart shape.

88. **B** The design is of a very thin square box.

89. **D** The flat design is for a cube box with two opposite sides shaded. The only answer choice that shows this figure is choice D.

90. **B** The design shows a box with a square base and curved sides that join with each other through slits in two of the opposing sides.

Reading Comprehension

1. **D** The passage states that most patients with stage III or stage IV tumors are candidates for treatment by a combination of surgery and radiation therapy. The best answer is D.

2. **C** The main routes of lymph node drainage are into the first station nodes: the buccinator, jugulodigastric, submandibular, and submental. The parotid is a second station node. The best answer is C.

3. **D** The final paragraph says that a dental exam should be performed in order to prevent late sequelae. The best answer is D.

4. **A** Early lesions (T1 and T2) of the anterior tongue may be managed by surgery or by radiation therapy alone. Both modalities produce 70 to 85 percent cure rates in early lesions. The best answer is A.

5. **A** The passage states that most primary cancers of the hard palate are of minor salivary gland origin. The best answer is A.

6. **E** Moderately advanced lesions of the anterior tongue have a local control rate of 65 percent. The best answer is E.

7. **A** While all of these choices are things a patient might consider, the passage only mentions the anticipated functional and cosmetic results of treatment and the availability of the particular expertise required of the surgeon or radiation oncologist for the individual patient. The best answer is A.

8. **B** Surgical treatment of cancer of the hard palate usually requires excision of underlying bone producing an opening into the antrum. The best answer is B.

9. **D** Early cancers of the lip have a cure rate of 90 to 100 percent. Small cancers of the retromolar trigone have a cure rate of as much as 100 percent, while moderately advanced lesions without evidence of spread to cervical lymph nodes have a cure rate of as much as 90 percent. Small cancers of the buccal mucosa have a cure rate of 90 percent. Moderately advanced lesions of the floor of the mouth without evidence of spread to cervical lymph nodes have a cure rate of as much as 70 percent, which is the lowest of the group. The best answer is D.

10. **C** According to the passage, stage III and IV patients should be considered for clinical trials because local recurrence and/or distant metastases are common in this group of patients. The best answer is C.

11. **E** Patients who smoke while on radiation therapy appear to have lower response rates and shorter survival durations than those who do not. The best answer is E.

12. **E** The passage states that a study of patients with head and neck cancers has shown that daily treatment of these patients with moderate doses of isotretinoin (13-cis-retinoic acid) for one year can significantly reduce the incidence of second tumors. The author would most likely agree that this is a sound course of treatment. The best answer is E.

13. **B** Small superficial cancers can be very successfully treated by local implantation using any one of several radioactive sources, by intraoral cone radiation therapy, or by electrons. The best choice is B.

14. **C** A hemiglossectomy is an excision of one side of the tongue. The best answer is C.

15. **A** With an extensive resection of the tongue, problems may include aspiration of liquids and solids and difficulty in swallowing in addition to speech difficulties. The best answer is A.

16. **D** More advanced lesions of the lower gingiva require segmental bone resection, hemimandibulectomy, or maxillectomy, depending on the extent of the lesion and its location. The best answer is D.

17. **A** All dental healthcare professionals are responsible for creating and maintaining a safe working environment. The best answer is A.

18. **A** Administrative controls include policies, procedures, and enforcement measures targeted at reducing the risk of exposure to infectious persons. The best answer is A.

19. **D** The passage states that immunization of DHCP before they are placed at risk for exposure remains the most efficient and effective use of vaccines in healthcare settings. The best answer is D.

20. **B** In addition to standard procedures, certain diseases, such as varicella, require transmission-based precautions. These might include patient placement (e.g., isolation), adequate room ventilation, respiratory protection (e.g., N-95 masks) for DHCP, or postponement of nonemergency dental procedures. The best answer is B.

21. **E** The second paragraph details the ways in which patients and DHCP can be exposed to pathogenic microorganisms. These ways include direct contact with blood, oral fluids, or other patient materials; indirect contact with contaminated objects (e.g., instruments, equipment, or environmental surfaces); contact of conjunctival, nasal, or oral mucosa with droplets (e.g., spatter) containing microorganisms generated from an infected person and propelled a short distance (e.g., by coughing, sneezing, or talking); and inhalation of airborne microorganisms that can remain suspended in the air for long periods. The best answer is E.

22. **A** The purpose of preventive practices is to reduce blood exposures. The best answer is A.

23. **C** Engineering controls eliminate or isolate hazards. They include using puncture-resistant sharps containers or needle-retraction devices. The best answer is C.

24. **E** Dental patients and DHCP can be exposed to pathogenic microorganisms including cytomegalovirus (CMV), HBV, HCV, herpes simplex virus types 1 and 2, HIV, *Mycobacterium tuberculosis*, staphylococci, streptococci, and other viruses and bacteria that colonize or infect the oral cavity and respiratory tract. The best answer is E.

25. **D** Hepatitis B, influenza, measles, mumps, rubella, and varicella are all vaccine-preventable. The best answer is D.

26. **B** CDC expanded the concept of universal precautions and changed the term to *standard precautions* because the relevance of universal precautions to other aspects of disease transmission was recognized. The best answer is B.

27. **B** The chain of infection requires that all of the following conditions be present: a pathogenic organism of sufficient virulence and in adequate numbers to cause disease; a reservoir or source that allows the pathogen to survive and multiply (e.g., blood); a mode of transmission from the source to the host; a portal of entry through which the pathogen can enter the host; and a susceptible host (i.e., one who is not immune). The best answer is B.

28. **D** A work-practice control is a behavior, such as wearing PPE, that helps to minimize the risk of infection. The best answer is D.

29. **A** The Advisory Committee on Immunization Practices (ACIP) provides national guidelines for immunization of HCP, which includes DHCP. The best answer is A.

30. **E** DHCP include dentists, dental hygienists, dental assistants, dental laboratory technicians (in-office and commercial), students and trainees, contractual personnel, and other persons not directly involved in patient care but potentially exposed to infectious agents (e.g., administrative, clerical, housekeeping, maintenance, or volunteer personnel). The best answer is E.

31. **C** The effectiveness of the infection-control program should be evaluated on a day-to-day basis and over time to help ensure that policies, procedures, and practices are useful, efficient, and successful. The best answer is C.

32. **B** Standard precautions apply to contact with blood; all body fluids, secretions, and excretions (except sweat), regardless of whether they contain blood; nonintact skin; and mucous membranes. The best answer is B.

33. **E** Occupational Safety and Health Administration (OSHA) provides practices and procedures for worker protection. The best choice is E.

34. **D** The passage states that the invasive nature of oral care might trigger violent and self-injurious behavior such as head banging. The best answer is D.

35. **C** Tooth eruption may be delayed due to phenytoin-induced gingival hyperplasia. The best answer is C.

36. **B** The mouth is always at risk during a seizure: patients may chip teeth or bite the tongue or cheeks. The best answer is B.

37. **A** Autism is a complex developmental disability that impairs communication and social, behavioral, and intellectual functioning. The best answer is A.

38. **C.** The passage repeatedly recommends talking to the caregiver as the best way to gather information. The best answer is C.

39. **D** The passage says that a provider should use a "tell-show-do" approach to providing care. The best answer is D.

40. **C** Damaging oral habits include bruxism; tongue thrusting; self-injurious behavior such as picking at the gingiva or biting the lips; and pica. The best answer is C.

41. **B** The passage advises providers to obtain and review the patient's medical history; consult with physicians, family, and caregivers; and determine who can legally provide informed consent for treatment. The best answer is B.

42. **E** While any of the five senses may present a problem for a patient with autism, the passage does not mention taste. The best answer is E.

43. **A** Some people have coexisting conditions such as intellectual disability or epilepsy. The best answer is A.

44. **E** If a seizure occurs during oral care, providers should remove any instruments from the mouth and clear the area around the dental chair, stay with the patient, turn him or her to one side, and monitor the airway to reduce the risk of aspiration. Objects should not be inserted between the teeth. The best answer is E.

45. **D** Obsessive routines, repetitive behaviors, unpredictable body movements, and self-injurious behavior may all be symptoms that complicate dental care. The best answer is D.

46. **B** Perseveration is a continuous, meaningless repetition of words, phrases, or movements. The best answer is B.

47. **C** The rate of caries in people with autism is the same as in the general population. The best answer is C.

48. **A** The purpose of a desensitization appointment is to help the patient become familiar with the office, staff, and equipment through a step-by-step process. The best answer is A.

49. **B** Immobilization techniques should be used only when absolutely necessary to protect the patient and staff during dental treatment. The best answer is B.

50. **E** Dental caries risk increases in patients who have a preference for soft, sticky, or sweet foods; damaging oral habits; and difficulty brushing and flossing. The best answer is E.

Quantitative Reasoning

1. **B** This diagram features a right angle, which means that we can use the Pythagorean theorem to solve the problem. The equation is $a^2 + b^2 = c^2$ where a and b are the lengths of the legs and c is the length of the hypotenuse (the leash). $5^2 + 7^2 = c^2$ so, $74 = c^2$ and $c = 8.6$.

2. **B** The slope of a line is $\frac{\Delta y}{\Delta x}$. A is at $(-3, 8)$ and B is located at $(3, 6)$. Substituting into the equation we get: $\frac{(6-8)}{3--3} = \frac{-2}{6} = -\frac{1}{3}$.

3. **B** If 55% voted for A then 45% voted for B. This equates to $(.45)(1860) = 837$ votes for B.

4. **C** Looking at the choices we see that when we FOIL the choices, choice C will yield $121 - x^2$. This can be confirmed knowing that choice C will have a $-11x$ and a $+11x$, which will cancel each other out.

5. **D** Cross multiplying, we get $6x - 9 = 2x - 8$. This equals $4x = 1$, $x = \frac{1}{4}$.

6. **E** Because the pentagon has five sides, we need to multiply the segments length by 5, so $5(x + 4) = 5x + 20$.

7. **E** Substituting the points into the equation we can see that $2(0) - 3(-3) = 0 + 9 = 9$.

8. **A** Together, the probability has to equal $\frac{3}{10}$ (30%). Sunday has a $\frac{3}{5}$ chance (60%). In order to have the 60% become 30% total, we must halve the probability. This is done by multiplying $\frac{3}{5}$ by $\frac{1}{2}$.

9. **D** Choice A shows a line with a positive slope according to $y = mx + b$. B shows a graph of an absolute value. C is a graph of a parabola. D does show the graph of an exponential relationship.

10. **B** The tangent of an angle is the length of the opposite side divided by the length of the adjacent side. $\frac{8}{15} = 0.5333$.

11. **C** Because the denominators are the same, we just need to focus on the numerators. $2 + x - (x - 2)$ is equal to $2 + x - x + 2 = 4$. The answer is $\frac{4}{5x}$.

12. **D** For the first letter there will be six choices. For the second letter there will be five, for the third, four, and for the fourth letter there will three choices. $6 \times 5 \times 4 \times 3 = 360$ combinations.

13. **E** This requires a number of steps:

$$-3\sqrt{48} =$$
$$-3\sqrt{2}\sqrt{2}\sqrt{12} =$$
$$-3(2)\sqrt{3}\sqrt{4} =$$
$$-3(2)\sqrt{3}(2) =$$
$$-12\sqrt{3}$$

14. **E** The volume of a cube is $l \times w \times h = 10 \times 2 \times 4 = 80$ cm³. The length of the edges is $40 + 8 + 16 = 64$ cm because there are four edges for each length. Finally, the surface area is the sum of the area of each face of the object $2(10 \times 2) + 2(4 \times 2) + 2(10 \times 4) = 136$ cm².

15. **A** The height of the balloon is opposite the given angle. We also know the length of the hypotenuse is 110 feet. Because we have the opposite side and the hypotenuse, we can say that sin $50° = \frac{x}{110}$. Sin $50° = 0.766$, so $0.766 = \frac{x}{110}$. $(0.766)(110) = x = 84.26$ feet.

16. **B** The equation of a circle is $(x - h)^2 + (y - k)^2 = r^2$. We can see immediately that the value of h has to be 0. The equation shows $y - 7$, meaning that k has a value of 7. To separate choice B from C, the value of 16 comes from the radius being squared, $4^2 = 16$, so r = 4.

17. **D** The equation for the length of a line segment is

$$d = \sqrt{(x_2 - x_1)^2 + (y_2 - y_1)^2}$$
$$d = \sqrt{(2 - -6)^2 + (-5 - 4)^2}$$
$$d = \sqrt{(8)^2 + (-9)^2}$$
$$d = \sqrt{(64) + (81)}$$
$$d = \sqrt{145}$$

18. **C** This equation will follow the form of $y = mx + b$. Dividing both sides by 2, we get $y = -3x + 4$. Because the line has to be perpendicular, we need to find the negative reciprocal, which is a slope of $\frac{1}{3}$.

19. **E** The value of x needs to be determined first. $2x + 2x + 3x + 5 + 3x + 5 = 360°$. $10x + 10 = 360°$. $x = 35°$. Angle ABC has a value of $2x$, or $70°$.

20. **D** Substituting, we get $3(35°) + 5° = 110°$.

21. **B** Remember that there are 360 degrees in a trapezoid. Keeping in mind that $x = 35°$ for this problem, and referring to question 19, $2x + 2x + 3x + 5 + 3x + 5 = 360$. $10x + 10 = 360$.

22. **C** Because line segment $\overline{HTP}$ has a total of $180°$, $180 - (6x + 20) = 180 - 6x - 20$.

23. **C** The total number of degrees in the triangle is 180, so now we add up all of the values of the angles and set them equal to 180.

$$180 = 180 - 6x - 20 + x + 40 + 4x - 5$$
$$0 = -x + 15$$
$$x = 15$$

24. **A** Two of the angles measure $55°$, so they are the same, whereas the third angle is $70°$. This means that the triangle is isosceles.

25. **D** The sum of the three angles of a triangle is the total number of degrees of the triangle. This equals $2x + 6 + x + 19 + 3x + 5 = 6x + 30$.

26. **E** We know that the sum of the angles is $6x + 30$. Setting this equal to $180°$, $6x + 30 = 180°$. $6x = 150$, $x = 25$.

27. **B** Segment BD is diagonal touching both line segment AB and line segment CD. Angle ABD is 44 degrees, as is angle BDC. Because they form alternate interior angles, the lines must be parallel.

28. **A** The $2x + 1$ is substituted for x in the equation $x^2 - 9$ giving: $(2x + 1)^2 - 9$. Multiplying it out gives $4x^2 + 2x + 2x + 1 - 9$. This comes out to be $4x^2 + 4x - 8$.

29. **C** This is the straightforward graph of $y = \csc x$, where two parabolas will not cross the asymptotes at whole number values of π.

30. **E** This is a straightforward, simple problem where the numerators are multiplied as are the denominators. $3 \times 1 = 3$ and $8 \times 2 = 16$. The answer is $\frac{3}{16}$.

31. **A** We first need a common denominator of 12. To do so, we need to multiply $\frac{5}{6}$ by $\frac{2}{2}$ and $\frac{1}{4}$ by $\frac{3}{3}$. This gives $\frac{10}{12} - \frac{3}{12} = \frac{7}{12}$.

32. **D** Cross multiplying first gives us $1x = 7x - 14$. $-6x = -14$, therefore $x = \frac{14}{16} = \frac{7}{3}$.

33. **D** This is a longer conversion problem that needs to be carefully drawn out. Remember that all units except seconds will need to cancel.

$$1 \; \cancel{\text{week}} \left(\frac{7 \; \cancel{\text{days}}}{1 \; \cancel{\text{week}}} \right) \left(\frac{24 \; \cancel{\text{hours}}}{1 \; \cancel{\text{day}}} \right) \left(\frac{60 \; \cancel{\text{minutes}}}{1 \; \cancel{\text{hour}}} \right) \left(\frac{60 \; \text{seconds}}{1 \; \cancel{\text{minute}}} \right) = 604{,}800 \; \text{seconds}$$

34. B There are 52 cards in a standard deck, and 13 of them will be hearts. $\frac{13}{52} = \frac{1}{4}$. One out of every four cards will be a heart.

35. C A great mnemonic device for mean is, "The average teacher is mean." To find the average, first add up all of the numbers and then divide by 7 because 7 values are present: $\frac{482}{7} = 68.9$. The median is 65 because when placed in order, 65 is the number in the middle of the set {45, 56, 60, 65, 78, 81, 97}. The mode is the most repeated number. None of the numbers are repeated.

36. B The range is the value of the highest number minus the value of the lowest number, $97 - 45 = 52$.

37. E When an equation is written as $y = ax^2 + bx + c$, the quadratic equation is needed to find the roots. This equation is shown below:

$$x = \frac{-b \pm \sqrt{b^2 4ac}}{2a}$$

38. B $\frac{(x_2 + x_1, y_2 + y_1)}{2}$ is the method for finding the midpoint between two points.

39. A $A = \frac{1}{2}(a + b)h$ is the equation for finding the areas of a trapezoid. Remember to add the two legs together first before any other calculations.

40. C II and IV are correct, but be careful of III. While III has the correct numerical value, the units are not correct as they need to be meters squared! I is incorrect because the diameter needs to be double the radius, 7.6 meters.

PART III
NATURAL SCIENCES

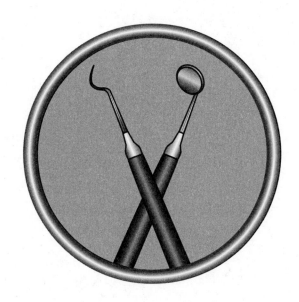

CHAPTER 4

The Cell and Molecular Biology

Read This Chapter to Learn About

➤ The Origin of Life

➤ Molecules of Life

➤ Prokaryotic and Eukaryotic Cells

➤ Organelles

➤ Movement of Substances Across the Cell Membrane

➤ Enzymes

➤ Energy

➤ Photosynthesis

➤ Cellular Respiration and Metabolism

➤ Cell Division and Chromosomes

THE ORIGIN OF LIFE

The origin of life encompasses an enormous number of detailed events. The major events will be briefly summarized in this section. Life began approximately four billion years ago when the solar system formed and the Earth cooled. The big bang theory is used to explain how the universe, including our solar system, might have come about. This theory supposes that a large, hot mass of material in the galaxy broke apart to distribute matter and energy throughout the universe. This distribution of material caused a major cooling of temperature. Nuclear fusion created many of the major elements that, over time, collided and condensed into stars that provided light and heat.

The primitive atmosphere of Earth consisted of a variety of organic and inorganic substances such as ammonia, methane, water, carbon monoxide, carbon dioxide, nitrogen gas, and hydrogen gas. What was lacking was oxygen gas. Water vapor formed rain, which collected into pools containing mineral runoff from rocks. A source of energy within these bodies of water, perhaps derived from lightning or sunlight, fueled the reactions needed to create organic molecules such as sugars, amino acids, nucleotides, and fatty acids. As these monomers collected in clay, they may have polymerized to form molecules such as proteins, carbohydrates, and nucleic acids.

Some proteins produced within clay had enzymatic properties, allowing them to interact with other molecules. The formation of a membrane around these primitive enzymes produced the first protocell that had the ability to self-replicate. An association of the protocell with RNA may have produced the first actual cell that resembled modern prokaryotes. These cells lacked organelles and lived in an anaerobic environment. Mutations that occurred in some populations of the first cells provided photoautotrophic abilities. The development of photosynthesis had an important impact in that it produced oxygen gas, making an aerobic environment in which aerobic cellular respiration evolved as the dominant energy-producing process.

Eukaryotic cells evolved from the prokaryotic-like cells. The theory of endosymbiosis explains the presence of organelles within eukaryotic cells. The engulfment of bacterial cells led to mitochondria, and the engulfment of photosynthesizing prokaryotes led to the development of chloroplasts, as seen in modern-day plants. Membrane infolding explains the presence of organelles such as the nucleus and endoplasmic reticulum in eukaryotic cells. Internalizing some of the cell membrane provided greater surface area for reactions to occur, and thus this adaptation was selected for. These early eukaryotic cells resembled protists in structure. Over time, symbiotic relationships occurred between eukaryotic cells that led to specialization and the division of labor needed to eventually produce multicellular organisms. All modern plants, animals, and fungi evolved from these primitive eukaryotic cells.

MOLECULES OF LIFE

The basic biochemicals of importance are a set of organic (carbon-containing) molecules called lipids, nucleic acids, amino acids, and carbohydrates. This is in addition to the inorganic (not containing carbon) molecules, such as water, that are also needed. We cannot go further without a discussion about the basic organic monomers that can become the complex polymers that make up life as we know it to be today.

Experimentation has shown that when a simulated early earth's atmosphere is recreated with nitrogen gas, methane, carbon dioxide, and water followed up with electricity being passed through these gases (to simulate lightning), amino acids were formed. Amino acids contain an amine group, $-NH_2$, and a carboxylic acid group, $-COOH$. There is also a varying part, $-R$, that can give the amino acid a range of acidities, polarities, and so on. In short, an amino acid has the general structure of: $HOOC-CHR-NH_2$. Because of the acidic properties of the carboxylic acid group and the basic properties of the amine group, an H^+ ion can be lost by the acid and gained by the amine group. The result is a zwitterion, an electrically neutral substance that contains both positive and negative charges: $^-OOC-CHR-NH_3^+$.

The bonding of amino acids involves the loss of water via a dehydration synthesis to give a protein. There are four levels of protein structure:

➤ The **primary structure** is nothing more than a sequence of amino acids. This can be an endless combination considering that there are 20 amino acids to be used. This helps to explain the diversity of tissue structure that living organisms can contain.

➤ The **secondary structure** is the formation of an alpha helix or beta pleated sheet. These structures can be held by the hydrogen bonds that form.

➤ The **tertiary structure** is the folding over of the secondary structure. Disulfide bridges (-S-S-) and hydrogen bonds also hold this structure together. If ions or non-polar portions of the molecule are present, there is also the possibility of ionic or dispersion forces.

➤ The **quaternary structure** is many tertiary structures put together.

Carbohydrates can range from a number of simple sugars, like glucose, to complex polysaccharides like starch or cellulose. The general formula for these simple sugars is $C_x(H_2O)_x$. Glucose can exist as a straight chain or as a ring. As a straight chain, glucose is said to be an aldose, because of the aldehyde functional group present. Some sugars, such as fructose, have a C=O more toward the interior of the molecule. These are called ketose sugars because the ketone functional group is present. The joining of simple sugars is completed by a dehydration synthesis to form disaccharides and then polysaccharides. These complex sugars can be stored and converted back to glucose as needed to provide energy.

Lipids are also a source of energy, in addition to being a source of protection and warmth. Lipids are formed from the esterification reaction between glycerol and a fatty acid. If the fatty acid has all single bonds, it will form a saturated fat. If the fatty acid has double bonds present, it is said to be an unsaturated fat.

PROKARYOTIC AND EUKARYOTIC CELLS

The cell is the basic unit of life. As a general rule, all cells are small in size in order to maintain a large surface area to volume ratio. Having a large surface area relative to a small volume allows cells to perform vital functions at a reasonably fast rate, which is necessary for survival. Cells that are too large have small surface area to volume ratios and have difficulties getting the nutrients that they need and expelling wastes in a timely manner.

The two major categories of cells are prokaryotic and eukaryotic. All organisms in the domains Bacteria and Archaea are composed of prokaryotic cells, while all members of the domain Eukarya are composed of eukaryotic cells. There are some similarities between the two cell types, but there are also significant differences. Table 4.1 depicts the major structural differences between prokaryotic and eukaryotic cells.

Table 4.1 Major Differences Between Eukaryotic and Prokaryotic Cells		
Characteristic	**Eukaryotic Cells**	**Prokaryotic Cells**
Cell size	Relatively larger	Relatively smaller
Organelles	Present	Absent
Organization of genetic material	Linear pieces of DNA organized as chromosomes housed within the nucleus	A single loop of DNA floating in the cytoplasm
Oxygen requirements	Generally need oxygen to produce energy during cellular respiration	May not require oxygen to produce energy during cellular respiration
Ribosomes	80S (made of 60S and 40S subunit)	70S ribosomes (made of 50S and 30S subunit)
Histone proteins	Present	Absent
Cell wall	Absent in animal cells, but present in fungi (made of chitin) and in plants (made of cellulose)	Mostly present in prokaryotes (composed of peptidoglycan in bacteria)
Mobility	More complex (9 +2) flagella; possibility of cilia and amoeboid movement	A simpler type of flagella

ORGANELLES

One primary factor that differentiates eukaryotic cells from prokaryotic cells is the presence of organelles. Organelles are membrane-bound compartments within the cell that have specialized functions. They help with cellular organization and efficiency by ensuring that specific reactions have specific organelles in which to occur. The structure of a typical eukaryotic cell can be seen in Figure 4.1.

The organelles and other structures, but not including the nucleus, are contained within the cytoplasm, which encompasses the space between the plasma membrane and the nucleus. The liquid portion of the cell is called the cytosol. It consists of water, nutrients, ions, and wastes, and it can be the site of a variety of chemical reactions within the cell.

All eukaryotic cells contain a membrane-bound nucleus. The nucleus houses the genetic material of the cell in the form of chromosomes. The outer boundary of the nucleus is referred to as the nuclear membrane (also termed the nuclear envelope), and it keeps the contents of the nucleus separate from the rest of the cell. The nuclear membrane has pores that allow certain substances to enter and exit the nucleus. Within the nucleus, there is a nucleolus. The job of the nucleolus is to make the ribosomal ribonucleic acid (rRNA) needed to produce ribosomes.

Ribosomes are made from rRNA (produced in the nucleolus) and protein. A ribosome consists of one large subunit and one small subunit that are assembled when protein synthesis is needed. Ribosomes can be found loose in the cytosol of the cell (free ribosomes) or attached to the endoplasmic reticulum of the cell (bound ribosomes). Free ribosomes and membrane-bound ribosomes are identical in structure and function but differ in the proteins that are being made in that free ribosomes make proteins that are destined to function either in the cytosol, mitochondria, chloroplast, or nucleus. Membrane-bound ribosomes will make proteins that will be translocated into the ER lumen or into the ER membrane (depending on the protein structure) and either function within the ER membrane or move through the endomembrane system and function within the lumen of an organelle or be released out of the cell. They can also be transported to function within the plasma membrane. The protein sorting is done with amino acid signaling sequences that are present on the nascent polypeptide and are eventually cleaved off by a signal peptidase and then rapidly degraded.

The endomembrane system consists of several organelles within the eukaryotic cell that work together as a unit to synthesize and transport molecules within the cell. This endomembrane system consists of: smooth endoplasmic reticulum, nuclear envelope, rough endoplasmic reticulum, Golgi complex, lysosomes, peroxisomes, and vesicles that transport materials within the system.

The endoplasmic reticulum (ER) is a folded network of membrane-bound space that has the appearance of a maze. The rough ER contains bound ribosomes on the surface,

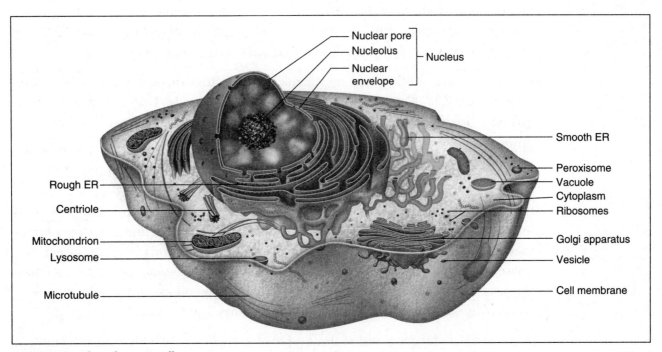

FIGURE 4.1 The eukaryotic cell.

while the smooth ER does not. While these two structures are connected, their functions are distinct.

In the smooth ER, the primary function is the production of lipids needed by the cell. In certain types of eukaryotic cells (such as the liver), the smooth ER plays a critical role in the production of detoxifying enzymes.

Since the rough ER has bound ribosomes, its function is related to protein synthesis. The ribosomes produce proteins that enter the rough ER. Once inside the rough ER, these proteins are chemically modified and moved to the smooth ER. The combined contents of the smooth ER and the rough ER are then shipped by vesicles to the Golgi complex for sorting.

Vesicles are tiny pieces of membrane that will break off and carry the contents of the ER throughout the endomembrane system. Vesicles from the ER arrive at the Golgi complex (also called the Golgi apparatus) and deliver their contents, which include proteins and lipids. These molecules will be further modified, repackaged, and tagged for their eventual destination. The contents of the Golgi complex leave via vesicles, and many of them will be moved to the cell membrane for secretion out of the cell.

Lysosomes are large, membrane-bound sacs that contain digestive enzymes used to break down any substances that enter the lysosomes. Cellular structures that are old, damaged, or unnecessary can be degraded in the lysosomes. Further, substances taken into the cell by endocytosis (the process of cells taking in molecules by enclosing them in a vesicle pinched off of the cell membrane) can be transported to the lysosomes for destruction. In order to function properly, the pH of the lysosomes must be acidic. Lysosomes contain ATP-driven H^+ pumps that pump H^+ ions into the lysosome, causing it to become more acidic, and their membrane proteins are highly glycosylated to protect them from the proteases. In some cases, cells purposefully rupture their lysosomes in an attempt to commit cellular suicide in a process known as apoptosis.

Peroxisomes are another type of vacuole found within the endomembrane system. They are capable of digesting fatty acids and amino acids. They also degrade toxic hydrogen peroxide, a metabolic waste product, to water and oxygen gas.

Mitochondria are the organelles responsible for energy production in the cell. They perform aerobic cellular respiration that ultimately creates adenosine triphosphate (ATP), which is the preferred source of energy for cells. Since all cells require energy to survive, the process of cellular respiration is a vital one for the cell. Mitochondria have some interesting and unusual features: they are bound by an inner and outer membrane, they contain their own DNA distinct from the nuclear DNA, and they can self-replicate. These unique features have led to the development of the endosymbiotic theory, which suggests that mitochondria are the evolutionary remnants of bacteria that were engulfed by other cells long ago in evolutionary time.

The cytoskeleton is composed of three types of fibers that exist within the cytoplasm of the cell. These fibers have a variety of functions including structural support, maintenance of cell shape, and cell division. Microtubules are one type of hollow fiber, made of the protein tubulin, that is responsible for structural support and the maintenance of cell shape. Microtubules also provide tracks that allow for the movement of organelles within the cell. During cell division, microtubules are used to help direct chromosomes through the cell. Microfilaments are made of the protein actin; they assist with cellular movement. The final type of fiber found in the cytoskeleton is intermediate filaments, the composition of which varies greatly from one cell type to the next. These filaments typically form a network throughout the cytoplasm and are anchored at the plasma membrane at specific points where the filament from one cell is in contact with the filament from another. There are four classes of intermediate filaments: keratin filaments, vimentin filaments, neurofilaments, and nuclear lamins. The primary purpose of the intermediate filaments is structural support for the cell.

Certain types of animal cells contain additional structures such as cilia and flagella. Cilia are hairlike structures on the surface of some cells that move in synchronized motion. For example, cilia on the surface of cells lining the respiratory tract constantly move in an attempt to catch and remove bacteria and particles that may enter the respiratory tract. Some animal cells, such as sperm, contain flagella, which essentially act as tails to allow for movement.

Plant cells are a particular type of eukaryotic cell that generally have all of the structures and organelles described to this point. However, there are a few additional structures that are unique to plant cells. These include a cell wall, chloroplasts, and a central vacuole. The cell wall is composed of cellulose (fiber) and serves to protect the cell from its environment and from desiccation. The chloroplasts within a plant cell contain the green pigment chlorophyll, which is used in the process of photosynthesis. Chloroplasts are similar to mitochondria in that they have their own DNA and replicate independently. Endosymbiotic theory is also used to explain their existence in plants. Finally, plant cells contain a large central vacuole that serves as reserve storage for water, nutrients, and waste products. The central vacuole typically takes up the majority of space within a plant cell.

The outer boundary of the cell is the cell membrane (plasma membrane); its purpose is to form a selectively permeable barrier between the cell and its external environment. The membrane itself is composed of a bilayer of phospholipids containing proteins scattered within the bilayer. Phospholipids are unique molecules because they have polar and nonpolar regions. The head of a phospholipid is composed of a glycerol and phosphate group (PO_4) that carries a charge and is hydrophilic. The tails of the phospholipid are fatty acids that are not charged and are hydrophobic. Phospholipids spontaneously arrange themselves in a bilayer where the heads align themselves toward the inside and outside of the cell where water is located, and the fatty acid tails are sandwiched between the layers. It should be noted that these phospholipids are not static when part of the membrane; rather they are quite dynamic and rapidly move laterally within one plane of the membrane. However, they will rarely flip to the opposite plane, since this would require the hydrophilic head portion of the phospholipid to move through the hydrophobic interior of the bilayer, which is energetically unfavorable. Regardless, there are proteins called flippases that will flip a phospholipid from one plane to the other if this is required by the cell.

Many molecules are capable of moving through the plasma membrane. Typically, these molecules will be small and nonpolar. However, it is not just nonpolar molecules that can cross the plasma membrane. For example, while O_2 and N_2 are both able to easily cross the membrane because they are small and nonpolar, ethanol and water are also able to cross the membrane rather easily even though they are polar. The more important factor in determining whether or not a molecule will cross the lipid bilayer, in addition to the size limitation, is the charge of the molecule. Charged molecules and ions will not pass through the bilayer, regardless of size. For example, K^+, Na^+, Ca^{2+}, and Cl^- will not pass through the membrane without the aid of a protein channel or transporter even though they are smaller than O_2, N_2, ethanol, and water. Charged molecules and ions are rather unwilling to pass through the lipid bilayer because it would force them to come in contact with the hydrophobic interior of the bilayer, which is energetically unfavorable.

In addition to the phospholipid bilayer, other substances are present in the cell membrane. The fluid mosaic model seen in Figure 4.2 shows the basic membrane structure. Cholesterol is found embedded within the interior of the membrane; its primary purpose is to regulate the fluidity of the membrane. Proteins are scattered within the bilayer; they may serve multiple purposes such as membrane transport, enzymatic

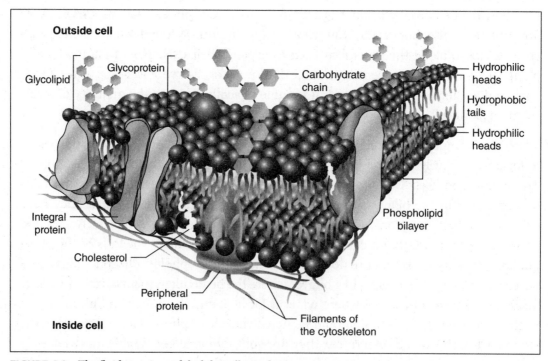

FIGURE 4.2   The fluid mosaic model of the cell membrane.

activity, cell adhesion, and communication; they may also serve as receptors for specific substances that may need to cross the membrane. Some proteins and lipids within the cell membrane contain carbohydrates on the exterior surface. These carbohydrates, or glycoproteins and glycolipids, often serve as identifying markers, or antigens, for the cell.

MOVEMENT OF SUBSTANCES ACROSS THE CELL MEMBRANE

There are a variety of ways that substances can cross the cell membrane. The three main membrane transports are passive transport, active transport, and bulk transport. Passive transport occurs spontaneously without energy, while active transport requires energy in the form of adenosine triphosphate (ATP).

Concentration gradients are a key consideration with movement across the cell membrane. The concentration gradient refers to a relative comparison of solutes and overall concentrations of fluids inside and outside the cell. Without the influence of outside forces, substances tend to move down their concentration gradient toward equilibrium. Only with an energy input can items move against their concentration gradient. Another important consideration for movement of molecules down a gradient is the electrical aspect if the molecules being moved are charged. This gradient is called the electrochemical gradient since it not only depends on the concentration gradient, which would be the difference in the amount of a molecule on either side of a membrane, but also on the charge being carried by a molecule and the membrane's electrical potential. For example, the interior of the plasma membrane (cytoplasmic side) has a negative potential when compared to the exterior face of the membrane (extracellular side). If Na^+ molecules were to be moved from the extracellular side of the cell into its interior and Na^+ concentration was greater outside the cell than inside, the molecules would move down their electrochemical gradients since there is a greater concentration of Na^+ outside the cell than inside (concentration gradient) and the positive charge of the sodium is attracted to the negative interior of the membrane (voltage gradient).

Passive transport mechanisms consist of diffusion and osmosis, both of which move a substance from an area of high concentration to an area of low concentration. Diffusion and osmosis are spontaneous processes and do not require ATP.

Diffusion is defined as the movement of small solutes down their concentration gradients. In other words, dissolved particles move from whichever side of the membrane has more of them to the side of the membrane that has less. Diffusion is a slow process by nature, but the following factors can influence its rate: temperature, the size of the molecule attempting to diffuse (large items are incapable of diffusion), and how large the concentration gradient is. Diffusion continues until equilibrium is met.

Osmosis is a very specific type of diffusion in which the substance moving down its concentration gradient is water. In an attempt to have equally concentrated solutions inside and outside the cell, osmosis will occur if the solute itself is unable to cross the cell membrane because it is too large. Simply put, osmosis moves water from the side of the membrane that has more water (and less solute) to the side of the membrane that has less water (and more solute).

When the concentrations of solutes inside and outside the cell are equal, the solutions are termed isotonic and there will be no net movement of water into or out of the cell. In most situations, isotonic solutions are the goal for cells. A solution that has more water and less solute relative to what it is being compared to is termed hypotonic, while a solution that has less water and more solute relative to what it is being compared to is termed a hypertonic solution. When cells are placed in hypertonic solutions, water will leave the cells via osmosis, which can cause the cells to shrivel. Cells placed in hypotonic solutions will gain water via osmosis and may swell and burst. The osmotic effects of each type of solution can be seen in Figure 4.3.

Active transport is in direct contrast to passive transport and is used to move solutes against their concentration gradient from the side of the membrane that has less solute to the side that has more. The solutes move via transport proteins in the membrane that act as pumps. Because this is in contrast to the spontaneous nature of passive transport, energy in the form of ATP must be invested to pump solutes against their concentration gradients.

The methods for membrane transport described thus far are limited by the size of molecules and do not affect the movement of large items (or large quantities of an item) across the membrane. Endocytosis and exocytosis are used to move large items across the cell membrane. Endocytosis is used to bring items into the cell. The membrane surrounds the item to form a vesicle that pinches off and moves into the cell. When liquids are moved into the cell this way, the process is termed pinocytosis. When large items, such as other cells, are brought into the cell, the process is termed phagocytosis.

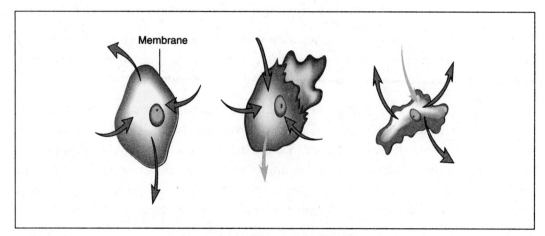

FIGURE 4.3 Osmosis in isotonic, hypotonic, and hypertonic solutions.

Exocytosis is used to transport molecules out of the cell. In this case, vesicles containing the substance to be transported move toward the cell membrane and fuse with the membrane. This releases the substance to the outside of the cell.

ENZYMES

Enzymes are a special category of proteins that serve as biological catalysts, meaning they speed up chemical reactions. Their names often end in the suffix *-ase*. They are essential to the maintenance of homeostasis within cells. Enzymes function by lowering the activation energy required to initiate a chemical reaction, thus increasing the rate at which the reaction occurs. Enzymes are unchanged during a reaction and are recycled and reused. Enzymes are involved in catabolic reactions that break down molecules, as well as in anabolic reactions that are involved in biosynthesis. Most enzymatic reactions are reversible.

As is true of all forms of proteins, the shape of an enzyme is critical to its ability to catalyze a reaction. The area on the enzyme where the substrates interact is termed the active site. Any changes to the shape of the active site will render the enzyme unable to function. Enzyme specificity is based on shape; a single enzyme typically only interacts with a single substrate or single class of substrates.

The induced fit model is used to explain the mechanism of action for enzyme function seen in Figure 4.4. Once a substrate binds loosely to the active site of an enzyme, a conformational change in shape occurs to cause tight binding between the enzyme and the substrate. This tight binding allows the enzyme to facilitate the reaction by orienting the substrates in such a way with respect to one another that would make the reaction more favorable. This leads to an increase in the rate of the reaction.

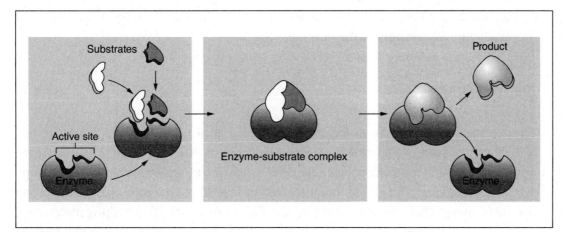

FIGURE 4.4 Enzyme function.

Some enzymes require assistance from other substances to work properly. If assistance is needed, the enzyme will have binding sites for cofactors or coenzymes. Cofactors are various types of ions such as Fe^{2+} and Zn^{2+}. Coenzymes are organic molecules usually derived from vitamins obtained in the diet. For this reason, mineral and vitamin deficiencies can have serious consequences on enzymatic functions.

There are several factors that can influence the activity of a particular enzyme. The first is the concentration of the substrate and the concentration of the enzyme. Reaction rates stay low when the concentration of the substrate is low, while the rates increase when the concentration of the substrate increases. Temperature is also a factor that can alter enzyme activity. Each enzyme has an optimal temperature for functioning. In humans, this is typically body temperature (37°C). At lower temperatures, the enzyme is less efficient. Increasing the temperature above the optimal point can lead to enzyme denaturation, which renders the enzyme useless. Extreme changes in pH can also lead to enzyme denaturation. The denaturation of an enzyme is not always reversible.

It is critical to be able to regulate the activity of enzymes in cells to maintain efficiency. This regulation can be carried out in several ways. Feedback or allosteric inhibition acts somewhat like a thermostat to regulate enzyme activity. Many enzymes contain allosteric binding sites and require signal molecules to function. As the product of a reaction builds up, repressor molecules can bind to the allosteric site of the enzyme, causing a change to the shape of the active site. The consequence of this binding is that the substrate can no longer interact with the active site of the enzyme and the activity of the enzyme is temporarily slowed or halted. When the product of the reaction declines, the repressor molecule dissociates from the allosteric site, which allows the active site of the enzyme to resume its normal shape. The enzyme is now capable of resuming its normal activity.

Another mechanism of enzyme regulation is the use of inhibitor molecules. A competitive inhibitor is a molecule that resembles the substrate in shape so much that it binds to the active site of the enzyme, thus preventing the substrate from binding. Noncompetitive inhibitors bind to allosteric sites, changing the shape of the active site and decreasing the functioning of the enzyme.

ENERGY

The preferred source of energy for cells is adenosine triphosphate (ATP). The structure of ATP can be seen in Figure 4.5. ATP is a hybrid molecule consisting of the nitrogenous base adenine (found in nucleotides), the sugar ribose, and three phosphate groups (PO_4). The breaking of the bond that attaches the last PO_4 to the molecule results in the release of energy that is used in a variety of cellular processes. The resulting molecule is adenosine diphosphate (ADP). The process of adding a PO_4 to ADP to convert it back to ATP for reuse is not a simple one. The chemical reactions of cellular respiration are used to achieve this goal.

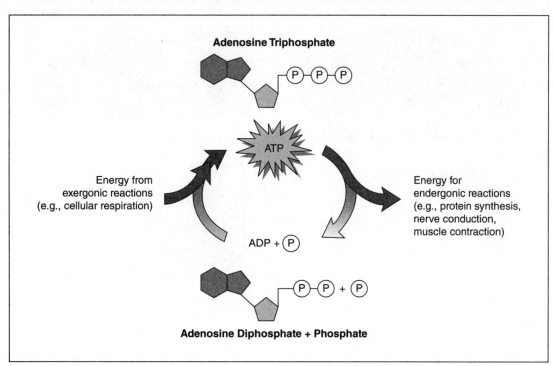

Adenosine Triphosphate

Energy from
exergonic reactions
(e.g., cellular respiration)

ATP

Energy for
endergonic reactions
(e.g., protein synthesis,
nerve conduction,
muscle contraction)

ADP + P

Adenosine Diphosphate + Phosphate

FIGURE 4.5 ATP/ADP cycle.

PHOTOSYNTHESIS

Since cellular respiration involves the breakdown of glucose to produce ATP, it is critical first to understand the synthesis of glucose that occurs during photosynthesis. Photosynthesis can be performed by traditional plants, algae, and certain types of bacteria. During this two-step process, solar energy is converted to chemical energy via a series of electron transfers that produce oxygen gas as a byproduct. This chemical energy is then used to fix carbon (from CO_2), ultimately to produce glucose for the plant. The overall equation for photosynthesis is:

$$6H_2O + 6CO_2 + \text{sunlight} + \text{energy} \rightarrow C_6H_{12}O_6 + 6O_2 + 6H_2O$$

The reactions of photosynthesis occur in the chloroplasts of the typical plant cell. This structure can be seen in Figure 4.6. The green pigment *chlorophyll* exists in the thylakoids; its job is to absorb solar energy. However, many wavelengths of visible light are reflected (and thus useless to the plant). The most valuable wavelengths of light for photosynthesis are those that correspond to blue and red light. The less useful green and yellow wavelengths are reflected, making plants appear green to our eyes.

Chlorophyll molecules and other pigments in the thylakoids arrange themselves as part of photosystems (abbreviated PS). The photosystems attract and absorb solar energy and facilitate the passage of electrons through carrier molecules. There are two types of photosystems: PSII (also called P680) and PSI (also called P700).

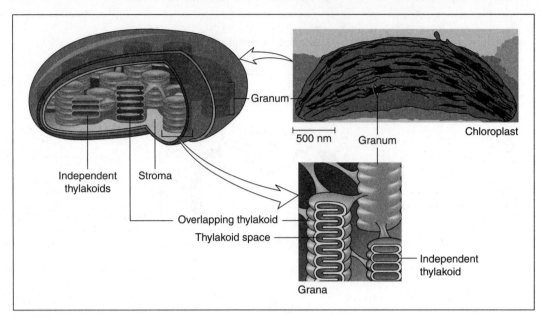

FIGURE 4.6 Chloroplasts.

During the light-dependent reactions, solar energy will be converted to chemical energy. This process happens in the thylakoid membrane of the chloroplasts. Solar energy will be used to split water molecules, which will provide a source of electrons for a series of redox reactions. A by-product of the splitting of the water molecules is that oxygen gas is released. The electrons from water will be moved to PSII, where they will be boosted to higher energy levels and passed through electron carrier molecules, ultimately resulting in the production of ATP that will be used in the light-independent reactions. Light energy provides the energy needed to boost the electrons to higher levels. The electrons then move to PSI, where they will again be boosted to a high energy level and passed through another set of electron carrier molecules. This time, NADP$^+$ will be reduced to NADPH, which will carry the energy of the electrons to the light-independent reactions. Figure 4.7 shows the steps involved in the light-dependent reactions.

The light-independent reactions are also known as the Calvin cycle. These reactions occur in the stroma of the chloroplast, as seen in Figure 4.8. Carbon dioxide is let into the plant by stomata on the surface of leaves, which are like pores that can open and close to regulate the entrance of CO_2 into (and the exit of water from) the plant. The first step of the Calvin cycle involves carbon fixation, where CO_2 is combined with RuBP with assistance from the enzyme rubisco. The remainder of the cycle involves ATP (produced in the light-dependent reactions) energizing molecules and NADPH (also from the light-dependent reactions) donating electrons to molecules. The eventual result is that a molecule of G3P is released from the cycle and the remaining molecules are used to regenerate RuBP (the starting point of the cycle). The significance of G3P is that two of these molecules can be joined to form glucose (food) for the plant. This glucose can be used to build molecules such as starch and cellulose in the plant, or it can be broken down to produce large amounts of ATP in the process of cellular respiration. The Calvin cycle needs to be performed three times in order to make one molecule of G3P, since only one molecule of CO_2 enters the cycle at a time.

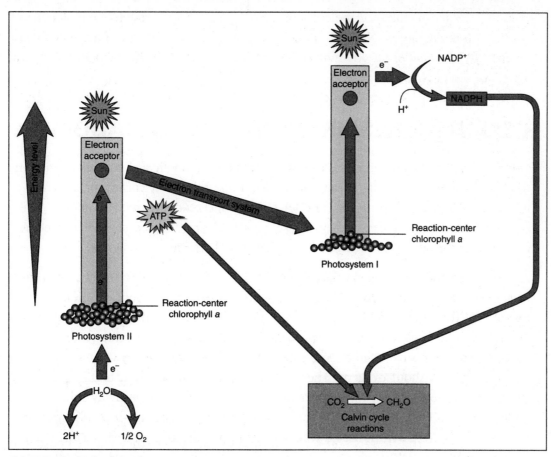

FIGURE 4.7 Light-dependent reactions.

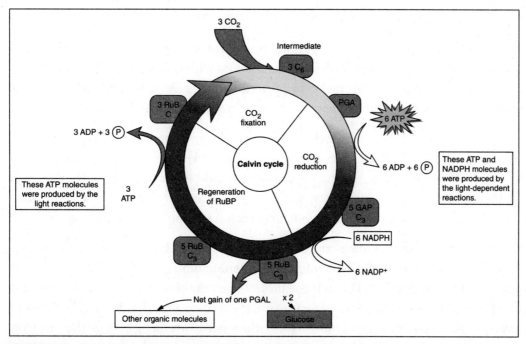

FIGURE 4.8 Light-independent reactions in the Calvin cycle.

Overall, in order to make one molecule of G3P, the Calvin cycle requires 9 molecules of ATP and 6 molecules of NADPH. Since two molecules of G3P form one molecule of glucose, the production of one molecule of glucose requires 18 molecules of ATP and 12 molecules of NADPH.

CELLULAR RESPIRATION AND METABOLISM

Cellular metabolism encompasses the sum total of all anabolic and catabolic reactions that occur within the cell. These critical reactions rely on a variety of enzymes to increase their rate to an appropriate level. Anabolic reactions require energy, while catabolic reactions release energy. These reactions are coupled so that the energy released from a catabolic reaction can be used to fuel an anabolic reaction.

A critical catabolic reaction in cells is the breakdown of glucose to release energy that is used to convert ADP back to ATP. This glucose is made in the anabolic reactions of photosynthesis that occurs in plants. In animals, the glucose is obtained from the diet. The breakdown of glucose occurs in the process of cellular respiration, which must be done by all living organisms. Cellular respiration can be done aerobically (using oxygen) or anaerobically (without oxygen). The aerobic pathway has a much higher ATP yield than the anaerobic pathway. The production of ATP in either pathway relies on the addition of a PO_4 to ADP. This can be achieved through substrate-level phosphorylation, in which ATP is synthesized by the transfer of a phosphate group from an intermediate molecule to ADP, or via oxidative phosphorylation, in which ATP is synthesized using the energy obtained by the transfer of electrons in the electron transport chain.

The aerobic pathway can be demonstrated by the following reaction in which glucose and oxygen interact to produce carbon dioxide, water, and ATP:

$$C_6H_{12}O_6 + 6O_2 \rightarrow 6CO_2 + 6H_2O + ATP$$

Aerobic cellular respiration begins with the process of glycolysis, followed by the Krebs cycle (also called the citric acid cycle), and concludes with the electron transport chain. The electron transport chain is fueled by protons (H^+) and electrons and is the step that produces the majority of ATP.

During glycolysis and the Krebs cycle, glucose will be systematically broken down and small amounts of ATP will be generated by substrate-level phosphorylation. Carbon dioxide will be released as a waste product. However, the most important part of these steps is that the breakdown of glucose allows for electron carrier molecules to accept electrons needed to run the electron transport chain in which ATP is produced in mass quantities.

Electron carrier molecules are a critical part of aerobic cellular respiration. These electron carrier molecules include nicotinamide adenine dinucleotide (NAD^+) and flavin adenine dinucleotide (FAD). When these molecules pick up electrons, they are reduced to NADH and $FADH_2$. The reduced forms of the carrier molecules deliver electrons to power the electron transport chain. Once these items are delivered to the electron

Table 4.2 A Summary of Aerobic Cellular Respiration

Step	Location in Cell	Starting Products	Ending Products
Glycolysis	Cytoplasm	Glucose, ATP, ADP NAD^+	Pyruvate, ATP, NADH
Krebs cycle	Matrix of mitochondria	Acetyl-CoA, ADP, FAD, NAD^+	CO_2, ATP, NADH, $FADH_2$
Electron transport chain	Inner membrane of mitochondria	NADH, $FADH_2$, O_2, ADP	NAD^+, FAD, H_2O, ATP

transport chain, the molecules return to their oxidized forms, NAD^+ and FAD. An overview of all the reactions of aerobic cellular respiration, including starting and ending points, is shown in Table 4.2.

Overall, the process of glycolysis breaks down glucose into two molecules of pyruvate. This happens in the cytoplasm of the cell and is the starting step for both aerobic and anaerobic cellular respiration. During the process, two ATP molecules are invested while four ATP molecules are gained via substrate-level phosphorylation. This leaves a net gain of two ATP for the process. In addition, NAD^+ is reduced to NADH that will be used in a later step (the electron transport chain) for oxidative phosphorylation. Figure 4.9 shows the major chemical reactions of glycolysis. At the end of glycolysis, the pyruvate molecules can be further broken down either aerobically or anaerobically. In the aerobic pathway, the subsequent reactions will occur in the mitochondria. The pyruvate from glycolysis must be moved to the mitochondria via active transport.

Mitochondrial Structure

A key feature of the mitochondrion is its double membrane. The folded inner membrane is called the cristae membrane; it is the site of the electron transport chain. The space between the inner and outer membrane is termed the intermembrane space. The space bounded by the inner membrane is a liquid called the matrix; it is the location of the Krebs cycle.

In aerobic respiration, the two pyruvate molecules remaining at the end of glycolysis will be actively transported into the matrix of the mitochondria. They will be modified in order to enter into the reactions of the Krebs cycle. This modification, termed pyruvate decarboxylation, involves the removal of the carboxyl group of pyruvate and its release as CO_2. The remnant of pyruvate is a two-carbon acetyl group. Coenzyme A (CoA) will be added to the acetyl group, creating acetyl-CoA, which is capable of entering the Krebs cycle. These modifications to pyruvate also allow for the reduction of NAD^+ to NADH that will be used later in the electron transport chain. Because there are two pyruvate molecules, this step produces two CO_2, two acetyl-CoA, and two NADH.

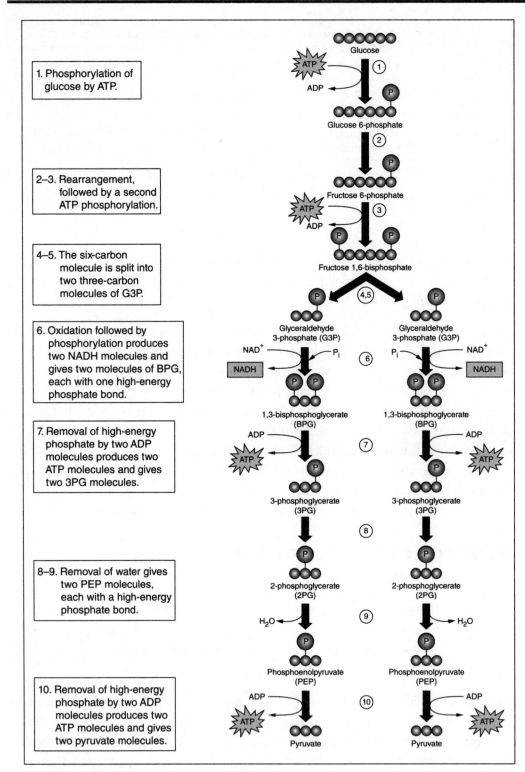

1. Phosphorylation of glucose by ATP.

2–3. Rearrangement, followed by a second ATP phosphorylation.

4–5. The six-carbon molecule is split into two three-carbon molecules of G3P.

6. Oxidation followed by phosphorylation produces two NADH molecules and gives two molecules of BPG, each with one high-energy phosphate bond.

7. Removal of high-energy phosphate by two ADP molecules produces two ATP molecules and gives two 3PG molecules.

8–9. Removal of water gives two PEP molecules, each with a high-energy phosphate bond.

10. Removal of high-energy phosphate by two ADP molecules produces two ATP molecules and gives two pyruvate molecules.

FIGURE 4.9 Glycolysis.

Now that acetyl-CoA has been formed, this molecule will enter the Krebs cycle by combining with a four-carbon molecule (oxaloacetate) to form the six-carbon molecule citric acid. The remaining reactions of the Krebs cycle are seen in Figure 4.10. The Krebs cycle involves the removal of the two carbons that entered as acetyl-CoA, which are released as CO_2, the production of one ATP molecule via substrate level

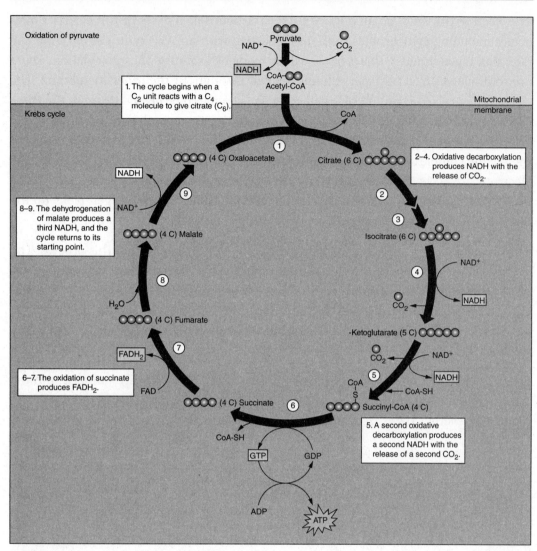

FIGURE 4.10 The Krebs cycle.

phosphorylation, and the rearrangement of the intermediate products to form the starting molecule of oxaloacetate. In this way, the cycle is able to continue. In addition, the rearrangement of intermediates in the process allows for the reduction of NAD^+ to NADH and FAD to $FADH_2$. Because there are two acetyl-CoA molecules, this cycle must turn twice. The end result is the production of four CO_2, two ATP, six NADH, and two $FADH_2$. At this point, glucose has been fully broken down into CO_2, which will be exhaled by animals and released through the stomata in plants or further used in photosynthesis. At this point, the process continues with the electron transport chain.

During glycolysis and the Krebs cycle, NAD^+ and FAD have been reduced to NADH and $FADH_2$. Once they are reduced, they will move toward the electron transport chains located in the inner membrane of the mitochondria. Here, they will be oxidized by releasing the electrons that they are carrying to the chain. At this point, the oxidized forms of NAD^+ and FAD will return to the glycolysis and the Krebs cycle to be used again.

The electron transport chain (Figure 4.11) is structurally a series of three carrier molecules including cytochromes that are associated with an ATP synthase enzyme. The ATP that is generated in this process will be made by oxidative phosphorylation. There are multiple electron transport chains located throughout the inner membrane. The electrons from NADH and $FADH_2$ will enter the chain and be passed through the three carrier molecules. NADH delivers its electrons to the first complex in the chain; those electrons are passed to the second and third complexes. $FADH_2$ delivers its electrons to the second complex and then passes the electrons to the third complex. Eventually the electrons are accepted by the terminal electron acceptor, which is the oxygen inhaled through the respiratory system (hence the aerobic label). As the oxygen picks up the electrons, it also picks up two protons (H^+); this process in turn creates water.

The chemiosmotic theory is used to explain how ATP is produced in this process. The energy from movement of the electrons donated by NADH and $FADH_2$ is used to pump protons into the intermembrane space. These protons build up, creating a proton gradient. The protons move through the ATP synthase enzyme via passive transport. As each proton moves through the ATP synthase enzyme, ADP is phosphorylated, producing one ATP.

For every NADH that donates electrons to the chain, 3 protons are pumped into the intermembrane space and 3 protons reenter through the ATP synthase; thus 3 ATP are made. For every $FADH_2$, 2 protons are pumped into the intermembrane space and

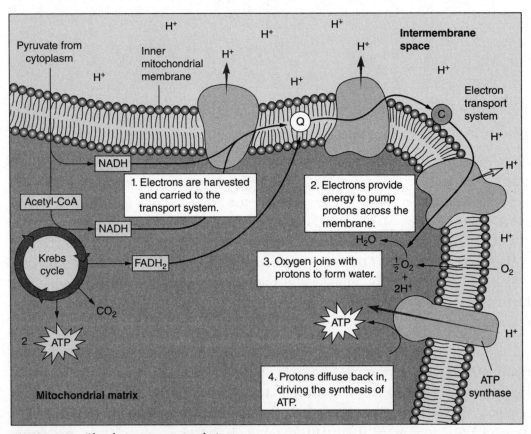

FIGURE 4.11 The electron transport chain.

Table 4.3 Summary of ATP Production in Aerobic Cellular Respiration

	Products of Previous Steps	ATP Made During Chemiosmotic Phophorylation in the Electron Transport Chain
Glycolysis	2 NADH 2 ATP	2 NADH = 6 ATP (however, the net gain will be 4 ATP due to the use of ATP to actively transport pyruvate to the mitochondria)
Krebs cycle	8 NADH 2 FADH$_2$ 2 ATP	8 NADH = 24 ATP 2 FADH$_2$ = 4 ATP
Total	4 ATP	32 ATP

2 protons reenter through the ATP synthase, so that 2 ATP are made. A total of 32 ATP are produced in the electron transport chain. Combining this number of ATP with the 4 ATP produced by substrate-level phosphorylation in glycolysis and the Krebs cycle leads to a grand total of 36 ATP per glucose molecule made in aerobic cellular respiration. A summary of ATP made throughout the process of aerobic respiration can be seen in Table 4.3.

If oxygen is not available to accept electrons, the electrons in the electron transport chain will build up, essentially shutting down the electron transport chain. Not only will ATP production drastically decline, but now that NADH cannot be oxidized to NAD$^+$ by the electron transport chain, there will not be enough NAD$^+$ to continue glycolysis. In this case, the use of fermentation will be necessary to complete the oxidation of NADH to NAD$^+$ in order to continue glycolysis.

There are times that oxygen is either not available or not utilized by cells to perform aerobic respiration. For animals, this may occur for brief episodes when the oxygen demands of the cells cannot be met. Unfortunately, the use of anaerobic respiration produces very little ATP as compared to aerobic cellular respiration, and thus cannot meet the ATP demands of larger organisms for extended periods of time. In other organisms, such as certain bacteria and yeasts that are single celled, anaerobic respiration is used permanently or for lengthy periods of time.

The first step in the anaerobic pathway is glycolysis. Once glycolysis occurs and pyruvate is generated, the anaerobic pathway continues with a second step, fermentation. Depending on the organism, fermentation can occur in one of two ways: lactic acid fermentation or alcoholic fermentation. The primary benefit of either type of fermentation is that it allows for the oxidation of NADH to NAD$^+$, which is necessary for glycolysis to continue in the absence of a functional electron transport chain. It is important to note that fermentation itself produces no ATP. The only ATP created during anaerobic respiration (glycolysis and fermentation) is from the glycolysis step. Therefore it is absolutely critical to regenerate the NAD$^+$ needed to continue with glycolysis. The total net gain of ATP from anaerobic respiration is 2 ATP as compared to 36 from complete aerobic respiration.

Lactic acid fermentation occurs in some types of bacteria and fungi, as well as in the muscle cells of animals when oxygen levels are not sufficient to meet the demands of aerobic respiration. In this step, pyruvate is reduced to lactic acid, thus regenerating the NAD+ needed to continue glycolysis. In humans, large amounts of lactic acid are responsible for muscle fatigue after major exertion.

Some organisms, such as certain bacteria and yeast, use alcoholic fermentation. In this step, pyruvate is decarboxylated, which produces CO_2 gas, and then reduced to form ethanol. As with lactic acid fermentation, NAD^+ is recycled so that glycolysis may continue.

CELL DIVISION AND CHROMOSOMES

Cell division in eukaryotes happens by one of two processes. Mitosis is normal cell division that takes place in growth and the replacement of cells. In mitosis, a parent cell is copied in order to produce two identical offspring (daughter) cells. However, there are times when the production of genetically identical offspring cells is not appropriate, such as in sexual reproduction. During the process of sexual reproduction, genetically diverse gametes must be created. These gametes will be produced by the process of meiosis. Mitosis and meiosis have many features in common.

During either form of cell division, it is critical that the chromosomes be replicated and properly allocated to each of the daughter cells. Chromosomes occur in homologous pairs. For each pair of chromosomes found in an individual, one member of the pair came from the maternal parent and the other member of the pair came from the paternal parent.

The total number of chromosomes found in an individual is called the diploid (2n) number. When individuals reproduce, this number must be cut in half to produce haploid (n) egg and sperm cells. The human diploid number is 46, and the human haploid number is 23. The process of mitosis begins with a diploid cell and ends with two identical diploid cells. In the process of meiosis, a diploid cell will begin the process and will produce four haploid gametes.

When a cell is not dividing, each chromosome exists in single copy called a chromatid. However, when the cell is preparing to divide, each chromosome must be replicated so that it contains two chromatids, sometimes called sister chromatids. Each chromosome has a compressed region called the centromere. When the chromosomes replicate, the sister chromatids stay attached to each other at the centromere.

Mitosis

Mitosis is the process of normal cell division in eukaryotic cells. It occurs in most cells except for gametes and mature nerve and muscle cells in animals. It begins with a single parent cell that replicates all components within the cell, divides the components into two piles, and then splits to form two genetically identical daughter cells. The most critical components for replication and division are the chromosomes, so particular care must be taken to ensure an equal distribution of chromosomes to each daughter cell.

Mitosis is necessary for the growth of organisms because it takes an increased number of cells for an organism to get bigger. When an individual has stopped growing, mitosis is only needed to replace cells that have died or been injured. For this reason, mitosis needs to be a regulated process that only occurs when new cells are needed. The cell cycle regulates the process of cell division in each individual cell. A normal cell cycle has the following stages, seen in Figure 4.12:

➤ **G_1.** This is the first gap phase of the cell cycle. In this stage, the parent cell is growing larger and is adding cytoplasm and replicating organelles.
➤ **S.** During this phase of DNA synthesis, the chromosomes are all being replicated. Once this stage is complete, each chromosome will consist of two sister chromatids connected at the centromere.
➤ **G_2.** This is the second gap phase. The cell will continue to grow in size and make final preparations for cell division.
➤ **M.** During the M phase, mitosis actually occurs. The replicated chromosomes and other cellular components will be divided up to ensure that each daughter cell receives equal distributions. The division of the cytoplasm at the end of the M phase is referred to as cytokinesis.

The first three phases of the cell cycle, G_1, S, and G_2, are collectively called interphase. Interphase simply means preparation for cell division. The actual cell division occurs during the M phase of the cycle.

Some cells lose the ability to progress through the cell cycle and are thus unable to divide. Mature human nerve and muscle cells are an example. Cells without the ability to divide are considered to be in the G_0 phase of the cell cycle where division will never resume.

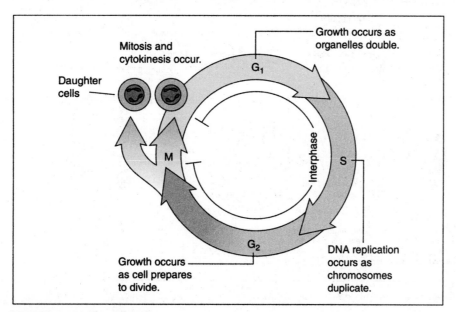

FIGURE 4.12 The cell cycle.

The M phase of the cell cycle is subdivided into five stages: prophase, prometaphase, metaphase, anaphase, and telophase. The primary concern in these stages will be alignment and splitting of sister chromatids to ensure that each daughter cell receives an equal contribution of chromosomes from the parent cell. A visual summary of the events of the M phase can be seen in Figure 4.13.

Chromosomes are located in the nucleus. Prior to division, the chromosomes are not condensed and thus are not visible. Leaving the chromosomes in an uncondensed state makes it easier to copy the DNA but makes the chromosomes very stringy and fragile. Once the DNA is replicated, the chromosomes must condense so that they are not broken as they are divided up into the two daughter cells.

During prophase, chromosome condensation occurs, making the chromosomes visible. The centrioles present in the cell replicate and move to opposite ends of the cell. Once they have migrated to the poles of the cell, they begin to produce a spindle apparatus, consisting of spindle fibers that radiate outward forming asters. The spindle fibers are made of microtubules that will ultimately attach to each chromosome at the kinetochore. The kinetochore appears at the centromere of each chromosome.

Following prophase is prometaphase, as shown in Figure 4.14. In this step, the nuclear envelope and lamina is broken down by the phosphorylation of the nuclear pore

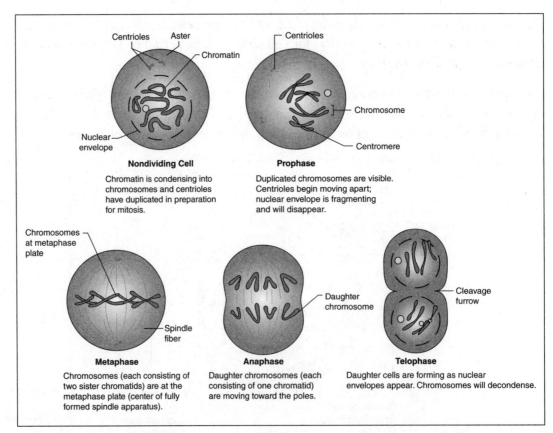

FIGURE 4.13 Events of M phase.

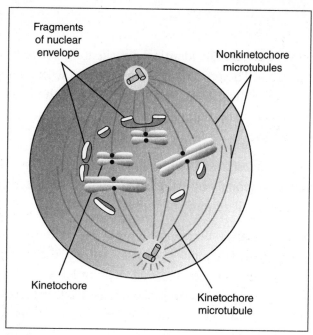

FIGURE 4.14   Prometaphase.

proteins and lamins. Once the nucleus breaks down, the spindle microtubules will attach to the chromosomes by binding to the kinetochore, which is a protein structure located on the centromere.

In metaphase, the chromosomes align down the center of the cell at the metaphase plate. This is a crucial part of mitosis, and the cell employs a checkpoint in order to ensure that all the chromosomes are properly lined up on the metaphase plate so that each of the daughter cells contains the correct number of chromosomes.

During anaphase, the centromere splits, allowing each chromatid to have its own centromere. At this point, the chromatids can be separated from each other and are pulled toward opposite poles of the cell, separating the chromosomes into two distinct piles—one for each daughter cell. The chromatids are moved to opposite poles by the depolymerization of the kinetochore microtubules.

The next step is telophase. Now that the chromosomes have been divided into two groups, the spindle apparatus is no longer needed and disassembles. The previously phosphorylated nuclear pore proteins and lamins are dephosphorylated, which allows the nuclear envelope and lamina to re-form around each set of chromosomes. The chromosomes uncoil back to their original state by the dephosphorylation of condensin, the protein responsible for the condensing of chromosomes during prophase. The final step of mitosis is cytokinesis, where the cytoplasm is divided between the cells. In animal cells, a cleavage furrow forms that pinches the cells apart from each other. In plant cells, a cell plate made of cellulose divides the two daughter cells. The end result is two daughter cells ready to begin interphase of their cell cycles.

Meiosis

Because mitosis produces genetically identical diploid daughter cells, it is not appropriate for sexual reproduction. The process of meiosis begins with a diploid parent cell in the reproductive system that has completed interphase and then follows stages similar to mitosis, twice. The result is four haploid gametes that are genetically diverse. A summary of the events of meiosis can be seen in Figure 4.15.

Meiosis I encompasses stages similar to mitosis with two major changes. The first involves genetic recombination between homologous pairs; the second involves the alignment of chromosome pairs during metaphase.

Prophase I of meiosis has many similarities to prophase of mitosis. The chromosomes condense, the centrioles divide and move toward the poles of the cell, spindle fibers begin to form, and the nuclear envelope breaks down. The unique event seen in prophase I is crossing over. Homologous pairs of chromosomes associate and twist together in synapsis. This configuration consists of two replicated chromosomes, or a total of four chromatids, and is often called a tetrad. At this point, crossing over can occur, where

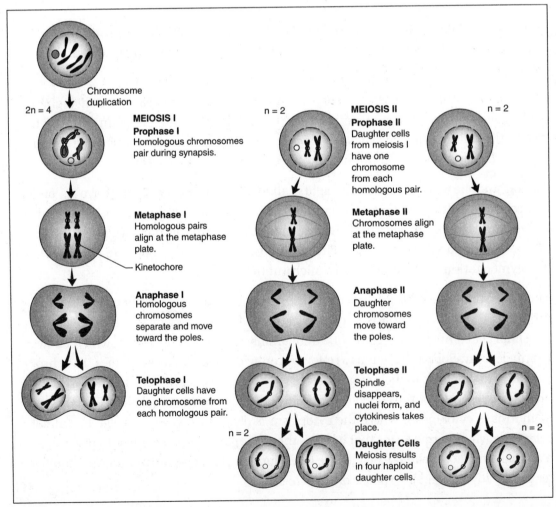

FIGURE 4.15 Meiosis I and II.

pieces of one chromatid break off and exchange with pieces of another. Crossing over can occur in more than one location and can unlink genes that were previously linked on the same chromosome. It is an important source of genetic diversity, creating combinations of alleles that were not seen previously.

In metaphase of mitosis, chromosomes align single file down the center of the cell. In metaphase I of meiosis, the chromosomes align as pairs down the center of the cell. This alignment of pairs is the critical factor in creating haploid daughter cells. Recall from your studies of genetics the law of independent assortment. The alignment of each member of the homologous pair during metaphase I is random, so each daughter cell will have a unique combination of maternal and paternal alleles.

The homologous pairs will separate from each other during anaphase I and be pulled to the poles of the cells. This separation is referred to as disjunction.

The events of telophase I are similar to mitosis. The spindle apparatus disassembles, nuclear envelopes form around each set of chromosomes, and cytokinesis occurs to form the two daughter cells. At this point, each daughter cell is genetically unique and contains half the number of chromosomes of the parent cell. However, these chromosomes are still in their replicated form, consisting of two chromatids.

Meiosis II is only necessary to split the chromatids present in the daughter cells produced during meiosis I. There will not be an interphase between meiosis I and II because the chromosomes are already replicated. The events of meiosis II are as follows:

➤ **Prophase II.** Centrioles replicate and move toward the poles of the cell, chromosomes condense, and the nuclear envelope breaks down. Chromosomal condensation and nuclear envelope breakdown only occur if the chromosomes were decondensed and the nuclear envelope re-formed during telophase I; these events do not occur in all species.
➤ **Metaphase II.** Chromosomes align down the center of the cell.
➤ **Anaphase II.** Sister chromatids are separated and move toward the poles of the cell.
➤ **Telophase II.** Nuclear envelopes re-form and cytokinesis occurs to produce daughter cells.

At the end of meiosis II, there are four daughter cells. Each is haploid with a single copy of each chromosome. Each cell is genetically diverse as a result of crossing over and independent assortment.

Gametogenesis

Meiosis results in four gametes. In men, all four of these gametes will become sperm. In women, only one of these gametes will become a functional egg cell; functional eggs are released once every 28 days, during ovulation. If all four gametes became functional eggs and were released each cycle, there would be the potential for four embryos. The three gametes that do not become functional eggs in women are termed polar bodies.

Mistakes that happen during meiosis can have drastic consequences. Because the gametes are used for reproduction, any chromosomal damage to the gametes will be passed on to the next generation. If chromosomes fail to separate properly during meiosis, a nondisjunction has occurred. This will lead to gametes that have the wrong number of chromosomes. If those gametes are fertilized, the resulting embryo will have the wrong diploid number. An example of this is Down syndrome, which often is the result of a nondisjunction in the female gamete that received an extra chromosome. This condition is referred to as a trisomy. When a gamete is missing a chromosome as the result of a nondisjunction and is fertilized by a normal gamete, the result is an embryo with 45 chromosomes. This is termed a monosomy. With the exception of Down syndrome, which is a trisomy of human chromosome 21 (which is very small) and certain trisomies and monosomies of the sex chromosomes (X and Y), most embryos with trisomies and monosomies do not survive development.

There are other forms of chromosomal damage that can occur in meiosis. They typically have serious, if not fatal, consequences. They are as follows:

➤ **Deletion:** This occurs when a portion of a chromosome is broken off and lost during meiosis. While the total chromosome number is normal, some alleles have been lost.

➤ **Duplication:** This occurs when a chromosome contains all of the expected alleles and then receives a duplication of some alleles.

➤ **Inversion:** This occurs when a portion of a chromosome breaks off and reattaches to the same chromosome in the opposite direction.

➤ **Translocation:** This occurs when a piece of a chromosome breaks off and reattaches to another chromosome.

Further aspects of the formation of gametes in humans, developmental biology, and genetics are covered in Chapters 6, 7, and 8.

BIOLOGY

CHAPTER 5

The Diversity of Life

Read This Chapter to Learn About

➤ Taxonomy

➤ Plantae

➤ Fungi

➤ Bacteria

➤ Viruses

➤ Animal Viruses

➤ Animalia

➤ Protista

➤ Archaea

➤ Bacteriophages

TAXONOMY

The categorization of living organisms based upon their differences and similarities is called taxonomy. This grouping, or ranking, allows for a classification based upon: kingdom, phylum, class, order, family, genus, and species. A mnemonic device for memorizing the classification is, "King Philip Came Over From Greenland Singing." This system of classification, however, has been subject to change and debate. The most recent change is the addition of a class that is larger than that of kingdoms, called domains. Let us examine this change further.

There are three domains in which living organisms are classified: Eukarya, Bacteria, and Archaea. All eukaryotic organisms are classified in the domain Eukarya, leaving all prokaryotic cells to be classified as either Bacteria or Archaea. While both of these latter domains share the characteristics of being single celled, absorbing their nutrients, having a single loop of DNA, and lacking organelles, there are some differences between the two groups. While Archaea used to be mistakenly classified as bacteria, their molecular and cellular structures were found to be quite different. They have unique cell walls, ribosomes, and membrane lipids. Archaea live in very diverse environments, and some species are termed extremophiles due to their habitats such as polar ice caps, thermal vents, and extreme salt concentrations. Most Archaea species are anaerobes, and none are known to be pathogens.

PLANTAE

Autotrophs and plants allow other organisms on earth to take advantage of the energy that the sun provides. If they did not capture this light energy and make it available to us, then life as we know it would not exist. In addition, plants have helped the atmosphere develop to contain 21 percent oxygen, which is vital to aerobic organisms. If that weren't enough, plants also make use of the carbon dioxide that is produced by other living organisms.

Plant cells vary from animal cells in that plant cells have cell walls. Plant cells have chloroplasts that contain chlorophyll, which is responsible for reflecting green light and absorbing wavelengths of red and blue light (optimally around 660 and 430 nm, respectively) for photosynthesis. Also, the central vacuole in plant cells is larger than that of animal cells.

The roots of the plant are responsible for anchoring the plant into the ground and for absorbing water and nutrients. The root hairs on the root dramatically increase the absorption surface area of the plant's roots. From the roots, the xylem carries water and minerals up to the leaves, whereas the phloem carries glucose from the leaves where it is synthesized. The leaves are where photosynthesis takes place. Their larger surface area allows for more direct contact with sunlight and for absorption of carbon dioxide. The gas exchange of carbon dioxide intake and oxygen output, in addition to transpiration, occurs through the stomata, whose opening is regulated by guard cells. The stomata of a plant will open when the guard cells that flank it become turgid through the osmosis of water into the cells. This is done by the buildup of K^+ in the interior of the guard cells. Potassium ions are moved into guard cells through specific membrane channels when H^+ ions are pumped out of the cell, thereby making the exterior of the cell more positive. This difference in membrane potential will drive K^+ to the more negative interior of the cell allowing it to accumulate within the cell. With the increase of potassium ions inside the cell, water will now enter by osmosis, causing the guard cells to become turgid and allowing the stomata to become open. The stomata will close when the K^+ is moved out of the cell, which will cause water to leave as well and make the guard cells flaccid.

Flowering plants, or angiosperms, have male reproductive organs called the stamen and female organs called carpel. The stamen is made up of the anther and filament, while the carpel is made up of the stigma, style, and, ovary. Inside the ovary are the ovule, embryo sac, and egg. Pollen can be carried from the stamen to the stigma by insects, wind, or other means, allowing pollination to occur. After fertilization has occurred, the ovary will develop into the fruit to protect the seeds that developed from the ovule.

FUNGI

Fungi constitute a diverse number of species within the Eukarya domain. Some fungi are unicellular, such as yeasts, while others are multicellular, such as mushrooms and molds. Many are harmless, while some are pathogenic. All are heterotrophs, gaining their nutrients from other organisms. They secrete enzymes that break down organic molecules to a small enough size that they can be absorbed through the cell membrane. They may do this by feeding on dead and decaying organisms or by parasitic relationships with living organisms.

While some fungi such as yeasts are unicellular, most are multicellular and fairly complex, as seen in Figure 5.1. Within a multicellular fungus, the mycelium is the structure that grows near food sources in order to obtain nutrients for the fungus. Within the mycelium, there are hyphae, filaments where the nucleus of each cell is located. Other structures such as those needed for reproduction are present, yet their structure will be different depending on the species of fungus. In fact, fungi are classified according to their reproductive structures and mechanisms of reproduction.

Life Cycles and Reproduction of Fungi

Depending on the species, fungi are able to reproduce sexually, asexually, or sometimes by both methods. During asexual reproduction, spores are formed in specialized structures in the fungus and perform mitosis to generate offspring. The structure of spores used for fungal reproduction is very different from that of the spores used as survival structures in certain species of bacteria. In some cases, fungal spores are not used at all and the cells fragment to form new cells in the process of budding.

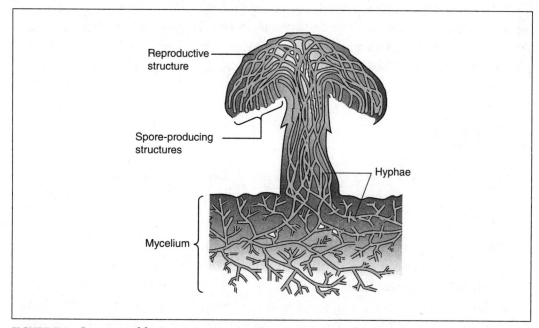

FIGURE 5.1 Structure of fungi.

Sexual reproduction is a less common means of reproduction in fungi and often occurs only when environmental conditions are poor. During sexual reproduction, gametes are made by specialized structures in the fungus. The two gametes fuse, leaving a diploid cell that performs meiosis and produces haploid spores.

Fungal Classification

Fungi are classified according to their method of reproduction. The following are the major groups of fungi:

➤ **Yeasts:** single celled, reproduce by budding.
➤ **Ascomycetes:** the "sac fungi" that contain asci, which are sacs that contain haploid spores; most yeasts and some molds fall in this group.
➤ **Basidiomycetes:** the "club fungi" that form basidia (club-shaped structures) that contain haploid spores; all reproduction is sexual via conjugation and nuclear fusion; mushrooms are an example.
➤ **Zygomycetes:** perform sexual reproduction by gamete fusion, meiosis, and the production of haploid spores; most bread molds fall into this group.
➤ **Chytrids:** produce flagellated spores; most species are parasites or decomposers that live in water.
➤ **Deuteromycetes:** the "imperfect fungi"; always reproduce asexually (or at least a sexual reproductive phase cannot be identified).
➤ **Lichens:** formed from an interaction between a fungus and a photosynthesizer such as algae.

Monera

The monera include organisms that have a prokaryotic cell that lacks a nucleus. This nonexistent kingdom now falls under the three-domain system and has been divided into the domains Archaea and Bacteria. Because of their importance in the medical field, it is worthy of looking into bacteria more closely as being model prokaryotes.

BACTERIA

Bacteria are extremely diverse. The classification of bacteria is generally based on the mechanisms used by the particular species to obtain nutrients from the environment. The following are the basic bacterial classifications:

➤ **Photoautotrophs:** These are bacterial species that produce their own nutrients through the process of photosynthesis, using carbon dioxide from the environment.
➤ **Photoheterotrophs:** Bacteria that perform photosynthesis but cannot use carbon dioxide from the environment are considered photoheterotrophs. In order to get the carbon needed for photosynthesis (which normally comes from carbon dioxide), they extract carbon from a variety of other sources.

➤ **Chemoautotrophs:** These species get their energy from inorganic compounds, and their carbon needs are obtained from carbon dioxide.

➤ **Chemoheterotrophs:** Energy is obtained for these species from inorganic substances, while carbon is obtained from a variety of sources other than carbon dioxide. These species are further subdivided based on the source of carbon they use. Some species can extract carbon through parasitic or symbiotic interactions with a host or through the decomposition of other organisms.

Bacteria can also be classified based on their oxygen requirements, or lack thereof, for cellular respiration. Some bacteria are **obligate aerobes**, always requiring oxygen for aerobic cellular respiration. Other bacteria are **obligate anaerobes**, never needing oxygen, generally not dividing, and in some cases being killed by exposure to oxygen. Finally, some bacteria are considered **facultative anaerobes**, requiring oxygen at times and not at other times.

Bacterial Shapes

Most bacteria have shapes that correspond to one of three typical conformations. These shapes and the organization amongst cells can be used as diagnostic features. The shapes exhibited by most bacteria are as follows:

➤ **Cocci** are circular in shape; they may exist singly, in pairs (diplococci), in clusters (staphylococci), or in chains (streptococci).

➤ **Bacilli** are rod or oblong shaped; they may occur in chains.

➤ **Spirilli** have a spiral shape.

Bacterial Structure

The bacterial cell is prokaryotic, meaning that it does not have a nucleus. As a result, its genome is located in the cytoplasm, in a region called the nucleoid, and is not bound by a membrane. The bacterial genome usually consists of a single, circular piece of DNA that does not contain many introns or exons, as opposed to eukaryotic cells, which will frequently contain introns and exons in their genomes.

A crucial component of a bacterial cell is its envelope, which includes the cell membrane, periplasm, cell wall, and outer membrane. However, not all bacteria contain these structures, and that allows us to separate bacteria into two groups depending on the structure of their envelope. In gram-positive bacteria (those bacteria that retain Gram's stain), the cell envelope consists of the cell membrane and a thick cell wall made of peptidoglycan. In gram-negative bacteria (those bacteria that do not retain Gram's stain), the envelope consists of a cell membrane, which in this case would be termed the inner membrane; the periplasm, which is the space between the inner membrane and outer membrane; a thin cell wall made of peptidoglycan; and an outer membrane. It is the thick cell wall of gram-positive cells that allows them to retain Gram's stain. As mentioned, this cell wall is made of peptidoglycan (murein), which is a polymer of disaccharides that are cross-linked with a chain of four to six amino acids. The disaccharide is composed of repeating units of N-acetylglucosamine and N-acetylmuramic acid, and the latter will form an amide link with the short chain of amino acids. A peptide cross-bridge will then form between two neighboring peptide chains, allowing the cell wall to increase in thickness as these cross-bridges form between other neighboring peptide chains as well. Because an intact cell wall is essential for the survival of bacterial cells, a common target of antibiotics, such as vancomycin and penicillin, is preventing proper synthesis of the cell wall. These antibiotics will interfere with a certain step of cell wall synthesis, such as cross-bridge formation, thereby preventing the peptidoglycan cell wall from fully forming, leading to death of the bacterial cell.

Gram-negative cells only contain a thin peptidoglycan cell wall, as opposed to the thick cell wall of gram-positive cells. However, the gram-negative cells contain an extra membrane in addition to the plasma membrane: the outer membrane. This membrane consists of two faces, as is typical of biological membranes. However, the face of the outer membrane that is pointed to the interior of the cell will contain lipoproteins that are attached to the cell wall, while the face of the outer membrane that is pointed to the exterior of the cell will contain lipopolysaccharides (LPS), which are lipids attached to polysaccharides. LPS are endotoxins and are not harmful so long as they are part of the cell. However, if the cell ruptures and LPS are released, they will begin to overstimulate the immune system of the host.

Table 5.1 gives an overview of some bacterial structures.

Table 5.1 Major Bacterial Structures	
Structure	**Function**
Cytoplasm	The space contained within the plasma membrane of the cell
Ribosomes	Protein synthesis
Chromosome	Contains the genes needed to produce proteins required for the cell. The bacterial chromosome consists of a single loop of DNA located in the nucleoid region of the cell.
Plasmids	Some bacterial cells contain small additional loops of DNA called plasmids. The plasmids often contain genes to code for resistance.
Cell wall	Most bacteria have a cell wall that contains peptidoglycan. The cell wall is found on the outer surface of the cell membrane. The cell wall typically can occur in one of two conformations, which can be identified using the Gram staining method. The gram-positive bacteria will have a thick cell wall made up of multiple layers of peptidoglycan, while the gram-negative will have a thin cell wall of only one layer of peptidoglycan.
Capsule and slime layers	The capsule is a layer of sugars and proteins on the outer surface of some bacterial cells. It forms a sticky layer that can help the cell attach to surfaces and can help keep bacterial cells from being phagocytosed.

Structure	Function
Flagella	Bacteria may have a single flagellum, multiple flagella, or no flagella. Those with one or more flagella are motile as the flagella rotate to propel the cell. The bacterial flagella are different from eukaryotic flagella in structure. Bacterial flagella consist of the protein flagellin in a hollow, helical conformation that anchors into the cell membrane. A proton pump in the membrane provides power to rotate each flagellum.
Pili	Pili are tiny proteins that generally cover the surface of some types of bacterial cells. They assist the cell in attaching to surfaces.
Spores	A few species of bacteria are capable of creating spores when environmental conditions are not favorable. When bacteria exist in spore form, they are capable of surviving adverse conditions for years. When conditions become favorable again, the spores germinate into the vegetative cell form again.

Table 5.1 Major Bacterial Structures (cont.)

Mechanisms for Bacterial Reproduction

Bacteria lack a nucleus and so cannot perform mitosis. Instead, bacteria divide by the process of binary fission. It involves the replication of the single loop of DNA, a copy of which is then provided to each of two daughter cells. This process can occur fairly quickly, in some cases as often as once every 20 minutes. Because bacteria are unicellular, creating a new cell means creating a new organism. This process qualifies as asexual reproduction, as each division produces genetically identical offspring. The only way to introduce variation into the population is by mutation, conjugation, or transformation.

Bacterial Conjugation

Some bacteria have another means of passing genetic material to other bacteria. During the process of conjugation seen in Figure 5.2, one bacterial cell may copy its plasmid to be passed to another cell. The most commonly studied type of plasmid to be passed is called the F plasmid or F factor (the F standing for fertility). In order to pass the plasmid to another cell, a physical connection must be established. This connection is referred to as the sex pilus, and it is made by the cell that contains the plasmid (termed the male or F^+). The sex pilus connects to a cell lacking the plasmid (the female or F^-) and serves as a bridge to pass a copy of the plasmid to the female. Once complete, both cells are male and contain the plasmid. Using conjugation provides a rapid mechanism to pass plasmids within a population. Occasionally, plasmids become integrated into the chromosome, and when the plasmid is transferred via conjugation, some of the bacterial chromosome may be transferred as well.

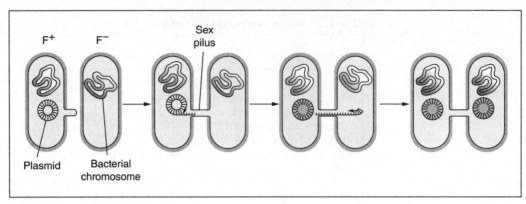

FIGURE 5.2 Bacterial conjugation.

Because many plasmids encode for resistance to things such as antibiotics, rapid conjugation can quickly render an entire bacterial population resistant to a particular antibiotic under the right selective pressures. This phenomenon has important medical significance, in that an antibiotic is used to kill bacteria causing infection, and if the bacteria are resistant to that antibiotic it is useless in stopping the infection. Some bacteria are resistant to multiple antibiotics as a result of picking up several plasmids via conjugation.

Bacterial Transformation

Another way that bacteria can pick up genetic variations is through transformation. Some bacteria are able to pick up DNA from their environment and incorporate it into their own chromosomal DNA. Bacteria that are able to pick up foreign DNA are termed competent. While some bacteria are naturally competent, others can be coerced to develop competence by artificial means within the lab.

Bacterial Gene Expression and Regulation

Just like other organisms, bacteria go through the processes of transcription and translation. The regulation of bacterial gene expression is primarily by operons, seen in Figure 5.3, which control the access of RNA polymerase to the genes to be transcribed primarily via repressor proteins. Many different operons have been described, but they all have certain basic features:

➤ A **promoter sequence** on the DNA where RNA polymerase must bind. If the promoter is inaccessible, the gene will not be transcribed.
➤ An **operator sequence** on the DNA where a repressor protein can bind, if present. When a repressor is bound to the operator, the promoter sequence will be blocked such that RNA polymerase cannot access the site.
➤ A **regulator gene** that produces a repressor protein when expressed.
➤ **Structural genes**, which are the actual genes being regulated by the operon.

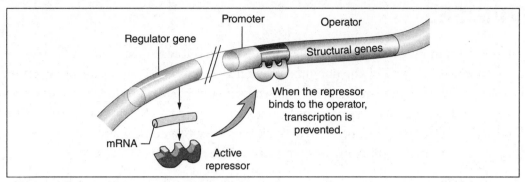

FIGURE 5.3 The operon system regulates gene expression.

Operons come in two basic categories: inducible and repressible. Inducible operons are normally "off," while repressible operons are normally "on." In an inducible operon, the repressor always binds to the operator so that transcription is always prevented unless an inducer molecule is present. When the inducer is present, it binds to the repressor, preventing the repressor from binding to the operator. This allows transcription to occur. In repressible operon systems, the repressor is always inactive such that transcription always occurs. Only when a corepressor is present to interact with the repressor can transcription be inhibited. When the repressor and corepressor are bound, they can then interact with the operator site and prevent access by RNA polymerase, thus turning off transcription.

The Bacterial Growth Cycle

Bacteria have a typical growth cycle that is limited by environmental factors as well as the amount of nutrients available. The growth cycle consists of the following stages:

➤ **Lag:** There is an initial lag in growth that occurs when a new population of bacteria begins to reproduce. This lag time is normally brief.

➤ **Logarithmic growth:** As bacteria begin to perform binary fission at a very rapid rate, logarithmic growth occurs. This can only last for a limited amount of time.

➤ **Stationary phase:** As the number of bacteria increase, resources such as food and space decrease, and while some bacteria are still dividing, some are dying, which evens out the population count.

➤ **Decline:** As the population hits its maximum, the lack of nutrients, along with the presence of a variety of toxins, means that the population will begin to decline—more cells will die than are being replaced by cell division. The few species of bacteria that are capable of making spores would do so at this point.

VIRUSES

Viruses are a unique biological entity in that they do not resemble typical cells nor are they classified into any of the domains previously discussed. There is debate whether viruses are living organisms at all because they are unable to reproduce without a host cell; nor can they perform many of the functions associated with living organisms without the help of a host. Because viruses lack typical cell structures such as organelles, they are much smaller than any form of prokaryotic or eukaryotic cells.

While some viruses contain more sophisticated structures, the only items required for a virus are a piece of genetic material, either DNA or RNA, and a protective protein coat for the genetic material, known as the capsid. Viruses are able to self-assemble in that if a viral genome and capsid proteins are mixed together, viral particles will form. The viral genome (a collection of all the genes present) can consist of only a few genes or can range up to a few hundred genes. Viruses are categorized as animal viruses, plant viruses, or bacteriophages.

Viral Life Cycles

Viruses are specific to the type of host cell that they infect. In order for a virus to infect a cell, that cell must have a receptor for the virus. If the receptor is absent, the cell cannot be infected by the virus. While it seems odd that cells would evolve receptors for viruses, it is usually a case of mistaken identity. The viruses can actually mimic another substance for which the cell has a legitimate need and thus has a receptor for. The process of viral infection is seen in Figure 5.4.

Once a virus binds to a receptor on the membrane of the host cell, the viral genetic material enters the host either by injecting itself across the cell membrane or by being taken in via endocytosis. At some point, the viral genes will be transcribed and translated by the host cell. The nucleic acid of the virus will also be replicated. Eventually new viruses will be produced and released from the host cell. Because each virus contains a copy of the original genetic material, they should all be genetically identical. Mutations are the primary way to induce variation into the viral population.

ANIMAL VIRUSES

As the name implies, animal viruses are designed to infect the host cells of various animals. Their genetic material may be DNA or RNA depending on the virus. Animal viruses are usually categorized according to the type of nucleic acid they possess, as well as whether the nucleic acid is single-stranded or double-stranded. Once the DNA or RNA of the virus is taken in by the host cell, the virus may immediately become active, using the host cell machinery to transcribe and translate the viral genes. New viruses are assembled and released from the host cell. The release of new viruses can be via lysis of the cell membrane, which immediately kills the host cell, or by budding, where

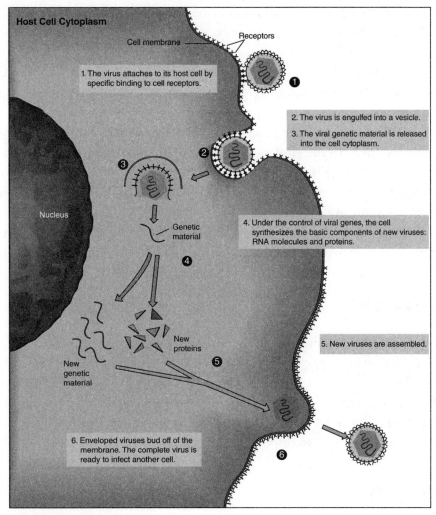

FIGURE 5.4 Viral infection.

the new viruses are shipped out of the host cell via exocytosis. Budding does not immediately kill the host cell but may eventually prove fatal to the host. Once the new viruses are released from the original host cell, they seek out new host cells to infect.

Alternatively, the virus may become latent, integrating itself into the chromosomes of the host cell, where it may stay for varying amounts of time. Eventually, the latent virus will excise from the host chromosome, and it will become active to produce and release new viruses. Some viruses are capable of alternating between active and latent forms multiple times. Infections caused by specific herpes viruses, such as cold sores and genital herpes, are notorious for alternating between active and latent forms.

RETROVIRUSES

Retroviruses are a unique category of RNA viruses. The human immunodeficiency virus (HIV) was the first retrovirus to be discovered. The key characteristic of retroviruses is that they enter the cell in RNA form that must be converted to DNA form. This is the opposite of the normal flow of information in the cell, which dictates that DNA produces RNA during transcription. The process of converting viral RNA backward into DNA is called reverse transcription and is achieved by an enzyme called reverse transcriptase, which is present inside the virus when it enters the host cell. The reverse transcriptase will produce a DNA copy of the RNA, thereby forming a DNA/RNA hybrid. The same reverse transcriptase enzyme will then convert the DNA/RNA hybrid into double-stranded DNA. The virus will then use the host's polymerase to make mRNA from this double-stranded DNA. In the case of HIV, the DNA then integrates into the host cell's chromosomes (in this case the host cell is a specific cell type in the immune system) and enters a latent phase that may last more than 10 years. When the viral DNA excises from the host chromosome, it becomes active and begins producing new viruses. When this happens on a mass scale, the death of host cells will signal the beginning of deterioration in the immune system, which causes acquired immunodeficiency syndrome (AIDS).

ANIMALIA

Animalia are eukaryotic, multicellular organisms. They are mostly motile heterotrophs that need to feed on other organisms. What is unique to animals is that the embryos go through a blastula stage that is not found in other kingdoms. Because of this, animals have differentiated tissues that can produce different organs. They also have muscles and nerves that allow them to move in response to their environment, as opposed to a plant that would use auxins to respond to sunlight.

PROTISTA

Protists are believed to have been the first eukaryotes to exist. While protists are eukaryotic, they are usually unicellular. If they are multicellular, they lack any specialization for the formation of tissues. Protists are found in aquatic environments and obtain nutrition autotrophically (like algae, dinoflagellates, euglena) or heterotrophically (like amoebae, apicomplexa, trypanosomes). The reproduction of protists can take place sexually and with the use of gametes or asexually via binary fission.

ARCHAEA

Archaea are single-celled organisms that lack a nucleus and do not contain membrane-bound organelles. They are considered to be prokaryotes. What makes them interesting is that they can inhabit the harshest environments on earth, making scientists believe that they were fit to survive the harsh conditions that existed on early earth.

Three microorganisms that fall under this domain are methanogens (methane generators), extreme halophiles (salt lovers), and extreme thermophiles (heat lovers). Methanogens are responsible for the methane gas that is produced in the intestines of animals and for producing "swamp gas" (methane gas) in wetlands. The extreme thermophiles

<table>
<tr><td colspan="4">**Table 5.2 Characteristics of Each Domain**</td></tr>
<tr><td></td><td>**Bacteria**</td><td>**Archaea**</td><td>**Eukarya**</td></tr>
<tr><td>Number of cells</td><td>Unicellular</td><td>Unicellular</td><td>Variable</td></tr>
<tr><td>Complexity of cells</td><td>Prokaryotic</td><td>Prokaryotic</td><td>Eukaryotic</td></tr>
<tr><td>Method of obtaining nutrients</td><td>Absorbed</td><td>Absorbed</td><td>Variable</td></tr>
</table>

Table 5.3 Characteristics of the Kingdoms of Eukarya				
	Plantae	**Animalia**	**Protista**	**Fungi**
Number of cells	Multicellular	Multicellular	Usually unicellular	Variable
Method of obtaining food	Made via photosynthesis	Ingested	Usually absorbed	Absorbed
Example organisms	Grass, trees, plants	Humans, starfish, birds, and fish	Algae, protozoa, slime molds	Yeasts, mushrooms, and molds

can be found in hot springs and hydrothermal vents where the water can reach as high as 80°C. These extremophiles can also thrive in a range of pH values as well. The diversity of the domains and within Eukarya can be seen in Tables 5.2 and 5.3.

BACTERIOPHAGES

Bacteriophages are DNA viruses that exclusively infect bacteria. They always inject their DNA into the host bacterial cell and then enter either a lytic cycle or a lysogenic cycle, as seen in Figure 5.5.

Lytic Cycle

A bacteriophage that uses the lytic cycle immediately activates once in its host to produce viral proteins and replicate viral nucleic acid. New viruses are synthesized and leave the host cell via lysis, always killing their bacterial host. The new viruses then go out and infect new host cells.

Lysogenic Cycle

The lysogenic cycle is a variation that some viruses use. Viral DNA injected into the host integrates into the bacterial chromosome. The viral DNA may stay integrated for varying lengths of time. Each time the bacterial cell divides by binary fission, the progeny receive a copy of the viral genome. Eventually, the viral DNA that has integrated into the chromosome will excise and enter the lytic cycle, releasing new viruses and killing the host.

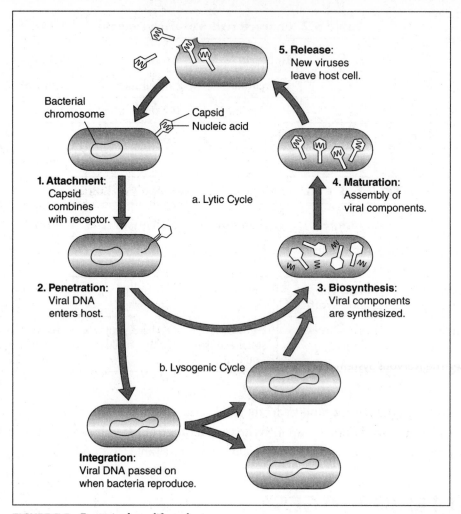

FIGURE 5.5 Bacteriophage life cycles.

Transduction

When new viruses are being packaged in a bacterial host, sometimes portions of the bacterial chromosome get packaged with the new viruses. When these viruses infect new bacterial hosts, they not only deliver the viral genome but also some bacterial genes that can recombine with the new host's chromosome. This is the process of transduction.

This chapter has provided a brief overview of the diversity of life on earth. The following chapter explores the structure and function of the complex systems of the human body.

CHAPTER 6

Structure and Function of Systems

Read This Chapter to Learn About

➤ The Nervous System

➤ Muscular Tissue

➤ The Skeletal System

➤ The Endocrine System

➤ The Cardiovascular System

➤ The Respiratory System

➤ The Digestive System

➤ The Urinary System

➤ The Lymphatic System

➤ The Immune System

➤ The Female Reproductive System

➤ The Male Reproductive System

➤ The Integumentary System

THE NERVOUS SYSTEM

The nervous system has the daunting task of coordinating all of the body's activities. The central nervous system (CNS) is composed of the brain and spinal cord. The peripheral nervous system (PNS) is composed of any nervous tissue located outside of the brain and spinal cord. Nerves are the primary structures within the PNS. In order to understand the functioning of the CNS and PNS, it is necessary to look at the detailed function of neurons.

The basic structure of neurons can be seen in Figure 6.1. Sensory (afferent) neurons exist in the PNS and direct their messages toward the CNS, while motor (efferent) neurons exist in the PNS and direct their messages away from the CNS. Interneurons are

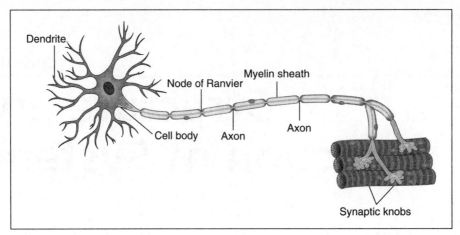

FIGURE 6.1 Neuron structure.

found only in the CNS. While neurons perform the critical function of transmitting messages throughout the body, there are also a large number of glial cells present in the nervous system. Glial cells provide support to neurons and are capable of mitosis, unlike mature neurons. The major structures within the neuron are as follows:

➤ **Dendrites:** projections that pick up incoming messages
➤ **Cell body:** processes messages and contains the nucleus and other typical cell organelles
➤ **Axon:** carries electrical messages down its length
➤ **Synaptic terminals:** occur at the ends of an axon; where electrical impulses are converted to chemical messages in the form of neurotransmitters
➤ **Myelin sheath:** produced by Schwann cells (specialized glial cells) in the PNS and oligodendrocytes in the CNS; surrounds the axon of some neurons; there are gaps between the myelin called nodes of Ranvier
➤ **Synapse:** the space between the synaptic terminals of one neuron and the dendrites of another neuron

Resting and Acting Potential

The resting potential is the state of the neurons when they are not generating messages. It requires the maintenance of an unequal balance of ions on either side of the membrane to keep the membrane polarized. The resting potential requires a great deal of ATP to maintain. During resting potential, sodium-potassium (Na^+/K^+) pumps within the membrane of the axon are used to actively transport ions into and out of the axon. The Na^+/K^+ pumps bring two K^+ ions into the axon while sending out three Na^+ ions. This results in a high concentration of Na^+ outside the membrane and a high concentration of K^+ inside the membrane. However, since three positive sodium ions are being pumped out but only two positive potassium ions are being brought back in, the membrane potential of the cell becomes more negative with each cycle of the Na^+/K^+ pump. There

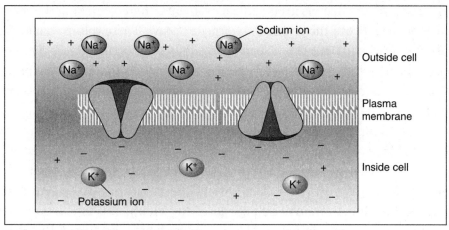

FIGURE 6.2   The sodium/potassium pump.

are also many negatively charged molecules, such as proteins, within the neuron, so that ultimately the inside of the neuron is more negative than the outside of the neuron. The resting potential typically has a voltage of about -70 mV. Figure 6.2 shows the resting potential in a neuron created by the sodium/potassium pump.

In order to transmit a message, the resting potential of the neuron must be disrupted and depolarized so that the inside of the cell becomes less negative. In order for this action potential to occur, a threshold voltage of about -55 mV must be achieved. Once the action potential has initiated, voltage-gated channels in the membrane of the axon will open. Specifically, Na^+ channels open, allowing Na^+ to flow passively across the membrane into the axon in a local area. The sodium ions do this passively because they are moving down their electrochemical gradient since there is a greater concentration of Na^+ outside the cell than inside and they are attracted to the negatively charged interior of the membrane. This local flow of Na^+ causes the next voltage-gated Na^+ channel to open since this area will also become depolarized. This continues down the length of the axon toward the synaptic terminals like a wave. While the speed of the axon potential can vary depending on the axon diameter and whether the axon is myelinated or not, its strength cannot. Action potentials are an all-or-nothing event: either the threshold voltage is reached and the action potential occurs, or it is not reached and no action potential occurs.

The events that occur in a typical neuron as a stimulus arrives to cause an action potential can be explained as follows: most voltage-gated Na^+ channels are closed while the neuron is at rest. However, when a stimulus arrives that causes the membrane to depolarize, voltage-gated Na^+ channels in the area of the depolarization open, allowing for an influx of Na^+. This influx further depolarizes the membrane, causing even more voltage-gated Na^+ channels to open as the membrane approaches the threshold voltage, if the original stimulus was strong enough, and generates an action potential. However, after these voltage-gated Na^+ channels open, they rather rapidly change conformation into an inactivated state, which will prevent any additional Na^+ from entering the cell. In addition, voltage-gated K^+ channels open, which causes K^+ to leave the cell as they flow down their electrochemical gradients, thereby making the membrane potential more negative as the positively charged K^+ leave. These voltage-gated K^+ channels will later close, and the cell will be able to achieve its resting potential once again. An important aspect of the voltage-gated Na^+ channels is the fact that they do not adapt a closed conformation after they are opened; rather they become inactivated and must go from an inactivated state to a closed state before they can open again. As a result, if a second stimulus arrives at this area that is capable of causing depolarization, it will not be able to generate an action potential since the voltage-gated Na^+ channels would be inactivated instead of closed. This time period, in which the neuron cannot generate a second action potential, is known as the refractory period. An additional consequence of the inactivation of voltage-gated Na^+ channels is that action potentials are transmitted in only one direction. This is because when one area of the membrane is depolarized, the area adjacent next to it becomes depolarized as well. However, the voltage-gated Na^+ channels in the initial area of depolarization will be inactivated, and so this area cannot generate another action potential since it cannot be depolarized. Only the membrane that is ahead of the action potential can be depolarized, which causes the action potential to move in only one direction and allows for proper transmittal of the electrical signal.

Each neuron specializes in specific types of neurotransmitters and contains vesicles full of them within its synaptic terminals. When an action potential reaches the synaptic terminals, the membrane in the area is depolarized, causing the opening of voltage-gated Ca^{2+} channels. This allows for Ca^{2+} to flow into the cell, causing the synaptic vesicles to fuse with the membrane and release the neurotransmitters they contained by exocytosis into the synapse. These neurotransmitters will diffuse through the synaptic cleft until they reach the neighboring neuron's dendrites and bind to ligand-gated ion channels, which will open and allow for an influx of ions. An action potential will be generated in this neuron if the conditions are right and the proper ions that will allow for membrane depolarization enter the neuron.

The central nervous system is composed of the brain and spinal cord. The brain and spinal cord both consist of many neurons and supporting glial cells. White matter within the brain and spinal cord consists of myelinated axons. Gray matter consists of clusters of cell bodies of neurons. Cranial bones and vertebrae protect the CNS, as do protective membranes called the meninges. Between the meninges, and within cavities of the brain, there is cerebrospinal fluid. This fluid has some critical functions, such as providing nutrients, removing wastes, and providing cushioning and support for the brain.

The Brain

The brain processes conscious thought and sensory information, coordinates motor activities of skeletal muscle and other organ systems within the body, and maintains vital functions such as heart rate and ventilation. The brain can be divided into the structures seen in Figure 6.3: cerebrum, cerebellum, brain stem, and diencephalon.

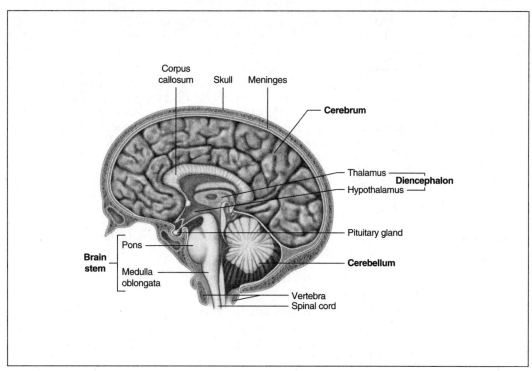

FIGURE 6.3 Major structures of the brain.

The cerebrum in particular has extremely diverse functions. The right and left hemispheres process information in different ways. The right side of the brain tends to specialize in spatial and pattern perception, while the left side of the brain tends to specialize in analytical processing and language. The connection of the two hemispheres via the corpus callosum is essential to integrating the functions of the two sides of the brain.

The functions of each of the parts of the brain including the cerebrum can be seen in Table 6.1.

Spinal Cord and Reflex Actions

The spinal cord serves as a shuttle for messages going toward and away from the brain. It also acts as a reflex center that can process certain incoming messages and provide an autonomic response without processing by the brain.

A reflex arc is a set of neurons that consists of a receptor, a sensory neuron, an interneuron, a motor neuron, and an effector. The receptor transmits a message to a sensory neuron, which routes the message to an interneuron located in the spinal cord. The interneuron processes the message in the spinal cord and sends a response out through the motor neuron. The motor neuron passes the message to an effector, which can carry out the appropriate response.

Table 6.1 Major Structures of the Brain	
Structure	**Function**
Cerebrum	The cerebrum is the largest portion of the brain; it is divided into a right and left hemisphere as well as into four lobes (frontal, parietal, occipital, and temporal). Within the cerebrum there are specific areas for each of the senses, motor coordination, and association areas. All thought processes, memory, learning, and intelligence are regulated via the cerebrum. The cerebral cortex is the outer tissue of the cerebrum.
Cerebellum	The cerebellum is located at the base of the brain. It is responsible for sensorimotor coordination for complex muscle movement patterns and balance.
Brain stem	The brain stem is composed of several structures; it ultimately connects the brain to the spinal cord. ➤ The **pons** connects the spinal cord and cerebellum to the cerebrum and diencephalon. ➤ The **medulla oblongata** (or medulla) has reflex centers for vital functions such as the regulation of breathing, heart rate, and blood pressure. Messages entering the brain from the spinal cord must pass through the medulla. ➤ The **reticular activating system** (RAS) is a tract of neurons that runs through the medulla into the cerebrum. It acts as a filter to prevent the processing of repetitive stimuli. The RAS is also an activating center for the cerebrum. When the RAS is not activated, sleep occurs.
Diencephalon	The diencephalon is composed of two different structures. ➤ The **hypothalamus** is used to regulate the activity of the pituitary gland in the endocrine system. In addition, the hypothalamus regulates conditions such as thirst, hunger, sex drive, and temperature. ➤ The **thalamus** is located near the hypothalamus and serves as a relay center for sensory information entering the cerebrum. It routes incoming information to the appropriate parts of the cerebrum.

The peripheral nervous system is composed of pairs of nerves that are bundles of axons. There are 12 pairs of cranial nerves branching off the brain stem and 31 pairs of spinal nerves branching off the spinal cord. The nerves that exist in the PNS are categorized into one of two divisions: the somatic nervous system or the autonomic nervous system.

The somatic nervous system controls conscious functions within the body such as sensory perception and voluntary movement due to innervation of skeletal muscle. The autonomic nervous system controls the activity of involuntary functions within the body in order to maintain homeostasis. The autonomic nervous system is further subdivided into the sympathetic and parasympathetic branches. Most internal organs are innervated by both branches. The sympathetic branch is regulated by acetylcholine, epinephrine, and norepinephrine. When activated, the sympathetic branch produces the fight-or-flight response, in which heart rate increases, ventilation increases, blood pressure increases, and digestion decreases.

The parasympathetic branch is antagonistic to the sympathetic branch and is the default system used for relaxation. Generally, it decreases heart rate, decreases ventilation rate, decreases blood pressure, and increases digestion. The neurotransmitter acetylcholine is the primary regulator of this system.

MUSCULAR TISSUE

Muscles provide structural support, help maintain body posture, regulate openings into the body, assist in thermoregulation via contractions (shivering) that generate heat, and contract to help move blood in veins toward the heart, assisting in peripheral circulation. Skeletal and cardiac muscle is striated, while smooth muscle is not. Cardiac and smooth muscles are involuntary, while skeletal muscle is under voluntary control.

The cells in skeletal muscle have multiple nuclei as the result of the fusing of multiple cells. The muscle cells also contain high levels of mitochondria to provide ATP needed for contraction and the protein myoglobin that acts as an oxygen reserve for muscles.

Muscles are a bundle of muscle cells held together by connective tissue, as seen in Figure 6.4. The muscle cells have sarcoplasm (cytoplasm), a modified endoplasmic reticulum called the sarcoplasmic reticulum, and a cell membrane called the sarcolemma that interacts with the nervous system via the transverse tubule system

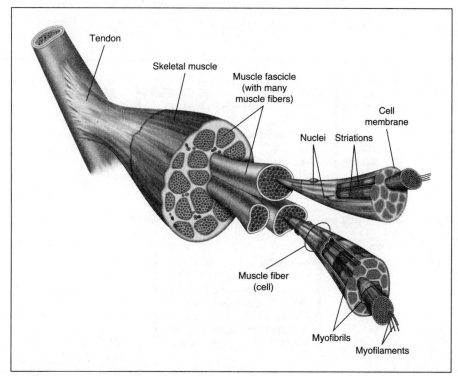

FIGURE 6.4 Skeletal muscle structure.

(T tubule). This system provides channels for ion flow through the muscle and has anchor points for sarcomeres. Within the muscle cells are bundles of muscle fibers called myofibrils made of the proteins actin, troponin, tropomyosin, and myosin. Actin fibers have a thin diameter and associate with the proteins troponin and tropomyosin to produce thin filaments. Myosin fibers have a thick diameter with protruding heads and are called thick filaments. In skeletal muscles, the actin and myosin fibers overlap each other in highly organized, repeating units called sarcomeres. The overlapping of the fibers is what leads to striation of the muscle. The shortening of sarcomeres is what causes muscle contraction. The structure of a sarcomere can be seen in Figure 6.5.

Muscle tissues have regions where the sarcolemma is in contact (via a synapse) with the synaptic knobs of a motor neuron from the somatic branch of the peripheral nervous system. This area is the neuromuscular junction. A neurotransmitter called acetylcholine is released from the motor neuron and binds to receptors on the sarcolemma, causing the initiation of an action potential that will result in shortening of the sarcomeres.

The action potential that occurs based on stimulation from the motor neuron will cause the release of calcium from the sarcoplasmic reticulum into the sarcoplasm. The calcium binds to the troponin in the thin filaments, which causes a conformational shift in the tropomyosin protein in the thin filament. This change in shape allows for the exposure of myosin binding sites on the actin. The myosin heads can now bind to the myosin binding sites on the actin forming crossbridges. Hydrolysis of ATP allows for the powerstroke to occur, which pulls the thin filaments toward the center of the sarcomere. The release of the myosin heads from the actin will occur when another ATP binds to the myosin heads. Calcium again exposes the myosin binding sites on actin so that the myosin heads can bind and the powerstroke can

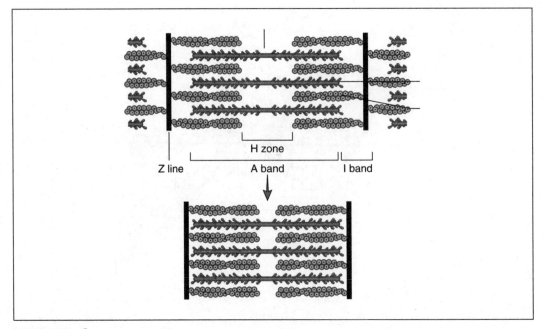

FIGURE 6.5 Sarcomere structure.

occur. The process repeats, each time pulling the thin filaments closer in toward the center of the sarcomere.

Smooth muscle can be found in many parts of the body, including the bladder, digestive tract, and reproductive tract, as well as surrounding blood vessels. The cells that compose smooth muscle contain a single nucleus, as opposed to the multiple nuclei found in skeletal muscle. Smooth muscle contains actin and myosin, but it is not organized as sarcomeres, which is why smooth muscle lacks striations. The actin and myosin slide over each other; this process is regulated by calcium and also requires energy provided by ATP. The autonomic branch of the peripheral nervous system innervates smooth muscle via sympathetic and parasympathetic stimulation, producing involuntary contractions. Smooth muscle can perform myogenic activity, meaning it can contract without stimulation from the nervous system.

Cardiac muscle is only found in the myocardium of the heart. It is striated due to the presence of sarcomeres, but is not multinucleated like skeletal muscle. Cardiac muscle is innervated by the autonomic branch of the peripheral nervous system. Like smooth muscle, it can also perform myogenic activity, contracting without stimulation from the nervous system.

THE SKELETAL SYSTEM

The human skeleton, shown in Figure 6.6, is an endoskeleton divided into two major parts: the axial skeleton and the appendicular skeleton. The skull, vertebrae, and rib cage compose the axial skeleton, while the pelvic and shoulder girdles and limbs in the body are part of the appendicular skeleton. The skeleton is used for protection of internal organs, support, storage of calcium and phosphates, production of blood cells, and movement. The skeleton itself is made of bones and associated cartilage.

Cartilage is a connective tissue. The matrix is termed chondrin and the primary cell type is the chondrocyte. During embryonic development, the skeleton begins as cartilage. During the developmental period, much of the cartilage is subject to ossification, whereby it is turned into bone by calcification. The primary areas where cartilage is found in the adult skeleton are the nose, ears, disks between vertebrae, rib cage, joints, and trachea. Cartilage is unique in that it contains no blood vessels, nor is it innervated.

Bone tissue occurs as compact bone and spongy bone. Compact bone is very dense, while spongy bone is less dense and contains marrow cavities. Within marrow cavities, there is yellow and red bone marrow. Red bone marrow contains the stem cells that differentiate into red blood cells, white blood cells, and platelets. Yellow bone marrow is primarily a reserve for adipose (fat) tissue.

Long bones within the body have a characteristic structure. The ends of the bone are typically covered in cartilage and are termed the epiphyses. The ends are made primarily of spongy bone covered in a thin layer of compact bone. The shaft of the bone (the diaphysis) is made of compact bone surrounding a marrow cavity. The epiphyseal plate is

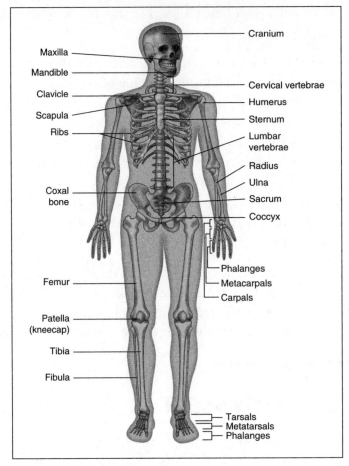

Maxilla
Mandible
Clavicle
Scapula
Ribs
Coxal
bone
Femur
Patella
(kneecap)
Tibia
Fibula

Cranium
Cervical vertebrae
Humerus
Sternum
Lumbar
vertebrae
Radius
Ulna
Sacrum
Coccyx
Phalanges
Metacarpals
Carpals
Tarsals
Metatarsals
Phalanges

FIGURE 6.6   The human skeleton.

a disc of cartilage that separates the diaphysis from each epiphysis; this is where bone lengthening and growth occurs. The periosteum surrounds the bone in a fibrous sheath and acts as a site for the attachment of muscles via tendons. The microscopic structure of bone consists of the matrix that is found within osteons, illustrated in Figure 6.7. There is a Haversian canal within each osteon that contains blood vessels, nerves, and lymphatic vessels. The canal is surrounded by lamellae, which are concentric circles of hard matrix. Within the matrix of the lamellae, there are small spaces called lacunae where mature bone cells reside.

Within the bone, there are three major cell types: osteocytes, osteoblasts, and osteoclasts. The osteocytes are found within the lacunae of osteons. They are mature bone cells involved in the maintenance of bone tissue. Osteoblasts and ostoeclasts are found within bone tissue as well, and are immature cells involved in bone remodeling. Osteo-blasts build bone by producing components of the matrix, while osteoclasts break down bone in the process of bone reabsorption. Eventually, osteoblasts and osteoclasts will become trapped within a matrix of bone tissue and become osteocytes. Osteoblasts are also responsible for bone growth and ossification during development. The hormones calci-tonin from the thyroid gland and parathyroid hormone from the parathyroid glands are

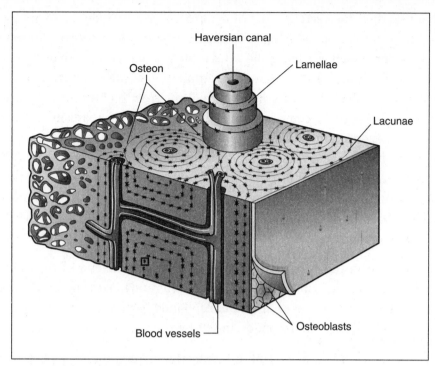

FIGURE 6.7 Bone tissue structure.

responsible for the process of bone remodeling. The levels of blood calcium must be carefully regulated, as calcium is needed for muscle contraction, nervous system communication, and other functions.

While on the topic of bone structure, it is important for a dentist-to-be to also review the important parts of the tooth. The tooth consists of the crown (the part that we see above the gums) and the root (the part that is below the gums). The enamel portion of the crown is mainly composed of hydroxylapatite, $Ca_5(PO_4)_3(OH)$. This is supported by the dentin, a softer layer that can absorb impact. The dentin is covered by the cementum, a bone that is connected to the jaw (alveolar bone). The cementum and alveolar bone are connected via elastic fibers called periodontal ligaments.

THE ENDOCRINE SYSTEM

In order to maintain homeostasis in the body, it is necessary to regulate the functioning of specific targets within the body. Hormones achieve this regulation. Hormones are chemical messengers secreted into the bloodstream that travel to a specific target in the body and change the functioning of that target. The target can be individual cells, tissues, or entire organs.

The secretion of hormones is usually regulated via negative feedback mechanisms. During negative feedback, the response of the endocrine system or a target is the opposite of a stimulus. For example, if the level of a specific hormone gets particularly high (the stimulus), then the secretion of that hormone will be reduced (opposite of the stimulus). It is not uncommon to see antagonistic hormones—two hormones with opposing functions, such as a hormone to raise blood sugar and another to lower blood sugar. Failure of the endocrine system to maintain homeostasis can lead to conditions such as diabetes, hyperthyroidism, hypothyroidism, growth abnormalities, and many others. While not nearly as common as negative feedback mechanisms, positive feedback mechanisms do exist. In this case, the stimulus causes actions in the body, regulated by hormones, that further amplify that stimulus, moving the body away from homeostasis. Positive feedback mechanisms are short-lived, and eventually homeostasis is regained via lack of stimulus. An example of a positive feedback mechanism in the body is that of childbirth, in which the body will continue to produce the hormone oxytocin to cause more uterine contractions until the infant is delivered.

The hypothalamus in the brain is the main link between the endocrine and nervous systems. The hypothalamus monitors body conditions and makes changes as needed. It produces regulatory hormones that influence glands such as the pituitary, which in turn regulates other glands in the endocrine system.

Hormones are generally secreted from an endocrine gland into the bloodstream. The endocrine system is composed of endocrine glands located throughout the body. The major endocrine glands can be seen in Figure 6.8.

The specificity of hormones is based on their interaction with a receptor on the target cells. Only cells that have a receptor for a specific hormone will be affected by that hormone.

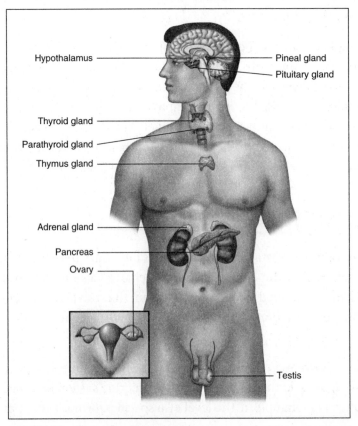

FIGURE 6.8 The endocrine system.

Once a hormone binds to the receptor, the cell's functioning will be changed in some way. These changes can involve gene expression, chemical reactions, membrane changes, metabolism, and so forth. Because the hormones must travel through the blood, making these changes is a relatively slow process. There are two major categories of hormones: steroids (which are lipid-soluble) and nonsteroids (which are water-soluble and classified as peptides). Steroid hormones are derivatives of cholesterol, while nonsteroid hormones are made of modified amino acids or small proteins. The target cell receptors for steroid hormones exist in the cytoplasm of the cell, while the receptors for nonsteroid hormones exist on the cell membrane of the cell.

A third category of chemical messengers is the prostaglandins. These are lipid-based molecules released from cell membranes. Prostaglandins function as a sort of local hormone involved in functions as diverse as regulation of body temperature, blood clotting, the inflammatory response, and menstrual cramping caused by uterine contractions.

Steroids are derivatives of cholesterol that are lipid soluble; they can easily cross the cell membrane. Once inside a cell, the steroid locates and binds to a cytoplasmic receptor. The steroid-receptor complex moves into the nucleus and interacts with DNA to cause activation of certain genes. This serves as the signal to initiate transcription and translation so that a new protein is expressed by the cell. This new protein will change how the cell is functioning in some way. A visual summary of steroid hormone action can be seen in Figure 6.9.

Nonsteroid hormones are composed of amino acid derivatives or small proteins; they do not cross the cell membrane. The hormone itself is termed a first messenger, since it will

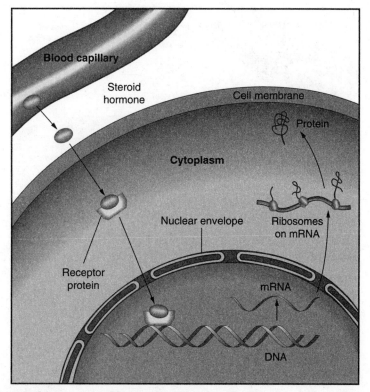

FIGURE 6.9 Steroid hormone mechanism of action.

never enter the cell; it only triggers a series of events within the cell, many of which are moderated by G proteins found on the cytoplasmic side of the plasma membrane. In a typical cell, these G proteins are in an inactive state with a molecule of GDP attached to them. When a signaling molecule, in this case a nonsteroid hormone, attaches to a G protein–coupled receptor in the plasma membrane, the receptor becomes active and changes conformation. This change allows the receptor to bind a G protein and activate it by causing it to release its GDP molecule and exchange it for a GTP molecule. The activated G protein will dissociate from the receptor and, usually, go on to activate an enzyme called adenylyl cyclase. When this enzyme is activated, it will convert ATP to cyclic AMP (cAMP), which will function as a second messenger in this signal transduction pathway. Second messengers are nonprotein molecules that change the function of the target cell by altering enzymatic activities and cellular reactions. In the case of cAMP, it will activate a protein called protein kinase A, which will proceed to activate other protein kinases by transferring phosphate groups from ATP to the protein, as is the function of a protein kinase. These activated protein kinases will then activate more protein kinases in a type of phosphorylation cascade until the proper protein needed to cause the cellular response to the initial first messenger is activated. This signaling pathway is shut down through the use of protein phosphatases that will remove the phosphate groups from the activated proteins, thereby deactivating them and stopping their kinase activity. In addition, phosphodiesterase will convert cAMP to ATP, thus deactivating cAMP. Also, the alpha subunits of G proteins have intrinsic GTPase activity, which will cause the bound GTP to be hydrolyzed to GDP, causing the deactivation of the G protein and stopping the further activation of adenylyl cyclase. A visual summary of nonsteroid hormone action can be seen in Figure 6.10.

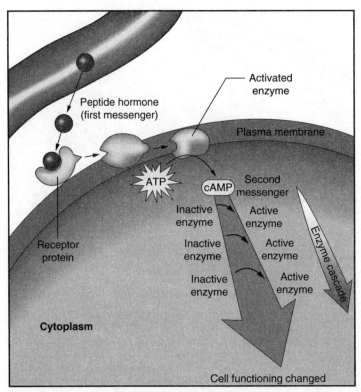

FIGURE 6.10 Nonsteroid hormone mechanism of action.

Major Endocrine Glands

The major endocrine glands of the body include the hypothalamus, pituitary gland (separated into the anterior lobe and posterior lobe), pineal gland, thyroid gland, parathyroid glands, and adrenal glands. Some organs within the body also have endocrine functions; these include the thymus gland, ovaries, testes, pancreas, heart, placenta, kidneys, stomach, and small intestine.

The hypothalamus and pituitary gland have a unique relationship based on their proximity to each other in the brain. The pituitary gland secretes many hormones, some of which influence the secretion of hormones from other endocrine glands. The regulatory hormones made by the hypothalamus control the secretion of hormones from the anterior pituitary. The hypothalamus produces releasing hormones that stimulate the release of anterior pituitary hormones, as well as inhibiting hormones that inhibit the release of hormones from the anterior pituitary. The hypothalamus also makes antidiuretic hormone and oxytocin, but both are stored and released from the posterior pituitary.

Table 6.2 lists the major hormones and the glands that produce them. Unless marked otherwise, each of these hormones is a nonsteroid.

Table 6.2 Endocrine Structures and the Hormones They Make	
Endocrine Structure	**Hormones and Function**
Anterior pituitary	➤ **Follicle stimulating hormone (FSH):** in women, stimulates the secretion of estrogen in the ovaries and assists in egg production via meiosis; in men, has a role in sperm production
	➤ **Luteinizing hormone (LH):** in women, stimulates the production of estrogen and progesterone by the ovaries and causes ovulation; in men, is involved in testosterone secretion from the testes
	➤ **Thyroid stimulating hormone (TSH):** stimulates the thyroid gland
	➤ **Growth hormone (GH):** stimulates growth of muscle, bone, and cartilage
	➤ **Prolactin (PRL):** stimulates the production of milk
	➤ **Adrenocorticotropic hormone (ACTH):** stimulates the cortex of the adrenal glands
	➤ **Endorphins:** act on the nervous system to reduce the perception of pain
Posterior pituitary	The following hormones are made by the hypothalamus but are released by the posterior pituitary.
	➤ **Antidiuretic hormone (ADH):** allows for water retention by the kidneys and decreases urine volume; also known as vasopressin
	➤ **Oxytocin (OT):** causes uterine contractions during childbirth; also stimulates milk ejection

(cont.)

Table 6.2 Endocrine Structures and the Hormones They Make (*cont.*)	
Endocrine Structure	**Hormones and Function**
Pineal gland	➤ **Melatonin:** influences patterned behaviors such as sleep, fertility, and aging
Thymus	➤ **Thymopoietin:** stimulates the maturation of certain white blood cells involved with the immune system (T cells); decreases with age as the thymus gland atrophies ➤ **Thymosin:** stimulates the maturation of certain white blood cells involved with the immune system; decreases with age as the thymus gland shrivels
Ovaries	➤ **Estrogen:** involved in the development of female secondary sex characteristics as well as follicle development and pregnancy ➤ **Progesterone:** involved in uterine preparation and pregnancy
Testes	➤ **Testosterone:** a type of androgen needed for the production of sperm as well as for the development and maintenance of male secondary sex characteristics
Pancreas	➤ **Insulin:** decreases blood sugar after meals by allowing glucose to enter cells to be used for cellular respiration; a lack of insulin or lack of response by cell receptors to insulin is the cause of diabetes mellitus; made by the beta islet cells ➤ **Glucagon:** increases blood sugar levels between meals by allowing for the breakdown of glycogen; antagonistic to insulin; made by the alpha islet cells
Heart	➤ **Atrial natriuretic peptide (ANP):** made by the heart to lower blood pressure
Kidneys	➤ **Renin/angiotensin:** Used to regulate blood pressure by altering the amount of water retained by the kidneys ➤ **Erythropoietin (EPO):** stimulates the production of red blood cells from stem cells in the red bone marrow
Stomach	➤ **Gastrin:** released when food enters the stomach; causes the secretion of gastric juice needed to begin the digestion of proteins
Small intestine	➤ **Cholecystokinin (CCK):** stimulates the release of pancreatic digestive enzymes to the small intestine; also stimulates the release of bile from the gallbladder to the small intestine ➤ **Secretin:** stimulates the release of fluids from the pancreas and bile that are high in bicarbonate to neutralize the acids from the stomach
Placenta (temporary organ during pregnancy)	➤ **Human chorionic gonadotropin (HCG):** signals the retention of the lining of the uterus (endometrium) during pregnancy ➤ **Relaxin:** releases ligaments attaching the pubic bones to allow for more space during childbirth ➤ **Estrogen:** needed to maintain pregnancy ➤ **Progesterone:** needed to maintain pregnancy

THE CARDIOVASCULAR SYSTEM

The cardiovascular system in humans consists of a four-chambered heart to pump blood and a series of vessels needed to transport blood in the body. Blood is a connective tissue used to deliver oxygen, nutrients, water, hormones, and ions to all the cells of the body. It is also used to pick up the carbon dioxide and wastes produced by cells and to move these to the appropriate areas for elimination. Further, it assists in thermoregulation in the body as well as fighting infectious agents. The cardiovascular system is closely linked to the following organ systems in the body:

➤ **Respiratory system** for the elimination of carbon dioxide, the pickup of oxygen, and assistance regulating blood pH.
➤ **Urinary system** for the filtration of blood, removal of nitrogenous wastes, regulation of blood volume and pressure, and regulation of blood pH.
➤ **Digestive system** for the pickup of nutrients to be distributed to the body.

The Blood

The critical functions of the cardiovascular system are achieved by blood transported through the system. For this reason, the composition of blood needs to be examined more closely. Blood consists of a liquid matrix, plasma, and formed elements or cells. Humans contain between four and six liters of blood; this entire volume can be circulated through the body in less than one minute. The pH of blood is 7.4 (slightly basic), and the temperature is slightly warmer than body temperature. Because blood is warmer than the body, changing patterns of circulation can help distribute heat to where it is needed in the body. Vasoconstriction decreases the diameter of vessels, keeping blood closer to the core to warm the body, while vasodilation increases the diameter of the vessels, allowing them to release heat toward the surface of the skin to cool the body.

Plasma is the liquid portion of the blood; it makes up approximately 55 percent of the total volume of blood. The primary component of plasma is water. In order to adjust the volume of blood in the body, the water levels of plasma can be altered. This is one role for the kidneys. They can retain or release water via urine to adjust the blood volume. An increase in blood volume will increase blood pressure, while a decrease in blood volume will decrease blood pressure. In addition to water, plasma also contains nutrients, cellular waste products, respiratory gases, ions, hormones, and proteins. There are three classes of plasma proteins produced by the liver: immunoglobulins are primarily used in the immune response, albumins are used to transport certain molecules within the blood, and fibrinogen is an inactive form of one protein that is needed to clot blood.

The formed elements or cells of the blood are all derived from stem cells in the bone marrow. The three types of cells that are found within the blood are erythrocytes (red blood cells), leukocytes (white blood cells), and thrombocytes (platelets). The hematocrit value of blood is a relative comparison of cell volume to plasma volume.

The percentage of blood occupied by cells is called the hematocrit value. It is generally about 45. Because red blood cells are by far the most abundant blood cell, hematocrit values are primarily influenced by red blood cells.

Erythrocytes are the most abundant type of blood cell. As they mature from stem cells in the bone marrow, they do something odd: they lose their organelles. Without organelles, these cells are unable to perform aerobic cellular respiration and they cannot perform mitosis to replace themselves. Further, they only live about 120 days, at which point they are destroyed by the liver and spleen. The end product of red blood cells' hemoglobin breakdown is bilirubin, which is ultimately excreted into the small intestine via bile from the liver. In order to make new red blood cells, more stem cells in the bone marrow must be coerced to differentiate into red blood cells by the hormone erythropoietin (EPO). Red blood cells also have an unusual biconcave disc shape that provides them with increased surface area and the ability to be flexible as they move through small vessels.

The critical component of red blood cells is the protein hemoglobin. Each cell contains about 250 million hemoglobin molecules. Functional hemoglobin consists of four protein chains, each wrapped around an iron (heme-) core. This molecule is capable of carrying four molecules of oxygen (O_2). In total, a single red blood cell can carry about a billion O_2 molecules.

As hemoglobin binds to one oxygen molecule, a conformational change in the shape of hemoglobin occurs to allow for the loading of the next three O_2 molecules. The same process occurs during the unloading of O_2. Once O_2 is unloaded in the capillary beds of the body, some of the CO_2 produced by the cells will be carried by hemoglobin. Carbon dioxide combines with water to produce carbonic acid, which dissociates into hydrogen ions and bicarbonate ions. The hemoglobin carries the hydrogen ions, while the bicarbonate ions are carried by plasma. The Bohr effect states that increasing concentrations of hydrogen ions (which decrease blood pH) and increasing concentrations of carbon dioxide will decrease hemoglobin's affinity for O_2. This allows O_2 to unload from hemoglobin into tissues of the body such as muscle when CO_2 levels are high in tissues. In the lungs, a high level of O_2 will encourage the dissociation of hydrogen ions from hemoglobin, which will join with bicarbonate ions in the plasma to form CO_2 and water. The CO_2 will be exhaled. The enzyme carbonic anhydrase catalyzes the formation and disassociation of carbonic acid.

Leukocytes are a diverse collection of cells, all of which are derived from stem cells in the red bone marrow; all of them function within the immune system. They are found in much lower levels than red blood cells; however, the white blood cell level can fluctuate greatly, particularly when a person is fighting infection. White blood cells can be categorized in the following manner, based on their microscopic appearance:

➤ **Granulocytes** have cytoplasm with a granular appearance. These cells include neutrophils, basophils, and eosinophils. Neutrophils are used to perform phagocytosis. Basophils and eosinophils are involved in inflammation and allergies.

➤ **Agranulocytes** have cytoplasm that does not have a grainy appearance. They include monocytes, which mature into macrophages, and lymphocytes, which are further subdivided into T cells and B cells. Monocytes and macrophages perform phagocytosis, while lymphocytes function as the specific defenses of the immune system.

➤ **Thrombocytes**, or platelets, are fragments of bone marrow cells called megakaryocytes.

Platelets only live 10 to 12 days once mature, so they are replaced often. During injury to blood vessels, a complex series of reactions is initiated. The platelets release thromboplastin, which converts an inactive plasma protein, prothrombin, to the active form, thrombin. Thrombin then converts fibrinogen to fibrin. Fibrin forms a meshwork around the injury that serves to trap other cells, forming a clot. The process of blood clotting requires multiple plasma proteins as well as calcium and vitamin K.

The Circulatory System

Blood flow progresses in unidirectional loops, as illustrated in Figure 6.11. One loop is the systemic circuit, which moves blood from the heart, throughout the body, and back to the heart. The other loop is the pulmonary circuit, which moves blood from the heart, to the lungs, and back to the heart.

Arteries are large blood vessels leaving the heart. The arteries have thick walls and are very elastic to accommodate blood pressure. As arteries leave the heart, they branch into smaller vessels called arterioles. The arterioles become more and more narrow, eventually forming the capillaries, which are the smallest vessels. Capillary beds are the site of gas exchange within tissues; they are so small that red blood cells have to line up

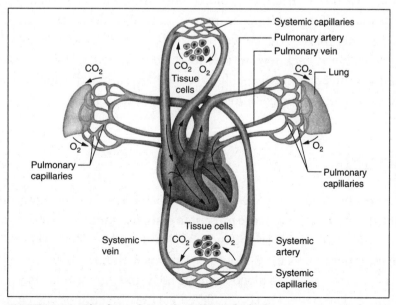

FIGURE 6.11 Blood circulation throughout the body.

single file to pass through them. Once gas has been exchanged, the capillaries widen and become venules that head back toward the heart. The venules become larger veins, which ultimately merge into the heart. Veins are not as thick-walled as arteries, since they do not have to deal with the forces exerted by blood pressure. While blood pressure pushes blood through arteries and arterioles, the movement of blood in venules and veins is facilitated by muscles that contract to push the blood along and valves that close to prevent backflow of blood. Vasoconstriction and vasodilation of arteries serves as a means to regulate blood flow, pressure, and temperature.

The arteries of the systemic circuit branch off the left side of the heart and carry oxygenated blood to the capillaries of the body where gas exchange occurs. As the blood is being moved from arteries to capillaries, there is a significant decrease in its velocity. Although it would be expected that blood moving from arteries that have a larger diameter to capillaries that have very small diameters would increase blood velocity, the key consideration that needs to be made is the number of capillaries in the body. Because there are very many capillaries throughout the body, the *total* cross-sectional area of the capillaries is much greater than that of the arteries. As a result, blood velocity actually decreases as it moves from arteries to capillaries. This decrease in velocity is essential in that it provides adequate time for gas exchange to occur between the blood and the interstitial fluid, which is the fluid that surrounds the cells. Deoxygenated blood returns to the right side of the heart via systemic veins. The pulmonary circuit involves pulmonary arteries that branch off the right side of the heart and carry deoxygenated blood toward the lungs. The pulmonary capillaries allow for gas exchange with the alveoli (air sacs) of the lungs. The newly oxygenated blood then moves back toward the left side of the heart via pulmonary veins.

A capillary bed is a collection of capillaries, all branching off a single arteriole, that serves a specific location in the body. The blood entering the systemic capillary bed is oxygenated and high in nutrients. As blood moves through the capillary bed, oxygen and nutrients must diffuse out into the interstitial fluid and carbon dioxide and wastes must diffuse in. After this has happened, the capillaries merge into a venule that carries the deoxygenated blood back toward the heart. In pulmonary circulation, deoxygenated blood enters the pulmonary capillary bed, where carbon dioxide diffuses out and oxygen diffuses in, causing oxygenation of the blood. Precapillary sphincters guard the entrance to the capillary beds.

The Heart

The structure of the heart can be seen in Figure 6.12. The myocardium is the cardiac muscle of the heart. Other tissues are present to compose supporting structures such as valves and chamber linings. The right and left sides of the heart have very distinct functions. Blood essentially flows in two loops or circuits within the body. The right side of the heart receives deoxygenated blood from the body and pumps this blood to the lungs to be oxygenated. The right side is considered part of the pulmonary circuit. The left side of the heart receives oxygenated blood from the lungs and pumps it to the body.

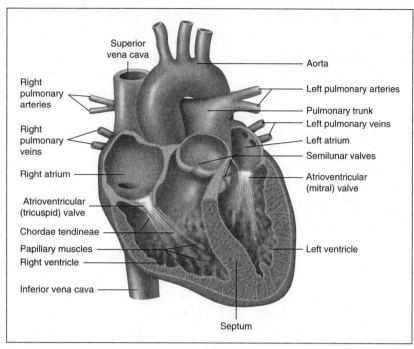

FIGURE 6.12 Structure of the human heart.

This is the systemic circuit. A fluid-filled sac called the pericardium surrounds the entire heart. The right and left sides of the heart must be kept separate from each other. This is achieved by the septum, which is a thick barricade between the two sides of the heart. Each side of the heart has two chambers. The upper chamber is the atrium, and the lower chamber is the ventricle. The atrium and ventricle are separated by atrioventricular (AV) valves: the tricuspid valve between the right atrium and right ventricle, and the bicuspid (mitral) valve between the left atrium and the left ventricle. Semilunar valves regulate the flow of blood out of the ventricles: the pulmonary semilunar valve for blood leaving the right ventricle and the aortic semilunar valve for blood leaving the left ventricle.

The pulmonary circuit begins when veins within the body merge into the venae cavae, which lie on the dorsal wall of the thoracic and abdominal cavities. The superior vena cava comes from the head and neck, while the inferior vena cava comes from the trunk and lower extremities. These vessels carry deoxygenated blood and merge into the right atrium of the heart. As the atrium contracts, blood will pass through the tricuspid valve into the right ventricle. As the ventricle contracts, blood passes through the pulmonary semilunar valve into the pulmonary arteries. These arteries carry blood to the lungs and are the only arteries in the body that do not carry oxygenated blood. The pulmonary arteries branch into capillaries that surround the alveoli (air sacs) in the lungs, where gas exchange occurs to oxygenate the blood.

Once gas exchange has occurred, pulmonary veins carry the oxygenated blood toward the left side of the heart into the systemic circuit. The pulmonary veins in the body are the only veins to carry oxygenated blood. Blood reenters the heart through the left atrium.

As the atrium contracts (in sync with contraction of the right atrium), blood is pushed through the bicuspid valve into the left ventricle. When the ventricle contracts (similarly in sync with the right ventricle) the blood is pushed into the aorta via the aortic semilunar valve. The aorta is the largest artery in the body, running along the dorsal wall of the body next to the inferior vena cava. The aorta splits into arteries, arterioles, and eventually capillaries, where the blood is once again deoxygenated and must be pushed back to the right side of the heart to begin the process all over again.

The first branches off the aorta are the coronary arteries, which serve to provide circulation to the surface of the heart. Blockage of the coronary arteries can stop blood flow to the cardiac muscle, causing death of that muscle. This is characteristic of a heart attack. After blood flows through the coronary arteries, deoxygenated blood is returned to the right side of the heart by coronary veins.

Cardiac muscle is involuntary and has the ability to contract on its own without stimulation from the nervous system. The impulses that generate heart contraction have to be spread through the conducting system of the heart. The sinoatrial (SA) node, also known as the pacemaker, is a bundle of conducting cells in the top of the right atrium that initiates contractions. The SA node sends electrical impulses through the two atria, causing them to contract. The impulse arrives at the atrioventricular (AV) node, where the impulse is delayed for a very short time. This delay ensures that all of the blood from the atria was moved to the ventricles and that the atria are empty when the ventricles contract. The impulse is then spread through the bundle of His and through Purkinje fibers in the walls of the ventricles, causing ventricular contraction.

Blood pressure is a measurement of the force that blood exerts on the walls of a blood vessel. Typically it is measured within arteries, which have enough pressure to overcome the peripheral resistance of the arterioles and capillaries. It is expressed with two values: a systolic pressure and a diastolic pressure. The systolic pressure is the higher value and is the pressure exerted on arteries as the ventricles contract. The diastolic pressure is the lower number and is a measurement of pressure on the arteries during ventricular relaxation. The primary means of regulation of blood pressure is by regulation of blood volume through the kidneys. The higher the blood volume, the higher the blood pressure is.

THE RESPIRATORY SYSTEM

The respiratory system has the primary jobs of providing the body with oxygen and eliminating carbon dioxide. Pulmonary arteries, coming off the right side of the heart, carry deoxygenated blood, which is low in oxygen and high in carbon dioxide, to the lungs. Oxygen that enters the lungs will be distributed to hemoglobin in the erythrocytes within the capillaries that branch off the pulmonary arteries that surround the alveoli. Carbon dioxide will diffuse into the alveoli from the pulmonary arteries to be exhaled. Now blood is oxygenated and will travel back to the left side of the heart via pulmonary veins. In addition to oxygenating blood, the respiratory structures are responsible for pH regulation, vocal communication, the sense of smell, and protection from infectious agents and particles.

The respiratory system is essentially a series of tubes that conduct air into the alveoli located in the lung tissues. The major structures of the system can be seen in Figure 6.13. Air is inhaled through the nose or mouth. Because the respiratory system is an open system, it is particularly vulnerable to infection. In the nose and pharynx (back of the throat), air is warmed to body temperature, moisturized so that gas exchange can occur, and filtered. Both areas are covered with a mucous membrane that helps prevent desiccation of the tissues and collects particles and microbes that may enter the system. The nose is particularly well suited to filtration because it has cilia and hair to help trap substances that enter the respiratory system. While filtration in the nose and pharynx will not catch all particles, it will catch many of them. The nose has the additional function of olfaction.

Air flows into the nose or mouth and through the pharynx, where there are two passageways: the esophagus and the larynx. During breathing, air will flow through the glottis, which is the opening of the larynx. The larynx is the voice box; it is made of cartilage and vocal cords that produce sound as they vibrate. Unless a person is swallowing, the esophagus will be closed off and the glottis will be open. But if a person is

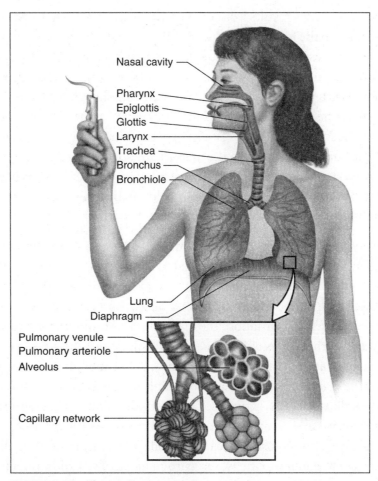

FIGURE 6.13 The respiratory system.

swallowing, a small piece of cartilage called the epiglottis will cover the glottis and stop food from entering the larynx. As air flows through the larynx, it eventually makes its way into the trachea and the lower respiratory tract. The trachea is supported by C-shaped rings of cartilage. The interior surface of the trachea is covered with mucus and cilia to trap any further materials that may not have been caught in the nose or pharynx.

The trachea branches off toward the left and right into bronchi. The two bronchi branch into smaller and smaller tubes called the bronchioles. Smooth muscles surrounding the bronchioles can adjust their diameter to meet oxygen demands. The bronchioles terminate in tiny air sacs called the alveoli. The alveoli are numerous, providing lots of surface area for gas exchange, and are made of simple squamous epithelium that allows for easy gas exchange with the capillaries that surround them.

The lungs are a collection of resilient tissue including the bronchioles and alveoli. In humans, the right lung has three lobes of tissue, while the left lung has only two lobes. Each lung is surrounded by a fluid-filled pleural membrane. A surfactant fluid produced by the tissues decreases surface tension in the alveoli. This keeps the alveoli inflated and functioning, which helps prevent alveolar collapse. Without surfactant to relieve surface tension, the lungs are unable to function.

Gas exchange in the lungs results from the flow of gases because of pressure gradients. In order to get air into the lungs, the volume of the chest cavity has to increase, decreasing pressure in the chest cavity. This allows air to flow from an area of greater pressure (outside the body) to an area with less pressure (the chest cavity). This is the process of inhalation (or inspiration) and it occurs when the diaphragm, the thin muscle that separates the thoracic cavity from the abdominal cavity, contracts and pushes down. The intercostal muscles of the rib cage also assist in inhalation by contracting to help move the rib cage up and out. When the diaphragm and intercostal muscles relax, the volume of the chest cavity decreases, which results in a higher level of pressure inside the chest cavity than outside it. This forces air to leave the lungs by the process of exhalation (expiration).

The rate of ventilation is controlled by the medulla oblongata of the brain. The diaphragm is innervated and neurally connected to the area of the medulla that controls breathing. Activity of these inspiratory neurons causes contraction of the diaphragm, which is followed by a period of inactivity that allows for relaxation of the diaphragm and exhalation. In a relaxed situation, the diaphragm is stimulated between 12 and 15 times per minute. During times of increased oxygen demand and excessive carbon dioxide production, this rate can increase significantly. While it might be expected that oxygen levels are the primary influence on breathing rate, it turns out that the primary trigger is carbon dioxide levels, monitored by chemoreceptors located in the brain and certain large blood vessels. As carbon dioxide levels increase, the pH decreases (remember carbonic acid levels increase as carbon dioxide levels rise) and thus the breathing rate must increase to eliminate the excess carbon dioxide, which in turn increases the oxygen levels.

The concentration of gases can be measured as partial pressures. After an inhalation, the amount of oxygen or partial pressure of oxygen in the alveoli is greater than the amount of oxygen or partial pressure in the capillaries surrounding the alveoli, which are branches of the pulmonary arteries. Gases will flow from an area of high concentration (partial pressure) to an area of low concentration (partial pressure), so oxygen will move from the alveoli into the capillaries and bind to hemoglobin. Further, immediately following inhalation, carbon dioxide levels will be low in the alveoli and high in the capillaries. Diffusion will move the carbon dioxide into the alveoli. At this point, the blood in the pulmonary capillaries is oxygenated and ready to move back to the left side of the heart via the pulmonary veins. The gases that diffused into the alveoli will be exhaled.

Carbon dioxide exchange has an important role in the maintenance of acid-base balance within the body. When carbon dioxide interacts with water, it forms carbonic acid. The carbonic acid is converted to the bicarbonate ion and hydrogen ions. The bicarbonate ions help buffer pH in the body. When the pH of the body becomes too alkaline, the reaction can be reversed. The bicarbonate and hydrogen ions join together to produce carbonic acid, which is then converted to water and carbon dioxide. The carbon dioxide is exhaled in order to adjust pH.

THE DIGESTIVE SYSTEM

The digestive system is designed to extract nutrients from food and eliminate wastes. The system is set up as a series of modified tubes to keep food and digestive enzymes sequestered from the body. It is also known as the gastrointestinal (GI) tract. In addition to the GI tract, there are several accessory structures (the liver, gallbladder, and pancreas) that perform functions vital to the digestive system. The GI tract and accessory structures can be seen in Figure 6.14.

The three primary components of the diet that require digestion are carbohydrates, proteins, and fats. The digestive system has the following functions: mechanical digestion of food achieved by chewing, chemical digestion of food achieved by assorted digestive enzymes, absorption of nutrients into the bloodstream, and elimination of waste products.

Any contact of the digestive enzymes with the rest of the body could result in the self-digestion of tissues. Further, the digestive system is an open system into which infectious organisms can enter. The contents of the system need to be kept away from the rest of the body. In order to ensure this, the digestive tubes are composed of four tissue layers, as follows:

➤ The **mucosa layer** is a mucous membrane that actually comes in contact with food. It serves as a lubricant and protects against desiccation, abrasion, and digestive enzymes. The mucosa lack blood vessels and nerve endings.
➤ The **submucosal layer** is below the mucosa. It contains blood vessels, lymphatic vessels, and nerve endings. Its primary function is to support the mucosa and to transport materials to the bloodstream.

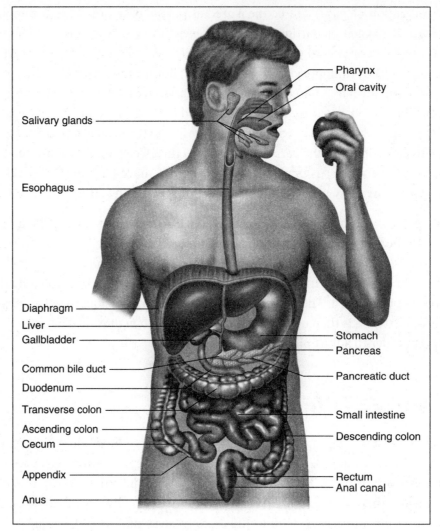

FIGURE 6.14   The digestive system.

> ➤ The **muscularis layer** is composed of two layers of smooth muscle that run in opposing directions. The nerve endings in the submucosa serve to stimulate the muscularis layer to produce contractions that propel food through the system. These muscular contractions are termed peristalsis.
> ➤ The **serosa** is a thin connective tissue layer that is found on the surface of the digestive tubing. Its purpose is to reduce friction with other surfaces in contact with the GI tract.

Food enters the digestive tract at the oral cavity. From there, it moves to the esophagus and then the stomach. Small bits of the stomach contents are released to the small intestine, which completes digestion with some help from secretions from the liver and pancreas. In the small intestine, nutrients are absorbed into the bloodstream. Finally, the waste products of digestion are solidified in the large intestine and are released.

As food is ingested and enters the mouth, three sets of salivary glands begin to secrete saliva. The teeth are responsible for mechanical digestion of food, breaking it into smaller pieces by chewing. As saliva mixes with the chewed food, chemical or enzymatic digestion begins. In addition to its lubricating function, saliva contains the digestive enzyme amylase, which begins the chemical breakdown of carbohydrates such as starch. Since food does not stay in the mouth for long, amylase rarely gets to complete its job in the oral cavity.

As food is ready to be swallowed, it must pass by the pharynx. Recall that the pharynx has two openings—one to the larynx and one to the esophagus. Normally, the esophagus is closed during breathing so that air passes through the larynx. When food touches the pharynx, a reflex action occurs that pushes the epiglottis over to cover the glottis of the larynx. This allows food to proceed down the esophagus. Once in the esophagus, muscular contractions will force the food toward the stomach by peristalsis.

The stomach is a relatively small, curved organ when empty but is capable of great expansion when full of food, due to the presence of many folds in its interior lining. The top and bottom of the stomach are each guarded by a muscular sphincter. The stomach is unique in that it has a very acidic environment; it must retain its own secretions. Tightly closing sphincters make sure this happens. The top sphincter opens to allow the bolus of food to enter. Once food is inside the stomach, it will be mixed with gastric juice for the purpose of liquefying it as well as initiating the chemical digestion of proteins. The hormone gastrin signals the gastric glands of the stomach to begin producing gastric juice as well as for the stomach to start churning. Gastric juice is composed of a mixture of mucus to protect the stomach lining from being digested itself; pepsinogen, which is an inactive form of the enzyme that digests protein; and hydrochloric acid, which is needed to activate the pepsinogen. The active form of pepsinogen is called pepsin. The hydrochloric acid secreted in the stomach provides an overall pH of 1 to 2, which is highly acidic. Normally, a pH this low would denature enzymes, but pepsin is unusual in that it is inactive except at a low pH. The low pH of the stomach also kills most infectious agents that entered the digestive tract with the food.

As the food mixes with gastric juice, the resulting liquid is called chyme. Depending on the size and nutritional content of the meal, it takes on average about four hours for the stomach to empty its contents into the small intestine. The chyme leaves the stomach in small bursts as the bottom sphincter (the pyloric sphincter) opens.

The small intestine is a tube approximately six meters in length. Its primary job is to complete the chemical digestion of food and to absorb the nutrients into the bloodstream. The small intestine relies on secretions from the liver and pancreas to complete chemical digestion. As the bottom sphincter of the stomach opens, small amounts of chyme enter the top region of the small intestine, the duodenum. It is important to neutralize the acidity from gastric juice by the secretion of sodium bicarbonate from the pancreas into the small intestine. In addition to receiving secretions made from the pancreas, the duodenum also receives secretions from the liver. These secretions help with chemical digestion, which occurs in the middle region of the small intestine (the jejunum) and the lower end (the ileum).

The liver is composed of several lobes of tissue and is one of the larger organs in the body. The liver has countless functions. In the case of the digestive system, the liver produces bile, which is a fat emulsifier. While bile is not an enzyme, it helps break fats into smaller pieces so that they are more susceptible to digestion by enzymes secreted from the pancreas. Bile contains water, cholesterol, bile pigments, bile salts, and some ions. Bile from the liver is stored in the gallbladder (a small structure on the underside of the liver) and is released to the small intestine, based on signals from the hormones secretin and cholecystokinin (CCK), via the common bile duct as food enters the small intestine.

The liver has some other functions within the digestive system. After the absorption of nutrients, blood from the capillaries of the gastrointestinal organs and spleen will travel directly to the liver via the hepatic portal vein. Once in the liver, the glucose levels of the blood will be regulated. When blood glucose levels get high, the liver will store the excess as glycogen under the influence of insulin. When blood sugar levels are low, the liver will break down glycogen to release glucose under the influence of glucagon. The liver will also package lipids in lipoproteins to allow them to travel throughout the body. The smooth endoplasmic reticulum within the liver can produce enzymes to detoxify certain harmful substances. The liver also stores vitamins A, E, D, and K (the fat-soluble vitamins). After these functions occur in the liver, the blood will leave via hepatic veins and empty into the inferior vena cava before entering general circulation. This type of circulation, in which blood from the gastrointestinal organs and spleen is moved through the liver, is known as hepatic portal circulation.

The pancreas secretes pancreatic juice into the small intestine via the pancreatic duct. While the pancreas has cells involved in endocrine functions, which are located in areas called islets of Langerhans, producing insulin and glucagon, it also has exocrine cells that produce pancreatic juice. The pancreas secretes pancreatic juice when food enters the small intestine as signaled by the hormones secretin and CCK. Pancreatic juice contains the following elements:

➤ **Bicarbonate ions:** act as a neutralizer of stomach acid
➤ **Amylase:** completes carbohydrate (starch) digestion that began in the oral cavity to release glucose
➤ **Proteinases:** complete protein digestion that was started in the stomach to release amino acids; three specific proteinases—trypsin, chymotrypsin, and carboxypeptidase—are found in pancreatic juice.
➤ **Lipase:** breaks down fats to fatty acids and glycerol
➤ **Nucleases:** break down DNA and RNA to nucleotides

Once the food has been exposed to the secretions of the pancreas, liver, and small intestine it is necessary to absorb the nutrients and eliminate the wastes. It can take anywhere from 3 to 10 hours for nutrients to be absorbed from the small intestine. The small intestine has an internal anatomy that makes it well suited for absorption because of its tremendous surface area. The mucosa in the small intestine are folded into villi, which form the brush border. The villi are then further folded into microscopic microvilli. Within each villus, there are capillaries and a lacteal (a lymphatic capillary).

Nutrients such as glucose and other simple sugars, amino acids, vitamins, and minerals diffuse into the capillaries within each villus, where they are carried into the bloodstream. The end products of fat digestion take another route. The fat products are assembled into a triglyceride and packaged in a special coating including cholesterol, which creates a chylomicron. These structures cannot diffuse into capillaries, so they enter the lacteals. The lymphatic fluids will carry the chylomicrons to the bloodstream at the thoracic duct (a merger between the two systems).

Now that the nutrients have been absorbed into the bloodstream, the remnants of digestion have made their way to the large intestine. Now water must be reclaimed by the body, which will in turn solidify the waste products. These waste products will be stored by the large intestine and released at the appropriate time. In addition, the large intestine contains a large population of normal flora or harmless resident bacteria. These bacteria are responsible for the synthesis of certain vitamins that the body needs.

The large intestine has a much larger girth than the small intestine, but it is shorter. The large intestine is about 1.5 meters long. There are four regions within the large intestine:

➤ The **cecum** is a small area where the large intestine connects with the small intestine on the right side of the body. There is an outgrowth of this area that constitutes the appendix. The appendix is a vestigial structure thought to play a noncrucial role in the lymphatic system.
➤ The **colon** constitutes the majority of the large intestine. The primary role of the colon is water absorption in order to solidify the feces. Vitamin absorption can also occur in the colon.
➤ The **rectum** is the ultimate destination for feces in the large intestine. Stretching of this area stimulates nerves and initiates the defecation reflex.
➤ The **anal canal** receives the contents of the rectum for elimination. There are two sphincters regulating exit from the anal canal. The first internal sphincter operates involuntarily, and the second external sphincter is under voluntary control.

THE URINARY SYSTEM

The urinary system consists of the kidneys, which produce urine, and supporting tubing to store and eliminate urine from the body. The kidneys are the main excretory organ of the body: however, the skin can also act as an excretory organ. In addition to producing urine as a means of eliminating nitrogenous cellular waste products, the urinary system also regulates blood pressure by means of blood volume, adjusts blood pH, and regulates the osmotic concentrations of the blood.

The two kidneys of the urinary system filter blood to produce urine. The urine then moves toward the bladder via two ureters, tubes that connect each kidney to the bladder. Once urine moves to the bladder, it will be stored. Eventually, urine will leave the body through the urethra. The anatomy of the urethra is different in males and females. In males, the urethra is relatively long and must be shared with the reproductive system

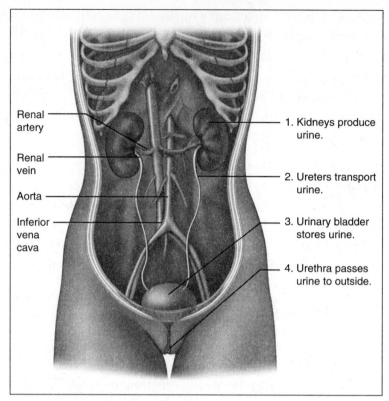

Renal
artery

Renal
vein

Aorta

Inferior
vena
cava

1. Kidneys produce
urine.

2. Ureters transport
urine.

3. Urinary bladder
stores urine.

4. Urethra passes
urine to outside.

FIGURE 6.15 The urinary system.

so that sperm can move through it when appropriate. In females, the urethra is shorter, and it is only used for urine passage. The structures of the urinary system can be seen in Figure 6.15.

Since the kidneys are the workhorse of the urinary system, their structure and function need to be examined in more detail. The kidneys are located above the waist and between the peritoneum (the membrane that lines the abdominal cavity) and the posterior wall of the abdomen. Their exact location can be described as being retroperitoneal because they are found posterior to the peritoneum. The kidneys are secured by several layers of connective tissue including a layer of fat, and each kidney has an adrenal gland that is located on top of it.

The outer region of the kidney is the renal cortex, the middle portion is the renal medulla, and the inner portion is the renal pelvis. The kidneys are responsible for filtering blood, so they have an excellent blood supply. The renal arteries are branches off the aorta and carry blood into the kidneys, while the renal veins carry blood away from the kidneys toward the inferior vena cava. The indentation where the ureter, renal artery, and renal vein attach to each kidney is the renal hilus.

Within the renal medulla of each kidney, there are triangular chunks of tissue called renal pyramids. Within these renal pyramids and extending into the renal cortex are about one million nephrons per kidney. The nephrons, shown in Figure 6.16, are microscopic tubules that actually produce urine. In reality a nephron is twisted along itself,

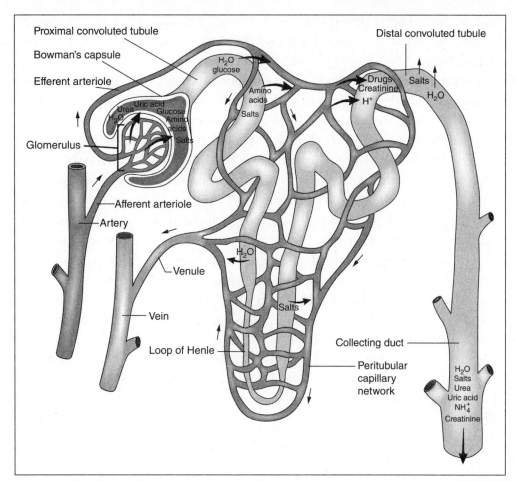

FIGURE 6.16 The structure of the nephron.

but for ease of viewing the nephron drawing presented here has been untwisted. Each nephron is surrounded by a network of capillaries. Any items leaving the nephron will be picked up by the capillaries and returned to the bloodstream. The important parts of the nephron are:

➤ The **renal corpuscle** has two parts. The first is the glomerulus, which is a network of capillaries. The glomerulus is surrounded by the Bowman's capsule. There is no direct connection between the glomerulus and the Bowman's capsule, but instead there is a space between the two. Afferent arterioles carry blood into the glomerulus, where blood pressure pushes certain components of the blood into the Bowman's capsule. Efferent arterioles carry blood out of the glomerulus. Only components of the blood that are small (plasma components such as water, ions, small nutrients, nitrogenous wastes, gases, and others) should enter the Bowman's capsule; blood cells and plasma proteins should not. The materials that enter the Bowman's capsule are referred to as filtrate and have approximately the same osmotic concentration as the plasma. A large percentage (approximately 99 percent) of filtrate that enters the nephron should be reabsorbed back into the bloodstream. Any components remaining in the nephron once filtration and reabsorption is complete will be lost as urine and will be much more concentrated than the plasma.

➤ The **proximal convoluted tubule** allows for the reabsorption of nutrients such as glucose and amino acids, water, salt, and ions. The majority of reabsorption occurs here.

➤ The **loop of Henle** also allows for reabsorption, primarily of salt (NaCl) and water by osmosis. A fairly complex countercurrent multiplier system is in effect in the loop of Henle. This area is a loop with a descending side and an ascending side located in close proximity to each other. Each limb of the loop has a different osmotic concentration. As salt is actively pumped out of the ascending limb, it creates a high osmotic pressure that draws water out of the descending limb via osmosis. Fresh filtrate then enters the loop of Henle, pushing the existing filtrate from the descending limb into the ascending limb. The process of pumping salt out of the ascending limb and the osmotic movement of water out of the descending limb is repeated several times.

➤ The **distal convoluted tubule** is where the fine tuning of filtrate concentration begins. Its activities are regulated by specific hormones described later in this section. The more water is reabsorbed in this section of the nephron, the more concentrated the urine, the lower the urine volume, and the higher the blood volume.

➤ The **collecting duct** can be shared by several nephrons. The remaining urine empties into the collecting duct, where it will move toward the renal pelvis and ultimately into the ureters to be carried to the bladder. Hormones can also be used in the collecting duct to allow for the reabsorption of more water, concentrating the urine even more.

Regulation of Blood Volume and Pressure

If antidiuretic hormone (ADH) is present, more water will be reabsorbed in the distal convoluted tubule and the collecting duct. This increases the concentration of urine and decreases urine volume. If aldosterone is present, more salt will be reabsorbed from the distal convoluted tubule and collecting ducts. Water will follow the movement of salt by osmosis. This results in an increased concentration of filtrate and a decrease in urine volume. Both ADH and aldosterone have the same effects on filtrate concentration. By increasing water reabsorption, blood volume is increased. The increase in blood volume is one way to increase blood pressure.

The secretion of ADH and aldosterone is regulated by renin produced by the kidneys. Renin secretion is triggered by low blood pressure in the afferent arterioles. Renin converts a protein made by the liver called angiotensin I into angiotensin II. Angiotensin II then triggers release of ADH by the posterior pituitary gland and aldosterone by the adrenal cortex.

One last hormone that alters nephron function is ANP (atrial natriuretic peptide), which is secreted by the heart. When the heart stretches due to elevated blood pressure, ANP is released. ANP decreases water and salt reabsorption by the nephrons. This results in less concentrated urine, a higher urine volume, and a lower blood volume. The reduced blood volume means a decrease in blood pressure.

As the kidneys filter blood, they also balance the pH of blood, which is one of their most important functions. Even a relatively minor change to blood pH can have drastic consequences, which is one of the reasons that kidney failure can be deadly. Luckily, dialysis methods are available to mimic normal kidney functions for patients whose kidneys do not work properly. Recall that carbon dioxide interacts with water to produce carbonic acid. Carbonic acid can then dissociate into hydrogen ions and bicarbonate ions, both of which influence pH. The pH of blood can be adjusted by changing the amount of bicarbonate ions reabsorbed and altering the amount of hydrogen ions retained in the nephron. When the blood pH drops and becomes acidic, more bicarbonate ions will return to circulation and hydrogen ions will be released in urine, which gives urine an acidic pH.

The substances remaining at the end of the distal convoluted tubule or collecting duct constitute urine. Urine will always contain water, ions (such as Ca^{2+}, Cl^-, Na^+, and K^+), and nitrogenous wastes. Depending on the diet and the functioning of other organs in the body, other components might be present in the urine. Because it was filtered directly from blood, the urine should be sterile. The presence of proteins, blood cells, or nutrients within the urine would be considered abnormal. The three primary nitrogenous wastes, all produced by cells, are as follows:

➤ **Urea:** As cells deaminate amino acids during protein metabolism, the resulting product is ammonia, which is highly toxic. The liver converts ammonia to a less toxic waste called urea. The kidneys concentrate urea and release it in the urine. Urea is the most abundant of nitrogenous waste products.

➤ **Uric acid:** During nucleic acid metabolism in the cell, uric acid is produced as the waste product.

➤ **Creatinine:** As muscle cells utilize creatine phosphate to produce ATP needed to fuel muscular contraction, creatinine is produced as a waste product.

In addition to their role in blood filtration and urine production, the kidneys have two additional jobs. First, the kidneys act to convert vitamin D from the diet into an active form that can be used by the cells. The kidneys are able to convert vitamin D to calcitriol, which helps the body absorb calcium and phosphorous. Second, the kidneys secrete the hormone erythropoietin (EPO), which is used to stimulate red blood cell production in the red bone marrow.

THE LYMPHATIC SYSTEM

The lymphatic system consists of a series of vessels running throughout the body, lymph, and lymphoid tissue, as seen in Figure 6.17. The system serves to return fluids that were unclaimed at the capillary beds to the circulatory system, picks up chylomicrons from the digestive tract and returns them to circulation, and fights infection via leukocytes. The vessels of the lymphatic system carry the fluid lymph, which has the same composition as plasma and interstitial fluid. Lymph moves through the vessels primarily due to the influence of muscular contractions that push it and valves that prevent its backflow.

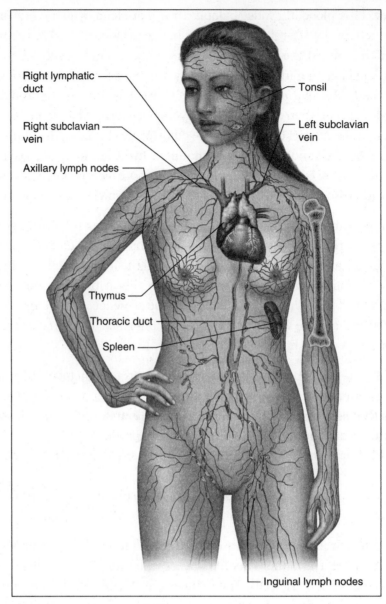

Right lymphatic duct

Tonsil

Right subclavian vein

Left subclavian vein

Axillary lymph nodes

Thymus

Thoracic duct

Spleen

Inguinal lymph nodes

FIGURE 6.17 The lymphatic system.

Lymph nodes are swellings along lymphatic vessels that contain macrophages for phagocytosis of pathogens and cancer cells, and lymphocytes for immune defenses. The lymph is filtered through the nodes before moving on in the system. Clusters of lymph nodes exist in the neck, under the arms, and in the groin. Swelling of the lymph nodes is a sign of infection. Tonsils resemble a lymph node in their ability to prevent infection by pathogenic organisms in the throat. Peyer's patches in the small intestine are clusters of lymphatic tissues that serve to prevent infectious organisms from crossing the intestinal wall into the abdomen. The thymus gland allows for the maturation of T cells, which are a form of lymphocyte needed for specific immune defenses. The spleen is located on the left side of the body and also acts as a blood filter. In addition, the spleen has an excellent blood supply and acts to destroy old red blood cells and platelets.

THE IMMUNE SYSTEM

The immune system exists anywhere white blood cells are found. This includes the blood, lymph, and tissues of the body. The job of the immune system is to differentiate "self" cells from "nonself" (foreign) cells and to eliminate both foreign cells and abnormal self cells. Immune defenses begin with nonspecific responses that try to prevent foreign cells from entering the body and attack them if they do enter, and later to move to specific responses if needed. A nonspecific immune defense always works the same way, no matter what the offending invader, while specific immune defenses are activated and tailor-made to a specific invader.

Nonspecific defenses come in several varieties:

➤ **Physical and chemical barricades** that prevent foreign cells from entering the body. The skin is an example of a barricade that generally prevents infection. Mucous membranes are another good barricade. Chemicals such as sweat, stomach acid, and lysozyme generally prevent infection.

➤ **Defensive leukocytes:** Neutrophils, monocytes, and macrophages (mature monocytes) are all capable of phagocytosis to destroy pathogens that may have entered the body. Eosinophils enzymatically destroy large pathogens such as parasitic worms that cannot be phagocytized. Finally, natural killer (NK) cells find self cells that seem to have odd membrane properties and destroy them. Cancerous cells are notorious for having altered cell membranes and are usually destroyed by NK cells.

➤ **Defensive proteins:** In the case of viral invaders, infected cells can secrete proteins called interferons. A virally infected cell releases these proteins as messengers to other cells that are yet to be infected. This limits the spread of the virus within the body by signaling uninfected cells to increase their defenses. Interferons are not specific to certain types of viruses—they work against all types of viruses. The complement system is a series of plasma proteins that are effective at killing bacteria by causing lysis of their cell membrane. The complement system also enhances phagocytosis within the area of invasion.

➤ **Inflammation:** When there is damage to tissues, the inflammatory response will initiate. It is characterized by redness and heat due to increased blood flow, swelling, and pain. Increased blood flow to the area is caused by the chemical histamine, which is secreted by basophils. This increased blood flow brings in other white blood cells, proteins, and other components needed to fight infection. Histamine makes capillaries more permeable than normal, which results in increased fluid in the area, causing swelling. This swelling can put pressure on pain receptors, creating the sensation of pain.

➤ **Fever:** When the body temperature is reset to a higher level by chemicals called pyrogens, fever is the result. Controlled fevers are beneficial, as they increase metabolism and stimulate other immune defenses. When fevers get too high, they are dangerous and can cause the denaturing of critical enzymes needed to sustain life.

When nonspecific defenses fail to control infection, specific defenses must be used. Since these are customized to the specific invader, they take at least a week to be created in order to respond strongly to a new antigen (a substance, including microbes, that elicits an immune response). There are two types of specific defenses, both of which use lymphocytes. Lymphocytes are derived from stem cells in the red bone marrow. B cells complete their maturation in the bone marrow, while T cells mature in the thymus gland. Both types of cells are designed to recognize foreign antigens and destroy invading microbes. Humoral immunity involves B cells, which ultimately secrete antibodies to destroy foreign antigens. Cellular (or cell-mediated) immunity involves the use of T cells to destroy infected or cancerous cells. A specific variety of T cell known as the helper T cell is the key coordinator of both humoral and cellular responses, which happen simultaneously.

Humoral immunity involves the production of specific antibody proteins from B cells that have been activated. Each B cell displays an antibody on its cell membrane, and each of the million or more B cells in the body has a different antibody on its membrane. The activation of a particular B cell by a specific antigen is based on shape recognition between the antibody on the B cell membrane and the antigen. The activation process is also dependent on chemicals from a helper T cell, which will be discussed in the next section. This activation causes proliferation of that B cell, which leads to a population of plasma cells (B cells that actively secrete antibodies) and memory B cells that produce the same type of antibody as the original cell from which they were derived. This is referred to as clonal selection; it is the key event of the primary immune response that leads to active immunity. It takes at least a week for this response to reach peak levels. Once antibodies are produced in large quantities by plasma cells, they circulate through blood, lymph, and tissues, where they seek out their antigen and bind to it, forming a complex. Once an antibody binds to an antigen, the complex will either be phagocytized or will agglutinate and later be removed by other phagocytic cells.

The primary immune response and active immunity can be achieved by natural exposure to an antigen or by vaccination. On secondary and subsequent exposures to the same antigen, the memory B cells that were created during the primary exposure can proliferate into plasma cells that produce antibodies, which provide a much faster response to the antigen. While antibodies do not circulate for long once an antigen has been destroyed, memory B cells can last for years if not for a lifetime.

Sometimes antibodies are passed from one person to another, which leads to passive immunity. This occurs during pregnancy, when maternal antibodies cross the placenta, and during breast-feeding. Breast milk contains antibodies that are transmitted to the newborn. Passive immunity can be induced by the injection of antibodies from one individual into another. Passive immunity is short-lived and declines within a few months.

Cellular immunity is based on the actions of T cells, which come in several varieties. T cells have a cell membrane receptor that, like antibodies on the surface of B cells, recognizes the shape of one particular antigen. However, T cells cannot be directly activated by contact with the antigen. The antigen must be presented to an activated cytotoxic T cell by a self cell that is infected or to a helper T cell by a macrophage, dendritic cell, or B cell that has engulfed the pathogen. The antigen presentation is done via cell-surface proteins known as the major histocompatibility complex (MHC). There are two different classes of MHC: Class I MHC molecules are found on the surface of all nucleated cells, while Class II MHC molecules are only found on professional antigen-presenting cells (macrophages, dendritic cells, and B cells). In the case of typical nucleated cells, when the cell becomes infected, the pathogen's proteins will be broken down into smaller pieces called antigen fragments. These pieces will be placed on the Class I MHC molecule and be presented to activated cytotoxic T cells. If an activated cytotoxic T cell with receptors for the presented antigen binds to the antigen that is being presented by the Class I MHC molecule, the cytotoxic T cell will release perforin molecules that will form pores on the infected cell's plasma membrane, as well as release granzymes, which will break down the infected cell's proteins. These actions will lead to the death of the infected cell, while the cytotoxic T cell will move on to attack other infected cells. It should be noted that proteins are regularly broken down by the cell and placed on Class I MHC molecules. However, these "self" proteins should not become bound to cytotoxic T cells since the T cells should not have receptors for these "self" proteins, as they are not foreign. Only when foreign peptide fragments are presented on the Class I MHC molecules should cytotoxic T cells bind to the cell.

Class II MHC molecules are only found on the professional antigen-presenting cells, which are macrophages, dendritic cells, and B cells. When these cells internalize a pathogen, they will present an antigen fragment on Class II MHC molecules that will bind to helper T cells that have receptors for the presented antigen. The cell presenting the antigen secretes the chemical interleukin-1 as it binds to the helper T cell. The helper T cell then secretes interleukin-2. This step is crucial for both humoral and cellular responses. The activation of the helper T cell and secretion of interleukin-2 allows for activation of B cells as well as the activation of cytotoxic T cells that can now bind to the antigen via Class I MHC. The cytotoxic T cell proliferates and produces effector cells by clonal selection that all have the ability to seek and destroy the foreign antigen. As with plasma cell activation, this primary response takes at least a week to occur. Memory T cells are also produced. Once the antigen has been completely destroyed, suppressor T cells are used to stop the response of cytotoxic T cells. Only memory T cells remain; they can be quickly activated to cytotoxic T cells on secondary and subsequent exposures to the same antigen.

THE FEMALE REPRODUCTIVE SYSTEM

The female and male reproductive systems have the common function of producing gametes for sexual reproduction. Egg cells in females and sperm cells in males are produced by the gonads. In addition, the female reproductive system has to be structured to accept sperm from the male system and to allow for embryonic and fetal development.

The female reproductive system is enclosed within the abdominal cavity and is open to the external environment. While having an opening to the outside environment is necessary for reproduction and childbirth, it presents some unique problems in terms of the ability of pathogens to enter the system.

The structures of the internal female reproductive system consist of the ovaries, where egg production occurs, as well as supporting structures, as seen in Figure 6.18. After an egg is released from an ovary, it is swept into the fallopian tube (oviduct) that is associated with that ovary. If sperm are present, they should meet with the egg in the fallopian tube, where fertilization will occur. The fallopian tubes merge into the uterus, which is composed of the muscular myometrium and the vascularized lining called the endometrium. If the egg has been fertilized, the embryo will implant into the endometrium, where development will continue. If fertilization has not occurred, the egg will be lost with the shedding of the endometrium, which occurs about every 28 days during menstruation. The vagina serves as an entry point for sperm to enter the system, an exit point for menstrual fluids, and the birth canal during childbirth. The pH of the vagina is acidic, which can discourage the growth of certain pathogens. The cervix regulates the opening of the uterus into the vagina and is normally very narrow.

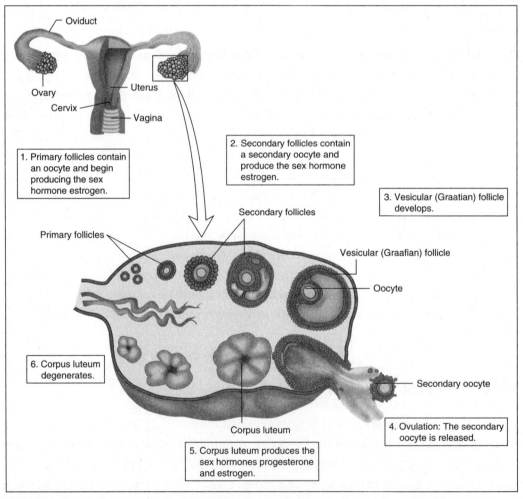

FIGURE 6.18 The female reproductive system.

The female reproductive cycle lasts about 28 days on average. There are characteristic changes within the uterus that occur during this time. These changes are referred to as the menstrual (or uterine) cycle, which goes through three phases as follows:

➤ **Menses:** During the first five or so days of the cycle, the existing endometrium is lost via menstrual fluid as arteries serving the endometrium constrict; this causes tissue death as the cells are cut off from oxygen and nutrients.

➤ The **proliferative phase:** During the second week of the cycle, the primary event in the uterus is the proliferation of cells to replace the endometrium that was lost during menstruation.

➤ The **secretory phase:** During the last two weeks of the cycle, hormones are secreted to prepare the endometrium for implantation, if an embryo is present. As the twenty-eighth day of the cycle approaches, the endometrium deteriorates and menses will soon begin as the cycle restarts.

Eggs are produced through the ovarian cycle (also seen in Figure 6.19), whose timing must be carefully choreographed to the menstrual cycle. The ovarian cycle also lasts 28 days and consists of the following phases:

➤ The **preovulatory phase:** This phase consists of the events prior to ovulation and lasts from days 1 to 13 of the cycle. This timing corresponds to menses and the proliferative phase of the menstrual cycle.

➤ **Ovulation:** The rupture of a follicle in the ovary and subsequent release of an egg to a fallopian tube constitutes ovulation. It occurs on day 14 of the cycle.

➤ The **postovulatory phase:** During this phase, the egg is released and may be fertilized. This phase lasts from days 15 to 28 and corresponds with the secretory phase of the menstrual cycle. Should fertilization occur, the embryo would implant into the endometrium during this phase. If fertilization has not occurred, the menstrual cycle restarts, causing the egg to be lost.

The events that lead to the ovulation of an egg are termed oogenesis and are regulated through the ovarian cycle. Within the ovaries of a female, the process of meiosis begins before her birth. This process results in the creation of primary follicles within the ovaries. A follicle consists of a potential egg cell (oocyte) surrounded by a shell of follicular cells to support the egg. The number of primary follicles is set at birth and is usually around 700,000. As the female is born and ages, many of these follicles will die. By the time a female reaches puberty at age 12 to 14, as few as 200,000 follicles remain. While the number has been drastically reduced and will continue to decline with age, there are still more than enough follicles to support the reproductive needs of a female, since only one egg will be released every 28 days. At birth, the oocytes are arrested in prophase I of meiosis, but will resume meiosis if they mature and will arrest again in metaphase II of meiosis; an oocyte will only complete meiosis if fertilization occurs. The ability to perform the ovarian cycle will end at menopause, when the ovaries are no longer sensitive to follicle-stimulating hormone (FSH) and luteinizing hormone (LH). The levels of estrogen and progesterone in the body then decrease and the ovaries atrophy.

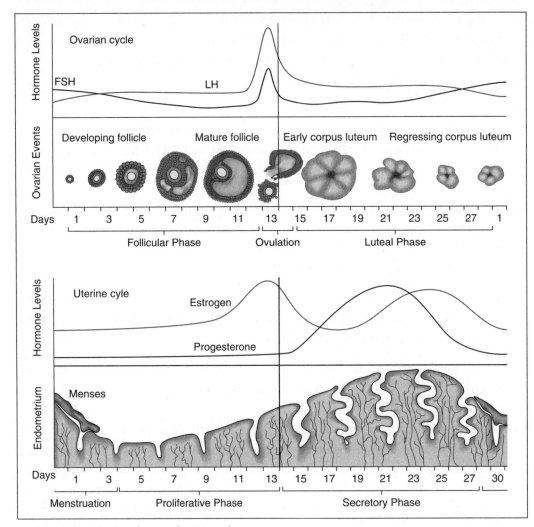

FIGURE 6.19 The female reproductive cycle.

During the preovulatory phase, a few primary follicles will resume meiosis and begin growing as primary oocytes. Starting at day 1 of the cycle, the anterior pituitary secretes FSH and LH. The hypothalamus produces gonadotropin releasing hormone (GnRH), which stimulates the release of FSH and LH. FSH causes the growth of several follicles that begin to produce estrogen. The more the follicles grow, the more estrogen is produced. Although several follicles begin to grow each month, typically only one will mature and be released. Estrogen is at its highest level during the second week of the cycle, which corresponds to the rebuilding of the endometrium after menstruation.

During the second week of the cycle, estrogen from the growing follicle continues to rise, stimulating the hypothalamus to release more GnRH. This leads to an increase in FSH and LH levels, thereby leading to a massive surge in LH. This surge causes the oocyte to complete meiosis I and arrest at metaphase of meiosis II, forming a secondary oocyte. It also causes the rupture of the follicle within the ovary. This is ovulation; it happens on day 14 of the cycle. The oocyte is released into the fallopian tubes, and the remnants of the follicle remain in the ovary. If the oocyte is fertilized, meiosis II will complete, resulting in a mature egg (ovum). Only one mature egg is needed during ovulation, so the remaining three cells produced during meiosis are termed polar bodies. They are much smaller than the egg and will be degraded. If more than one egg is released on a given cycle, the potential exists for multiple fertilizations and multiple embryos, which results in fraternal twins or triplets.

The remains of the follicle in the ovary become the corpus luteum, which will secrete estrogen and progesterone under the stimulation of LH. However, the estrogen and progesterone combination will inhibit the hypothalamus and anterior pituitary and suppress FSH and LH production so that no more eggs are released during this cycle. These hormones also keep the endometrium prepared to receive an embryo during the secretory phase (third and fourth weeks) of the menstrual cycle.

At the end of the fourth week of the cycle, if an embryo has not implanted into the endometrium, the cycle needs to restart. At this point, the corpus luteum degrades. Without the corpus luteum, the levels of estrogen and progesterone decline. The lack of these hormones, particularly progesterone, is the cause of menstruation, which can only occur when these levels are low. Further, the lack of estrogen and progesterone allows the pituitary gland to begin secreting FSH and LH again to begin the process of a new cycle.

Because estrogen and progesterone have the ability to suppress the actions of FSH and LH, they are the hormones of choice for use in birth control methods such as pills, patches, injections, rings, or implants. Synthetic estrogen and/or synthetic progesterone can be used to manipulate the ovaries into not ovulating, since FSH and LH are suppressed.

THE MALE REPRODUCTIVE SYSTEM

In contrast to the female system, the male reproductive system is not housed completely within the abdominal cavity. It is a closed system, as seen in Figure 6.20. The male gonads or testes produce sperm. The remaining reproductive structures serve as a means to transport sperm out of the body and into the female system.

Sperm begin their development in the seminiferous tubules of the testes, where they are nourished by Sertoli cells. The testes are housed in the scrotum outside of the abdominal cavity, where the temperature is a few degrees cooler than body temperature. Oddly enough, sperm require a temperature cooler than normal body temperature to survive their development. As sperm develop in the testes, they move into the epididymis associated with each testis, which is also located in the scrotum. Once in the epididymis, the sperm acquire motility and are stored.

When ejaculation occurs, the sperm must be moved toward the male urethra. The sperm enter the vas deferens, which are tubes that move up into the abdominal cavity.

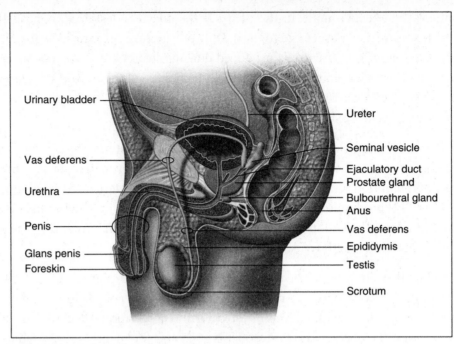

FIGURE 6.20 The male reproductive system.

From there, the two vas deferens merge into the ejaculatory duct and into the urethra. Recall that the urethra is also used for urine passage. When sperm are moving through, the urethra is unavailable to the bladder. Once the sperm are in the urethra, three types of glands add their secretions to the sperm as they pass by. This creates semen, which is a mixture of sperm and secretions. The urethra progresses through the length of the penis where it can be introduced into the female vagina.

The associated glands of the male reproductive system that provide secretions to semen are as follows:

➤ The **seminal vesicles** provide a fluid rich in nutrients to serve as an energy source for the sperm.
➤ The **prostate gland** wraps around the urethra and deposits a secretion that is alkaline, to balance the acidic environment of the vagina.
➤ The **bulbourethral glands** secrete a fluid prior to ejaculation that may serve to lubricate the urethra for sperm passage.

The process of spermatogenesis produces sperm through meiosis. Unlike meiosis in females, which produces one egg and three polar bodies, meiosis in men results in the production of four sperm cells. While women only need to release one egg per reproductive cycle, men need millions of sperm per fertilization attempt. While the one egg produced in oogenesis is quite large, the sperm produced in spermatogenesis are quite small. This is because the egg cell must contain additional components needed to support embryonic development.

Spermatogenesis requires the hormonal influence of testosterone and begins at puberty. Testosterone is secreted during embryonic development to cause the development of male reproductive structures, but testosterone development is then halted until puberty. Diploid cells in the testes called spermatogonia differentiate into primary spermatocytes, which undergo meiosis I, producing two haploid secondary spermatocytes. The secondary spermatocytes undergo meiosis II to produce four mature sperm (spermatozoa). The spermatozoa then move to the epididymis to mature. The process takes between two and three months to complete.

Mature sperm contain an acrosome that contains digestive enzymes used to penetrate the egg, a head that contains the nucleus the sperm will contribute to the egg, and the tail (a flagellum) that is propelled by ATP produced by large numbers of mitochondria.

Some of the same hormones that are used in the female reproductive system are also used to regulate spermatogenesis. GnRH from the hypothalamus allows for the secretion of LH from the anterior pituitary. LH causes the production of testosterone by cells in the testes. The secretion of GnRH from the hypothalamus also results in the release of FSH from the anterior pituitary. While testosterone is needed to stimulate spermatogenesis, FSH is also needed to make the potential sperm cells sensitive to testosterone. The levels of testosterone regulate sperm production in a manner that resembles a thermostat.

THE INTEGUMENTARY SYSTEM

The major functions of the skin are to make our brain aware of our surroundings and to protect the inner body parts. One way in which skin can communicate with the brain is by transmitting information regarding the temperature of the surroundings. The brain can then tell the sweat glands to produce sweat in an effort to cool the body, helping to maintain homeostasis via thermoregulation. The nerves in the skin will also communicate with the brain to move the muscles away from harm by signaling pain via nerves. In addition to this there is also the sense of touch, which can signal a range of emotions or reactions between two organisms.

The skin also acts as a first line of defense against pathogens. When the skin is intact, pathogens have almost no chance of entering the body. However, if the skin is compromised by a cut or open wound, the body is susceptible to infection. Keep in mind that even when this layer of defense has been compromised, there are still two more levels of defense to fight infections. (The body can fight the infection or memorize the infectious material for a quicker response the next time it is encountered.)

The two major parts of the skin are the dermis and the epidermis (*epi* meaning "over"). The uppermost layer of the epidermis is made up of dead cells that are routinely lost and replaced. Underneath the several layers of the epidermis are the following components of the dermis:

➤ **Arteries and veins** for blood circulation.
➤ **Nerves** to transmit signals to the brain regarding environmental conditions.

➤ **Sweat (sudoriferous) glands** to produce sweat and regulate body temperature.
➤ **Hair roots and follicles** for producing hair.
➤ **Oil (sebaceous) glands** for releasing sebum to lubricate the hair and skin.

While we have studied much detail, keep in mind that all of the body's systems are interdependent and rely upon one another for proper functioning, health, and—most of all—maintaining homeostasis.

CHAPTER 7

Developmental Biology

Read This Chapter to Learn About

➤ Fertilization

➤ Embryonic Development

➤ Fetal Development and Birth

FERTILIZATION

As the haploid nucleus of a sperm cell is contributed to an egg cell (also containing a haploid nucleus) during fertilization, the resulting cell is termed a zygote. The zygote begins cell division by mitosis, which produces a ball of identical cells—the embryo. In humans, the first eight weeks of development constitute embryonic development, and all development after eight weeks constitutes fetal development. The human gestation period is 266 days. These nine months are divided into trimesters. Embryonic development is complete within the first trimester.

Sperm have the ability to survive about 48 hours in the female system, while an egg cell only survives about 24 hours. Sperm deposited prior to or right after ovulation are capable of fertilizing the egg, which should happen in the upper third of the fallopian tube. While 200 to 500 million sperm are typically released during ejaculation, only about 200 will make it to the egg cell. Secretions from the female system will change the membrane composition of the sperm near its acrosome. In this way, when the sperm bumps into the egg, the contents of its acrosome will be released due to membrane instability. This will allow the sperm to penetrate the corona radiata (outer layer) of the egg. Next the sperm must pass through the next layer of the egg, the zona pellucida. The first sperm to pass through the zona pellucida will pass its nucleus into the egg. This will cause a depolarization in the membrane of the egg that will make it impenetrable to fertilization by other sperm. The nuclei of the egg and sperm fuse, creating the zygote.

EMBRYONIC DEVELOPMENT

About one day after fertilization, the zygote performs its first mitotic division, becoming an embryo. This initiates cleavage, which is the rapid cell division characteristic of early embryonic development. Within about four days, the embryo reaches the morula stage, in which it consists of a ball of cells. During early cleavage, the embryo may split into two, which results in identical twins. By about six days, the center of the embryo hollows out and becomes filled with fluid. The embryo is now termed a blastula or blastocyst. The outer cells of the blastocyst are the trophoblast, which will aid in implantation and the development of extraembryonic membranes and the placenta. The inner cell mass is the source of embryonic stem cells, which have the ability to differentiate into any cell type. Implantation of the embryo begins about one week after fertilization and completes by the second week. The events of early embryonic development can be seen in Figure 7.1. The blastocyst produces a critical hormone that is important in the maintenance of pregnancy. Human chorionic gonadotropin (HCG) is the signal to the corpus luteum not to degrade. Normally, the degradation of the corpus luteum would cause a decline of estrogen and progesterone and would trigger menstruation. At this point in development, menstruation would mean a loss of the embryo, resulting in a spontaneous abortion. HCG ensures that the corpus luteum will continue to secrete estrogen and progesterone so that menstruation is delayed.

The next event of embryonic development is the gastrula stage. During gastrulation, three primary germ layers are formed as the cells in the embryo shift into layers. Once a

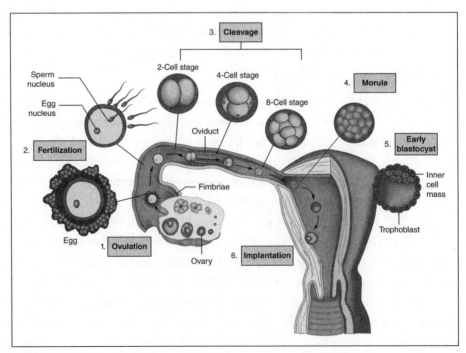

FIGURE 7.1 Early embryonic development.

cell enters a germ layer, its ability to differentiate into specific cell types is limited. The three germ layers and the fates of cells in these layers are as follows:

➤ **Ectoderm:** cells in this layer will express the genes needed to become skin cells and cells of the nervous system.
➤ **Mesoderm:** cells in this layer will express the genes needed to become muscles, bones, and most internal organs.
➤ **Endoderm:** cells in this layer will express the genes needed to become the lining of internal body cavities as well as the linings of the respiratory, digestive, urinary, and reproductive tracts.

Once the germ layers are complete, neuralization begins the development of the nervous system. Mesoderm cells form the notochord. Ectoderm above the notochord starts to thicken and folds inward, forming neural folds that continue to deepen and fuse to produce a neural tube that will eventually develop into the central nervous system. At this point, a head and tail region have been established in the embryo.

As differentiation continues, certain cells can influence the gene expression of other cells in the process of induction via chemical messengers. Communication between cells is also used to establish positional information in the embryo, which is critical to the formation of internal organs as well as the limbs. Homeobox genes produce proteins that are essential for guiding the development of the shape of the embryo. The proteins produced by the homeoboxes are transcription factors that serve to turn on specific genes within cells at specific times.

Induction helps ensure that the right structures occur in the right places. An additional process that is necessary during embryonic development is apoptosis of certain cells. While it seems odd to talk about cell death during development, it is necessary. For example, the separation of fingers and toes is the result of apoptosis of the cells that at one time joined the structures.

The remainder of embryonic development deals with organogenesis and refining the shape of the embryo. Organ systems are developed on an as-needed basis with the most critical organs being produced first. By the fourth week, the heart is working and limbs are established. By the end of embryonic development (the eighth week), all major organs are established and most are functioning.

While the embryo is in the process of implanting into the endometrium, four membranes will be formed outside of the embryo:

➤ The **amnion** surrounds the embryo in a fluid-filled sac that serves a protective function and provides cushioning for the embryo and fetus.
➤ The **allantois** is a membrane that will ultimately form the umbilical cord, which is the connection between the embryo and the placenta (the organ that will deliver nutrients and oxygen and remove carbon dioxide and wastes).
➤ The **yolk sac** is where the first blood cells develop. In other species, it serves as a source of nutrients.
➤ The **chorion** will eventually become the embryo's side of the placenta.

The placenta develops from the chorion and grows in size during development. It provides nutrients and oxygen to the embryo and removes wastes. Recall that fetal hemoglobin has a greater affinity for oxygen than adult hemoglobin. The placenta produces HCG, estrogen, and progesterone to maintain the pregnancy. It also produces the hormone relaxin to release the ligaments that attach the mother's pubic bones to provide more space in the birth canal. It takes about three months for the placenta to develop fully.

FETAL DEVELOPMENT AND BIRTH

Fetal development is primarily a refinement of the organ systems that are already established during embryonic development. The fetus enlarges and the organ systems are refined so that they are all functioning or capable of functioning at the end of gestation.

Labor is triggered by the hormone oxytocin, which is produced by the posterior pituitary gland. Oxytocin causes contractions of the uterus that intensify with time. Initially, the cervix must dilate, which can take hours. The amnion usually ruptures during the dilation stage. Once the cervix is dilated, contractions continue, leading to expulsion of the baby. After the baby is delivered, the umbilical cord is clamped and cut, which severs the connection to the placenta. Finally, the placenta is delivered at the end of labor.

CHAPTER 8

Genetics

Read This Chapter to Learn About

➤ DNA

➤ Protein Synthesis

➤ The Genetic Code

➤ Regulation of Gene Expression

➤ Mendelian Genetics

DNA

Deoxyribonucleic acid (DNA) is the genetic material of the cell. The information encoded in DNA ultimately directs the synthesis of particular proteins within cells. These proteins determine all of our biological characteristics. When a cell divides, DNA will self-replicate to ensure that progeny cells receive the same DNA instructions as the parent cell.

DNA Structure

DNA is a nucleic acid polymer consisting of nucleotide monomers. A nucleotide is a hybrid molecule consisting of deoxyribose (a sugar), a phosphate group (PO_4), and a nitrogenous base. There are four nitrogenous bases used to make nucleotides: adenine (A), thymine (T), cytosine (C), and guanine (G). Each nucleotide differs only by the nitrogenous base used, so there are four possible nucleotides used in DNA. The nitrogenous base of each nucleotide can be classified as a purine or pyrimidine based on the chemical structure. A purine is a double-ringed structure, while pyrimidines are single-ring structures. The nitrogenous bases A and G are purines, while C and T are pyrimidines.

James Watson and Francis Crick, with the help of Rosalind Franklin, proposed their famous model for DNA structure in 1953. By using information from other studies, they knew that DNA existed in a double-stranded conformation and that the amount of A and T in a DNA molecule was always the same, as was the amount of C and G. Using this information, they developed the model of DNA structure seen in Figure 8.1. A single strand of DNA has a sugar-phosphate backbone. Two strands of DNA are hydrogen-bonded together via their nitrogenous bases. The idea of complementary base pairing is essential to this model. This means that a purine must pair with a pyrimidine. An A on one strand of DNA will always bond to a T on another strand of DNA, using two hydrogen bonds. A C on one strand will always bond to a G on another strand, using three hydrogen bonds. This base pairing holds together the two strands of DNA, which then twist around themselves to take on the double helix conformation. Each strand of DNA has a specific polarity or direction in which it runs. This polarity is referred to as 5' and 3', referring to particular carbon atoms in the ribose molecule. The complementary strand of DNA always runs antiparallel, in the opposite direction of the original strand. So if one DNA strand runs 5' to 3', the other strand of the double helix runs 3' to 5'.

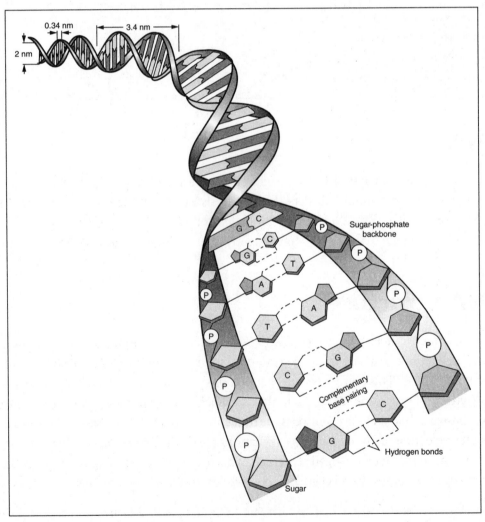

FIGURE 8.1 DNA double helix.

Chromosome Structure

In eukaryotic cells, DNA is organized in linear chromosomes. Humans have 23 pairs or a total of 46 chromosomes per somatic (nonreproductive) cell. A single chromosome consists of one DNA double helix wrapped around specialized histone proteins that form chromatin. Each of these chromosomes consists of an enormous amount of DNA, all of which must fit into the nucleus of the cell. Organizing the DNA around histones and other specialized proteins helps compact the DNA. During cell division, the chromatin coils even more to form a compact chromosome. When chromosomes replicate in preparation for cell division, the new copies stay attached to the original copies at a location called the centromere.

DNA Replication

During normal cell division, it is essential for all components of the cell, including the chromosomes, to replicate so that each progeny cell receives a copy of the chromosomes from the parent cell. The process of replicating DNA must happen accurately to ensure that no changes to the DNA are passed on to the progeny cells.

The process of DNA replication is termed semiconservative replication. One double helix will need to be replicated so that two double helices result—one for each progeny cell. Because the DNA double helix has two strands, each strand can serve as a template to produce a new strand. The process of semiconservative replication has three basic steps. First, the original DNA double helix must unwind. This process is achieved using the enzyme helicase. Next, the hydrogen bonds that hold the nitrogenous bases together must be broken. This "unzips" the double helix in a localized area of the chromosome called the origin of replication. Finally, each template strand will be used to produce a complementary strand of DNA using the normal rules of complementary base pairing. DNA polymerase binds to the DNA template and chemically reads the nucleotide sequence while assembling the complementary nucleotides to produce the new strand. The synthesis of DNA occurs in both directions, moving outward from the origin of replication in replication forks.

As DNA is synthesized during replication, the DNA polymerase reads the template DNA strand from the 3' to 5' direction, which means that the new DNA being synthesized will run in the 5' to 3' direction. Since one DNA template runs in the 3' to 5' direction, DNA polymerase will be able to read it and produce a continuous complementary strand called the leading strand. However, the other DNA template runs in the 5' to 3' direction, so the complementary strand (the lagging strand) will be synthesized in a discontinuous manner since the replication fork is moving against the direction of DNA synthesis. In order to synthesize the discontinuous strand of DNA, a primer (a short sequence of nucleotides) must bind to the DNA; DNA polymerase will begin to synthesize the new DNA strand until it runs into the next primer. This results in small pieces of DNA termed Okazaki fragments that must eventually be linked together. The primers will eventually be degraded and the Okazaki fragments will be linked using the enzyme DNA ligase.

DNA Repair

During the process of DNA replication, it is possible for DNA polymerase to make mistakes by adding a nucleotide that is not complementary to the DNA template or by adding or deleting nucleotides on the new DNA strand. Luckily, DNA polymerase has a proofreading ability that usually detects these errors and repairs them. However, if these errors are not corrected, there will be a permanent change to the DNA. This change is termed a mutation. In some cases, the mutation that cannot be successfully repaired will trigger the process of cellular suicide (apoptosis) to destroy the damaged cell. When this mechanism does not initiate, the mutation remains and can be passed on to progeny cells.

PROTEIN SYNTHESIS

A gene is a segment of DNA located on a chromosome that has information to encode for a single protein. Proteins are made in the cytoplasm of the cell with assistance from ribosomes. The DNA and genes of a cell are located in the nucleus. Unfortunately, the DNA cannot leave the nucleus, nor can the ribosomes enter the nucleus. To get around this problem, the DNA message in the nucleus is converted to an intermediate ribonucleic acid (RNA) message that can travel to the cytoplasm and be read by the ribosomes to produce a protein. Protein synthesis is a two-step process: the conversion of DNA to RNA is transcription, and the conversion of RNA to a protein is translation. The central dogma of molecular biology describes the flow of genetic information in the cell:

$$DNA \rightarrow RNA \rightarrow protein$$

RNA is another form of nucleic acid and is a critical player in the process of protein synthesis. RNA molecules are another form of nucleic acid; they are very similar to DNA, with the few exceptions seen in Table 8.1. Within the cell, there are three types of RNA: ribosomal RNA (rRNA), transfer RNA (tRNA), and messenger RNA (mRNA). Each type has a specific role in the process of protein synthesis. The functions of each type of RNA can be seen in Table 8.2.

Table 8.1 Differences Between DNA and RNA		
	DNA	**RNA**
Number of strands	2, double helix	Single
Sugar used in the nucleotide	Deoxyribose	Ribose
Nitrogenous bases used	Adenine, thymine, guanine, cytosine	Adenine, uracil, guanine, cytosine

Table 8.2 Types of RNA	
Type of RNA	**Function**
Ribosomal: rRNA	rRNA is made in the nucleolus of the nucleus. It is a structural component of ribosomes.
Transfer: tRNA	tRNA is located in the cytoplasm of the cells. It is used to shuttle amino acids to the ribosome during the process of translation.
Messenger: mRNA	mRNA is copied from DNA in the nucleus and serves as the messenger molecule to carry the DNA message to the ribosomes in the cytoplasm.

The first step of protein synthesis is to produce mRNA from the DNA. The process of transcription initially resembles the process of semiconservative DNA replication. At the point where transcription is to begin, the DNA double helix must unwind. In this local area, the hydrogen bonds holding together the base pairs must break. Since only one strand of mRNA needs to be produced, only one strand of the DNA will serve as a template. The enzyme RNA polymerase will recognize sequences of DNA called promoters and bind to them. The RNA polymerase will chemically read the sequence of DNA and assemble the complementary RNA nucleotides in the 5' to 3' direction. The rules of complementary base pairing during transcription are similar to those of DNA replication, with one major change: RNA uses the base uracil (U) instead of thymine (T). If the DNA molecule contains the base A, then the complementary RNA molecule will contain the base U, while C and G will pair. RNA polymerase will continue to synthesize the complementary RNA strand until it reaches a termination sequence on the DNA. At this point, the RNA molecule will be released and the DNA double helix will re-form. The process of transcription can be seen in Figure 8.2.

Once RNA has been produced from the DNA template, it must be modified before it can be translated into a protein. First, a 5' cap will be added to the 5' end of the RNA. This cap is a chemically modified nucleotide that will help regulate translation. Next, a poly-A tail will be added to the 3' end of the RNA. This tail consists of many A nucleotides placed on the end of the RNA. The purpose of the tail is to prevent degradation of the RNA molecule. While some of the chromosomal DNA has information that is needed to code for proteins, the majority of the DNA does not. The coding DNA molecules are termed exons, and the noncoding DNA molecules are termed introns or "junk DNA." Unfortunately, the introns are located within the exons, disrupting their sequence.

During transcription, the RNA that is copied from the DNA contains the sequences of both the introns and the exons. Prior to translation, the introns must be removed, and the exons must be spliced together to form functional mRNA. Several unique RNAs can be produced by splicing the same exons in different sequences. This RNA splicing occurs in the nucleus. Once the splicing is complete, the mRNA molecule moves through the nuclear pores to the cytoplasm, where translation will occur.

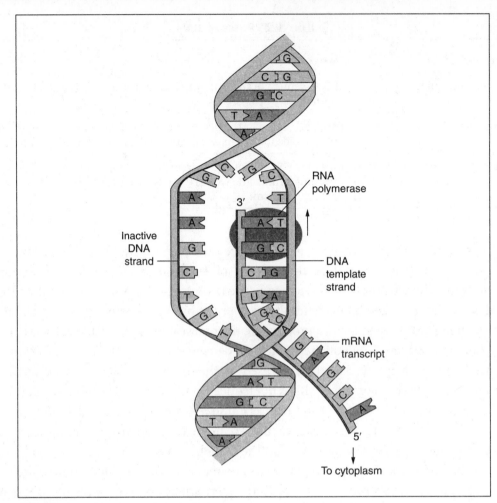

FIGURE 8.2 The process of transcription.

THE GENETIC CODE

Now that the mRNA has been produced, it must be translated into a protein. The mRNA will be read as codons, 3 nucleotides at a time. Each codon has the information to specify for one amino acid. Mathematically, there are 4 nucleotides in the mRNA, and if every combination of 3 letters is used, there will be 64 possible codons, all of which are listed in the genetic code seen in Figure 8.3. Since there are only 20 amino acids used to make proteins, there is an overlap or redundancy in the code in that more than one codon can code for the same amino acid.

Knowing the sequence of codons on the mRNA makes it possible to use the genetic code to decipher the sequence of amino acids that will be used to build the protein in translation. Any change to the DNA, which in turn changes the mRNA codons, can potentially change the order of amino acids and thus the shape and function of the intended protein.

The process of translation occurs in the cytoplasm. The codons on the mRNA will be read, and the appropriate amino acids needed to produce the protein will be assembled. This process will require assistance from various enzymes, ribosomes, and tRNA.

		U	C	A	G	
	U	UUU } Phe UUC } UUA } Leu UUG }	UCU } UCC } Ser UCA } UCG }	UAU } Tyr UAC } UAA Stop UAG Stop	UGU } Cys UGC } UGA Stop UGG Try	U C A G
	C	CUU } CUC } Leu CUA } CUG }	CCU } CCC } Pro CCA } CCG }	CAU } His CAC } CAA } Gln CAG }	CGU } CGC } Arg CGA } CGG }	U C A G
	A	AUU } Ile AUC } AUA } AUG Met or start	ACU } ACC } Thr ACA } ACG }	AAU } Asn AAC } AAA } Lys AAG }	AGU } Ser AGC } AGA } Arg AGG }	U C A G
	G	GUU } GUC } Val GUA } GUG }	GCU } GCC } Ala GCA } GCG }	GAU } Asp GAC } GAA } Glu GAG }	GGU } GGC } Gly GGA } GGG }	U C A G

Second letter (columns), First letter (rows left), Third letter (right)

FIGURE 8.3 The code for amino acids.

Eukaryotic ribosomes are composed of two subunits, one large and one small, of rRNA and various proteins. Once the ribosome assembles on the mRNA, there will be two RNA binding sites inside the ribosome: the peptidyl (P) site and the aminoacyl (A) site.

The purpose of the tRNA molecules is to shuttle the appropriate amino acids to the ribosomes, as dictated by the codons on the mRNA. The tRNA itself is a piece of RNA folded into a specific configuration. On one end, the tRNA contains an anticodon. This sequence is complementary to the codon on the mRNA. On the other end of the tRNA, a specific amino acid will be attached.

Translation occurs as a three-step process. First, the ribosome must assemble on the mRNA. Next, the amino acids dictated by the codons must be brought to the ribosome and bonded together. Finally, the resulting protein must be released from the ribosome. The entire process of translation can be seen in Figure 8.4.

The process of translation begins when the ribosome assembles on the mRNA. The location for ribosomal assembly is signaled by the start codon (AUG) found on the mRNA. The small ribosomal subunit then binds to the mRNA. The first tRNA will enter the P site of the ribosome. This tRNA must have the appropriate anticodon (UAC) to hydrogen bond with the start codon (AUG). As seen in the genetic code, the amino acid specified by the start codon is methionine. Thus the first amino acid of every protein will be methionine. Now, the large subunit of the ribosome can assemble on the mRNA.

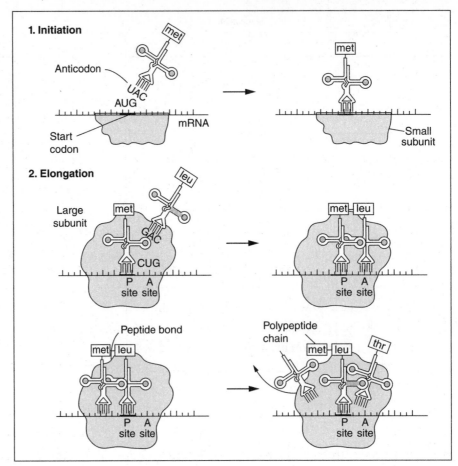

FIGURE 8.4 Translation.

At this point, the P site of the ribosome is occupied but the A site is not. A tRNA bearing the appropriate anticodon to bind with the next codon of the mRNA will enter the ribosome and hydrogen bond to the codon. A key enzyme, peptidyl transferase, will be used at this point to form a peptide bond between the two amino acids in the P and A sites. The two amino acids will now be attached to the tRNA in the A site. The tRNA in the P site will break off (leaving behind its amino acid) and leave the ribosome. The ribosome will now move over one codon to the right, putting the remaining tRNA in the P site and leaving an empty A site. This process—a new tRNA entering, a peptide bond forming between amino acids, the tRNA in the P site leaving, and the ribosome shifting over by one codon—will occur over and over again.

There are three mRNA codons (UAA, UAG, and UGA) that act as stop codons and do not code for amino acids. When one of these codons reaches the A site of the ribosome, no more tRNAs enter and the protein will be released from the ribosome. The ribosomal subunits will dissociate. This signals the end of translation. In some cases, it is necessary for the released protein to be modified before it can be functional. This often occurs in the endoplasmic reticulum or the Golgi complex.

Mutations

Mutations change the coding sequence of DNA from that which was originally intended. When the DNA changes, the mRNA codons change, and the amino acid sequence of the protein made may change. This may produce a protein that functions better than the one coded for by the original sequence of DNA (thus providing an advantage), one that functions equivalent to the intended protein, or, in the worst case, a protein that functions worse than the intended protein or does not function at all. Recall that mutations happen spontaneously and that the rate of mutation is increased by exposure to mutagens.

When a single nucleotide is swapped for another, this is termed a point (substitution) mutation. This will ultimately change a single codon on the mRNA. In some cases, this mutation will be silent; that is, if the codon is changed and still codes for the intended amino acids, there will be no detectable consequence. However, sometimes even a single point mutation can have major consequences. If the new codon codes for a different amino acid than what was intended (a missense mutation), the new protein may not function properly. This can lead to a genetic disease such as sickle-cell anemia. It is also possible for a change in a single nucleotide to produce a stop codon in a new location, causing a nonsense mutation. In this case, the protein produced would be too short and most likely nonfunctional.

A frameshift mutation is the result of the addition or deletion of nucleotides. Unlike the point mutation, in which the overall number of nucleotides does not change, adding or deleting changes the number of nucleotides. Since mRNA is read in codons, an addition or deletion will alter all of the codons from the point of the mutation onward. This disrupts the reading frame of the mRNA. Since many codons are changed, the frameshift mutation generally produces a damaged or nonfunctional protein.

REGULATION OF GENE EXPRESSION

Gene expression refers to the process that controls which genes are transcribed and translated. Each cell has many genes, and it is not necessary for every cell to express every gene it has. In order to be efficient, cells are selective about which genes they express, making only the proteins that are necessary at a given time.

Gene expression can be regulated on a permanent level due to a process called differentiation. Because nearly all of the cells within the body are specialized, it makes sense that these cells really only need to express the genes related to that cell's particular function. Even though all cells have the same genes, each specialized cell is only capable of expressing a small subset of those genes. So while brain cells have the gene to produce the protein insulin, they are unable to express this gene; it is not needed for the functioning of a brain cell, and it would be inefficient to make an unnecessary protein. The process of differentiation happens early in development and is thought to be irreversible. Cells that have yet to differentiate are referred to as stem cells.

Once a cell has differentiated and committed to a set of genes that it needs to express, genes within this set can be regulated on a minute-to-minute basis. There are a number

Table 8.3 Mechanisms for Regulating Gene Expression

Stage at Which Regulation Occurs	Mechanisms Used
Transcriptional regulation	Coiling of chromosomes to physically prevent or allow the access of transcription factors and RNA polymerase to the promoter regions of DNA
Posttranscriptional regulation	mRNA splicing and control over the rate at which mRNA leaves the nucleus via nuclear pores
Translational regulation	Lifespan of mRNA, which is influenced by the length of the poly-A tail added during RNA modification in the nucleus
Posttranslational regulation	Degradation of protein immediately following synthesis or failure to properly modify the protein, rendering it useless

of ways to regulate the process of transcription and translation. These methods can completely prevent gene expression. If gene expression does occur, there are methods to control the rate of the process, in turn influencing the amount of protein that is produced. Table 8.3 summarizes the major mechanisms for the control of gene expression.

MENDELIAN GENETICS

The basic principles of genetics were proposed by Gregor Mendel in the 1860s. His work with traits in pea plants led him to propose several theories of inheritance. Mendel did all his work and postulated his theories at a time when the genetic material had not even been discovered, so the fact that his theories hold true today could be considered quite a stroke of luck.

Several pieces of terminology are essential in order to discuss genetics. The exact genetic makeup of an individual for a specific trait is referred to as the genotype, while the physical manifestation of the genetic makeup is referred to as a phenotype for a specific trait. A gene has information to produce a single protein or enzyme; however, genes can exist in different forms termed alleles. In some cases, mutations can cause the production of alleles that produce faulty versions of the enzymes needed for metabolism, leading to a class of genetic disorders known as inborn errors of metabolism.

Mendel's Law of Segregation

Several important ideas are found in Mendel's law of segregation. These ideas can be summarized in the following way:

➤ For every given trait, an individual inherits two alleles for the trait.
➤ As an individual produces egg and sperm cells (gametes), the two alleles segregate so that each gamete contains only a single allele per trait. During fertilization, each gamete contributes one allele per trait, providing the offspring with two alleles per trait.

There are exceptions to the law of segregation. These include the alleles carried on sex chromosomes in males. Because males contain one X chromosome and one Y chromosome, the male will not have two alleles per trait for genes on the sex chromosomes.

Individuals can inherit two of the same allele (homozygous individuals) or two different alleles (heterozygous individuals) for any given trait. In the heterozygous individual, only one allele is normally expressed, while the other allele is hidden. The dominant allele will be the one expressed; the recessive allele will be hidden in the presence of a dominant allele. When an individual is heterozygous for a particular trait, his or her phenotype will appear dominant, yet the individual will still carry and can pass on the recessive allele via his or her gametes. A recessive phenotype is only observed when the individual is homozygous for the recessive allele. Keep in mind that dominant traits are not necessarily more common or more advantageous than recessive traits. Those labels only refer to the pattern of inheritance that the allele follows. The most common allele in the population is usually referred to as wild type. By convention, a single letter is selected to represent a particular trait. The dominant allele is always notated with a capital letter, while the recessive allele is notated with a lowercase letter.

A monohybrid cross is a breeding between two parents (the P generation) where a single trait is analyzed. The offspring of this cross are called the F_1 generation. A breeding between two F_1 offspring will produce the next generation, F_2, and so on. When the genotypes of parents are known for a specific trait, a Punnett square can be used to predict the genotypes of the offspring. In order to use a Punnett square, the genotypes of both parents must be known. The potential gametes of each parent are determined, and every possible combination of gametes is matched up in a matrix in order to determine every genotype of the potential offspring. A ratio of the phenotypes of the offspring is expressed as dominant:recessive.

Mendel worked with many traits in the pea plant. He found that when he crossed a true-breeding (homozygous) plant of a dominant phenotype to a true-breeding plant of a recessive phenotype, 100 percent of the F_1 offspring had the dominant phenotype. However, when he bred two of the F_1 offspring, he found that 75 percent of the F_2 offspring had the dominant phenotype, while 25 percent had the recessive phenotype. While the recessive phenotype had disappeared in the F_1 generation, it had reappeared in the F_2 generation. The F_1 offspring were all heterozygous. When two heterozygotes are bred to produce the F_2 generation, the offspring will always show Mendel's observed 3:1 phenotypic ratio. A cross between two heterozygotes that results in a 3:1 phenotypic ratio can be seen in Figure 8.5.

Using a testcross (also called a backcross) is a method to determine the genotype of a parent with a dominant phenotype. An organism with the dominant phenotype may be either homozygous or heterozygous. In the testcross, the parent with the dominant phenotype is always crossed to a homozygous recessive mate. The outcome of the phenotypic ratio of the offspring will reveal the genotype of the unknown parent. If 100 percent of the offspring have the dominant phenotype, then the unknown parent

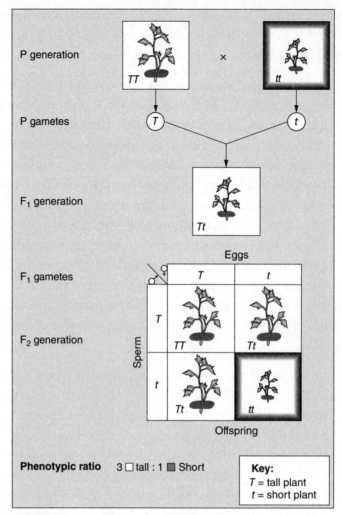

FIGURE 8.5 Cross between two heterozygotes.

was homozygous dominant. If the offspring display a 1:1 ratio, the genotype of the unknown parent was heterozygous.

Mendel's Law of Independent Assortment

A dihybrid cross considers the inheritance of two different traits at the same time. The rules of the monohybrid cross apply as long as the traits involved meet certain criteria. Mendel's law of independent assortment states the following:

➤ The alleles must assort independently during gamete formation, meaning that the distribution of alleles for one trait has no influence on the distribution of alleles for the other trait.

➤ If two genes are linked—that is, they occur on the same chromosome—they will not assort independently and thus will be inherited together, changing the expected outcomes in the offspring.

Two unlinked traits can be considered together in a Punnett square. When two traits are involved in a dihybrid cross, each trait is assigned a different letter. In order to predict the possible offspring, all possible gamete combinations of each trait for the parents must be considered. A Punnett square is used as a matrix to match up all possible gamete combinations for the offspring. Suppose two parents have the genotypes AABB and aabb. All F$_1$ offspring will be AaBb. If two F$_1$ offspring are bred, a 9:3:3:1 phenotypic ratio will be seen in the F$_2$ generation. See Figure 8.6 for an example of a dihybrid cross.

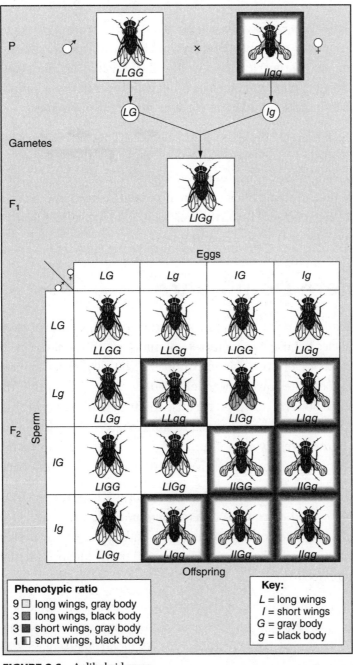

FIGURE 8.6 A dihybrid cross.

While Mendel's laws tend to be good predictors of inheritance for some genetic situations, sometimes these laws do not apply. Not every trait operates according to a simple dominant/recessive pattern or in a completely predictable manner.

The location of a gene on a chromosome is referred to as the locus of the gene. Genes that are linked occur on the same chromosome, which means that if one allele is found in a gamete, the other will be too. In the case of linkage, the combination of gametes produced will not be as diverse as would be the case with nonlinked alleles. In some cases, the loci of the alleles are so close together that they will always be inherited together. However, if the loci of the alleles are far away from each other on the chromosome, then there is a possibility for crossing over or genetic recombination to occur.

For the traits Mendel observed with pea plants, there were always two alleles. One was dominant and one was recessive. However, while an individual can only inherit two alleles (one from each parent) for any given trait, there may be more than two alleles to select from in the gene pool that consists of all genotypes in the population. These new alleles arise due to mutation and increase diversity in the population.

Human blood type is an example of multiple alleles. The ABO system has three alleles: I^A, I^B, and i. The alleles I^A and I^B are dominant, while the allele i is recessive. Each allele codes for either the presence or absence of particular antigens on the surface of red blood cells. Any time multiple alleles are involved with a trait, more than two potential phenotypes will be expected. This is the case in blood type, where four phenotypes can be observed: type A, type B, type AB, and type O.

Incomplete Dominance

According to Mendelian rules, a heterozygous individual always expresses the dominant phenotype. If alleles behave by incomplete dominance, this will not be the case. Using flower color in snapdragons is a classic example. If the allele R codes for red flowers and the allele r codes for white flowers, Mendelian rules would suggest that the heterozygote (Rr) would have red flowers. However, because this trait behaves according to incomplete dominance, both alleles will be expressed to some degree, leading to a pink (intermediate) phenotype in the heterozygous offspring. In the case of incomplete dominance, only two alleles are involved, yet there are three potential phenotypes that can arise.

Codominance is similar to incomplete dominance. For this to occur, the trait involved must have multiple alleles and more than one of them must be dominant. If a heterozygous individual inherits two different dominant alleles, both alleles will be expressed, leading to an individual that has both phenotypes (as opposed to the blended phenotype seen with incomplete dominance).

Human blood type is an example of codominance as well as multiple alleles. Should an individual inherit the genotype of $I^A I^B$, he or she will express the A phenotype as well as the B phenotype. In this case, the result is type AB blood. See Table 8.4 for more details on human blood type.

Table 8.4 The Genetic Basis of Human Blood Types		
Blood Type	**Potential Genotypes**	**Antigens on Red Blood Cell Surface**
Type A	I^AI^A or I^Ai	A
Type B	I^BI^B or I^Bi	B
Type AB	I^AI^B	A and B
Type O	Ii	None

Polygenic Traits

Generally, a single gene influences one trait. Polygenic traits involve gene interaction. This means that more than one gene acts to influence a single trait. Skin color and hair color are both examples of polygenic traits. Because more than one gene is involved, the number of potential phenotypes is increased as a result of continuous variation.

Epistasis is a unique genetic situation in which one gene interferes with the expression of another gene. In many cases, epistasis can lead to the masking of an expected trait. An example is coat color in Labrador retrievers. These dogs have black, chocolate, or yellow fur. In addition to the gene that controls fur color, the B gene, there is another allele that controls how pigment is distributed in the fur, the E gene. The B gene produces an enzyme that processes brown pigment to black pigment. Dogs that have the genotype BB or Bb will produce black pigment, while those with the genotype bb will produce brown pigment. The E gene allows the pigment to be deposited into the hair follicle. If the Labrador is EE or Ee, it will be able to deposit the pigment. However, dogs with the genotype ee will not. Therefore, the gene B determines if a dog will produce black or brown pigment, but these phenotypes can only be expressed if the dog is homozygous dominant or heterozygous for the E gene. Any dog that is homozygous recessive for the E gene, ee, will be yellow.

Pleiotropy occurs when a single gene influences two or more other traits. Most frequently, the effects of pleiotropy are seen in genetic diseases. In sickle-cell disease, the mutation in the hemoglobin gene results in the production of hemoglobin protein with a reduced oxygen-carrying ability. In turn, this affects multiple organ systems in the body, explaining the multiple symptoms of the disease.

When alleles are found on the X and Y sex chromosomes, the normal rules of genetics may not apply. While the sex chromosomes do contain genes to influence gender, there are other traits found on these chromosomes that have nothing to do with gender. Women inherit an XX genotype, while men inherit an XY genotype. In men, traits that occur on the sex chromosomes are the exception to the normal rule of always having two alleles per trait. Because the sex chromosomes in men are not a true pair, they do not have two alleles per trait on their sex chromosomes. The Y chromosome in men is always inherited from the father and contains relatively few genes compared to the X chromosome.

When a recessive trait is located on the X chromosome, women must receive two copies of the recessive allele (one from each parent) to express the recessive trait. However, men who inherit a recessive allele on their only X chromosome will express the recessive phenotype. Color blindness and hemophilia are examples of traits that are sex linked. While women can express these traits, they must receive the recessive alleles on both X chromosomes (meaning they must receive these alleles from both of their parents). Therefore, these traits are more commonly observed in men, who need only receive the recessive trait on their single X chromosome.

Women who are heterozygous for a trait on the X chromosome do not express the trait, yet they are carriers for the trait and can pass it to their sons. Since women are genotypically XX, every egg cell they make contains the X chromosome. Men are XY, and thus half their sperm contain the X chromosome and half contain the Y. In males, the Y chromosome must come from the father; the X comes from the mother.

Environmental Influences on Genes

While some genes behave according to very predictable rules, there are many cases where some external or internal environmental factor can interfere with the expression of a particular genotype. Penetrance of a genotype is a measure of the frequency with which a trait is actually expressed in the population. If a trait has 80 percent penetrance, 80 percent of the people with the genotype for the particular trait have the phenotype associated with the genotype. While some traits always show 100 percent penetrance, others do not. Within an individual, expressivity is a measure of the extent of expression of a phenotype. This means that in some cases expression of a phenotype is more extreme than in others.

There are many examples of how the environment affects the expression of a particular phenotype. Hydrangea plants may have the genotype to produce blue flowers, but depending on the acidity of the soil they are grown in (an environmental factor), they may express a different phenotype than expected (for example, they may produce pink flowers). Women who have the BRCA 1 and 2 alleles are at a high but not guaranteed risk for developing breast cancer, meaning that something other than the allele determines the expression of the allele.

There are many traits that cannot be predicted by genotype alone, such as intelligence, emotional behavior, and susceptibility to cancer. In many cases, the interaction of genes and the environment is a complicated relationship that is impossible to predict. Factors in humans such as age, gender, diet, and so forth are all known to influence the expression of certain genotypes.

CHAPTER 9

Evolution, Ecology, and Behavior

Read This Chapter to Learn About

➤ Genetic Change

➤ Natural Selection

➤ Genetic Basis for Evolution and the Hardy-Weinberg Equation

➤ Types of Natural Selection

➤ Types of Evolution

GENETIC CHANGE

Evolution simply means change. The changes referred to are genetic ones; thus the concept of mutation is at the center of the process of evolution. Evolution is something that occurs over generations of time; thus a single individual does not evolve, but populations of individuals do evolve. Microevolution deals with genetic changes to a specific population of individuals in a given area, while macroevolution is concerned with changes that occur to a species on a larger scale over a longer period of time.

There are a variety of factors that are responsible for the microevolution of a particular population. Natural selection, based on mutation, tends to be the major driving force for evolution, while genetic drift and gene flow can also influence the process.

New alleles are created by mutation. Some of these new alleles code for proteins that are beneficial, neutral, or detrimental as compared to the original protein intended by the allele. New alleles that code for beneficial proteins can provide advantages that are ultimately selected for by natural selection and are passed to the next generation, while detrimental alleles will be selected against.

NATURAL SELECTION

A central concept to the explanation of how evolution occurs is that of Darwin's natural selection. Natural selection explains the increase in frequency of favorable adaptations from one generation to the next. This results from differential reproductive success, in which some individuals reproduce more often than others, thus selecting for particular traits and increasing the frequency of their alleles in the next generations. Those that reproduce less decrease the frequency of their alleles in the next generation.

The concept of evolutionary fitness is key to natural selection. In this context, fit refers to the reproductive success of an individual and its contribution to the next generation. Those individuals that are more fit are more evolutionarily successful in that their genetic traits will be passed to the next generation; this increases the frequency of specific alleles in the gene pool.

Over generations, selective pressures that are exerted on a population can lead to adaptations. When selective pressures change, some organisms that may have been considered marginally fit before may now be extremely fit under the new conditions. Further, those individuals that may have been very fit previously may no longer be fit. Their genetic adaptations will be selected against. While an individual cannot change its genetics, over time, the population has changed genetically, which is termed adaptation.

Competitive interactions within a population are another critical factor for natural selection. The ability to outcompete other individuals for resources, including mates, is a key feature of fitness. In any given population, some individuals are better able to compete for resources and are considered more fit than others, leading to differential reproductive success. This concept assumes that mating in the population is random. In some cases, such as with humans, mating is nonrandom, which leads to another form of selection to be discussed shortly.

Competition between species can also influence the evolutionary progression of all species involved. In some cases, symbiotic relationships exist in which two species exist together for extended periods of time. In mutualistic relationships, both species benefit from the association. In parasitic relationships, one species benefits at the expense of the other species. In commensalism, one species benefits while the other species is relatively unharmed. When two species are competing for the same ecological requirements or niche, the reproductive success and fitness, as well as the growth, of one or both populations may be inhibited based on their ability to compete for resources. This will change the microevolutionary course of the population.

When individuals leave a population, they take their alleles with them, resulting in gene flow. This can decrease genetic variation within the gene pool, ultimately affecting the evolution of the population. Outbreeding occurs with the individuals that left the population. The new populations that these individuals enter can increase diversity in their gene pool by adding new alleles to it. Genetic drift involves changes to the allelic frequencies within a population due to chance. While this is generally negligible in large populations, it can have major consequences in smaller populations. The bottleneck effect and the founder effect are examples of genetic drift to be discussed shortly.

GENETIC BASIS FOR EVOLUTION AND THE HARDY-WEINBERG EQUATION

The Hardy-Weinberg equation can be used to calculate allelic frequencies within a population given that the population is large and microevolution is not occurring, which is not necessarily a realistic situation. In the equation, p represents the frequency of a dominant allele and q represents the frequency of a recessive allele, such that $p + q = 1$. Further, the equation $p^2 + 2pq + q^2 = 1$ can be used to show the frequency of homozygous dominant individuals (p^2), heterozygotes ($2pq$), and homozygous recessive individuals (q^2). Given information on the frequency of a single allele, all other pieces within the equation can be determined. While these frequencies are accurate at a given time, any evolution occurring within the population would shift these predicted values.

Violations of Hardy-Weinberg

In order for Hardy-Weinberg allelic frequencies to hold true, it is necessary for certain criteria to be met. If any of these criteria are violated, the allelic frequencies will change over time. Any of the following will negate Hardy-Weinberg equilibrium:

➤ Nonrandom mating
➤ Gene flow
➤ Populations with a small number of individuals
➤ Mutations
➤ Bottleneck effect
➤ Founder effect

The bottleneck effect is a form of genetic drift in which catastrophic events wipe out a large percentage of a population. When the population is small, the few remaining alleles in the gene pool may not be characteristic of the larger population. Generally, genetic diversity is lost due to inbreeding by the remaining members of the population. The founder effect is a form of genetic drift that occurs when a small number of individuals leave a larger population and form their own small population where inbreeding is necessary. The new population only has the diversity brought to it by the founding members.

TYPES OF NATURAL SELECTION

For any given trait, there can be several different phenotypes. If two phenotypes are present for a particular trait, dimorphism is the case. If three or more phenotypes are seen for a particular trait, polymorphism is at work. For example, flower color in snapdragons exhibits polymorphism with red, white, and pink phenotypes. Some phenotypes can be considered intermediates (like pink flowers); others are extremes from either end

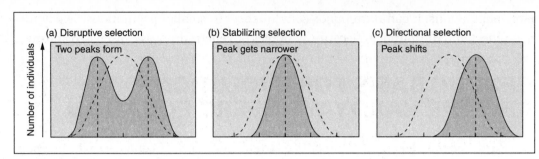

FIGURE 9.1 Types of natural selection.

of the intermediate phenotype (like red and white flowers). When natural selection occurs, it may select for intermediate phenotypes, either extreme phenotype, or both extreme phenotypes, as seen in Figure 9.1.

In directional selection, an allele that is considered advantageous is selected for. The allelic frequency continues to shift in the same direction generation after generation. In this case, one allele that produces an extreme phenotype is selected for. The selection of antibiotic resistance alleles in bacteria is an example of directional selection. Over time, selective pressures can result in an entire population possessing the same alleles for a particular trait.

Stabilizing selection leads to favoring of the alleles that produce an intermediate phenotype. Human birth weight would be an example of stabilizing selection. Babies of an intermediate weight are favored over those that are too small to survive or too large to be easily delivered.

In some cases, the environment favors two extreme phenotypes at the same time. In this case, disruptive selection occurs. Individuals with either extreme phenotype are favored, while those with the intermediate forms of the alleles are selected against. Over time, the continued selection of both extremes may lead to the evolution of two distinct species.

When particular alleles are purposely selected for through nonrandom mating, artificial selection occurs. The breeding of domesticated dogs is an excellent example of the results of artificial selection. All breeds of dogs are members of the same species, having been selectively bred from wolves for specific traits that are appealing to the breeder. Both toy poodles and Great Danes are examples of the extreme phenotypes that can be selected for when artificial selection is used. Traits that are artificially selected for are not necessarily the result of the most fit alleles. Many breeds of dog have medical conditions or predispositions as a result of artificial selection and inbreeding.

TYPES OF EVOLUTION

The evolutionary process can proceed in a variety of directions or patterns: convergent, divergent, and parallel evolution. When two populations exist in the same type of environment that provides the same selective pressures, the two populations will evolve in a similar manner via convergent evolution. While the populations may not be closely related, they may develop similar, analogous structures to allow them to function in similar environments. Fish in Antarctica have evolved the ability to produce specialized glycoproteins that serve as a sort of antifreeze to prevent their tissues from freezing in the low-temperature water. Fish on the opposite side of the world, in the Arctic, have evolved the same kind of antifreeze protection mechanism. Genetic studies show that the two species of fish produce antifreeze proteins that are very different from each other, which strongly suggests that two independent events led to the evolution of these mechanisms.

In an individual population, groups within the population may evolve differently. Over time, this may lead to the development of new species via divergent evolution. In many cases, changes to the population or geographic isolation may cause different adaptations within the population. This sort of evolution can lead to homologous structures. Vertebrate limbs are an excellent example of divergent evolution. The forearms of different vertebrate species have different structures and functions; however, they all diverged from a common origin.

When two species share the same environment, the evolution of one species can affect the evolution of the other species. This is called parallel evolution or coevolution. Any changes to one species will require adaptations to the other species in order for them to continue to exist in the same environment. An example might be how the predation patterns of birds influence the evolution of butterfly species sharing the same space. Some butterflies have evolved the ability to store poisonous chemicals that deter birds from eating them, while other butterflies simply mimic the poisonous ones to avoid being preyed upon.

Evidence for Evolution

There is a large body of evidence to support evolutionary theory. Most evidence comes from studies of paleontology, biogeography, molecular biology, comparative anatomy, and comparative embryology.

➤ **Paleontology:** The field of paleontology provides evidence for evolution in the form of the fossil record. Fossilization occurs when a whole organism or parts of an organism become embedded in sediments and petrified over thousands of years. These fossils serve as physical evidence of organisms that lived in the past.

➤ **Biogeography:** The study of the natural distribution of organisms, biogeography, can also lend credence to evolutionary theory. Looking at similarities and differences between different organisms living in different locations can help decipher evolutionary relationships between organisms as well as common ancestors.

➤ **Molecular biology:** The ability to compare DNA and other molecules, such as proteins, made by various organisms also helps support evolutionary theory. Organisms that are more closely related share more DNA similarities than organisms that are distantly related. Evolutionary time can be measured by genetic changes over time. Comparisons of mutation rates in conserved gene sequences can be used to construct molecular clocks, which can be used to estimate when specific lineages emerged.

➤ **Comparative anatomy:** An analysis of anatomical features in organisms can be used to make comparisons between different species. Homologous structures, such as the forelimbs of mammals, are similar in structure between various organisms, and they share a similar function, indicating that these structures came from a common ancestral species. Analogous structures have similar functions between various organisms, but these structures have different lines of descent. Vestigial structures seen in organisms have no functional value, yet are evolutionary remnants from ancestral species. Examples of vestigial structures are the human appendix, bone structure for hind limbs in whales, and the coccyx (tailbone) in humans. Since these structures remain, even without apparent functions, they are evidence of prior evolutionary forces at work.

➤ **Comparative embryology:** While many organisms look distinctly different in their adult forms, they may share striking similarities during their developmental periods. Comparative embryology is used to study these similarities during the developmental process. A modification of Haeckel's theory that ontogeny recapitulates phylogeny (or recapitulation) suggests that species that have an evolutionary relationship generally share characteristics during embryonic development.

Cladistics

Species in existence today all have relations to their ancestors. Cladograms are diagrams that show the relationship between species and their common ancestors. Species of organisms can be classified into groups called clades based upon the branch that they have been assigned to in an evolutionary tree. Keep in mind however, that the classification of organisms has been modified over time. What differentiates a cladogram from a phylogeny (an evolutionary history) is that cladistics focuses on shared characteristics and derived traits. For example, our four limbs (tetrapod) is an ancestral (shared) trait. We share it with all the terrestrial vertebrates and with the ancestor to them all. On the other hand, our opposable thumb is a derived character. It isn't something we share with the ancestor of the terrestrial vertebrates; it evolved later. We are in the middle of a taxonomic revolution because our ability to sequence DNA and compare sequences is unprecedented (DNA sequence comparisons are the gold standard of quantifying relatedness). We have sequenced thousands of genomes and are sequencing more every day. We also have the supercomputing power to analyze and compare all the sequences.

Populations and Communities

A population is a group of species in a given area. The area is usually confined by the species' ability to interbreed with others of the same population. For example, one could define the rats that live in a New York City subway station as a population. This would be much more realistic than calling all of the rats in the United States a population. When all of the populations in a given area are considered together (from all domains, kingdoms, etc.) it is called a community.

A niche is the role an organism plays in the ecosystem through its use of all biotic and abiotic factors. Keeping in mind that only one species can occupy a particular niche, should another similar species migrate into the same area and try to occupy a niche that is already occupied, either resource partitioning or competition will follow. Should there be competition, remember that only the best obtainer of resources will be successful and have a higher likelihood of passing on the genes that made it more successful.

Succession is the change in the composition of species in an area over time. It occurs when no life previously existed in an area or when there is a major disturbance. For example, wildfires do cause destruction and do invade the lives of humans, but the biotic factors will make a comeback, and usually in a fairly specific order. Eventually, a climax community results, where the composition of biotic factors remains fairly constant even though individuals may come and go. However, it may take an extremely long time for such a climax community to form due to the chance of environmental change upsetting the rising climax community. As a result, the likelihood of a climax community in the wild is very small.

Competition

Key resources that are in limited supply will always result in competition between species and among the members of a species. All ecosystems are limited by the biomass and productivity of the autotrophs, the organisms that convert light energy into energy for other organisms. But don't be fooled: the producers (typically plants) are limited by the amount of water and sunlight they can obtain. For example, taller trees can block the sunlight from reaching the rain forest's floor and, therefore, the autotrophs that rely on the sunlight to grow. The cutting down of just a few tall trees in the Amazon rain forest sounds like a negative behavior, but it will allow sunlight to reach the organisms living on the ground, thereby helping them grow.

Predation

All carnivores eat other organisms. These species will be found higher up on the food energy pyramid. We typically think of a predator as something that eats another animal, although, technically an herbivore can be a considered a predator of a plant.

Symbiosis

There are different kinds of relationships between two organisms that live in very close association. For example, there are birds that follow certain animals, and there are bacteria that live in our intestines. The relationship can be mutualistic and benefit both (mutualism). A good example of this is the protozoans living in the intestines of termites that help in the digestion of cellulose. Commensalism is when one organism can benefit one without helping or harming the other. Finally, there is parasitism, where one organism benefits at the expense of another. An example of parasitism is a flea or tick living on your cat or dog.

Ecosystems

The sum of all living and nonliving things that coexist in an area or community is called an ecosystem. This includes organisms from all domains and kingdoms living in the particular area in addition to the abiotic factors such as air and water that these organisms interact with. Ecosystem areas can include some common settings such as forest, desert, tundra, coral reef, and taiga. What is most important is how energy flows from one organism to another in the ecosystem. This energy flow can be diagramed with the use of a food chain or a food web.

Let us first begin with an energy pyramid (Figure 9.2). Because it is the photosynthetic producers that can capture the sun's energy and make it available to other species, they are given the biggest portion at the bottom of the pyramid (trophic level A). On top of the producers are what we call the primary consumers. These are herbivores that can consume the producers (trophic level B). The next level up presents the secondary consumers, which are carnivores. The secondary consumers are predators who feed upon the herbivores (trophic level C). An example would be a cheetah that preys upon a gazelle. Finally, on top, are the tertiary consumers that eat other carnivores (trophic level D).

A food chain diagrams a monophagous pathway. A series of these pathways can be put together to show a food web, which is considered to be polyphagous. An example of a food chain is shown in Figure 9.3.

Finally, within the ecosystem there is the continuous recycling of materials that are not living. Some of these cycles can include the carbon cycle, nitrogen cycle, and oxygen cycle. Another such cycle is the water cycle. This cycle can include situations such as the following:

➤ Water is stored in the ocean but evaporates into the air.
➤ Moisture in the air can condense and precipitate.
➤ Precipitation can come in the form of rain and run off into the ocean.
➤ Precipitation can come in the form of ice or snow and be stored at higher altitudes.
➤ Snow and ice at higher altitudes can seasonally melt and become runoff.
➤ Water can filter into the ground and become water storage.

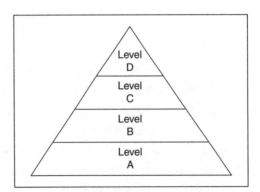

FIGURE 9.2 A sample energy pyramid.

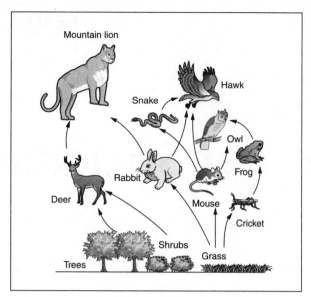

FIGURE 9.3   A sample food web for a particular ecosystem.

Animals and Social Behavior

Ethology is the study of animal behavior. Animals that live in complex societies show behaviors that allow them to thrive as a population. This is especially important in eusocial (truly social) animals like humans, ants, big cats, and primates. For example, we as humans are trained to hold doors open for others and give up a seat on the bus for the elderly or for pregnant women. These examples of social behaviors help to keep order and help our species survive and even thrive. Each organism has to recognize the balance between being able to get what it needs as an individual and cooperating for the betterment of the group. Along with this there is kin selection, the concept that we are more likely to behave altruistically toward those who are related to us. This helps to keep the population safe and thriving. An example is a human jumping in a lake to save a family member who is drowning. Hamilton's equation $br - c > 0$ takes into account the number of offspring involved and the degree of relatedness between an altruist and the recipient of aid. In general, a higher degree of relatedness means a greater degree of altruistic behaviors.

CHAPTER 10

Atomic and Molecular Structure

Read This Chapter to Learn About

➤ Basic Atomic Theory
➤ The Modern Theory of the Atom
➤ Detailed Atomic Structure
➤ Electron Configurations

BASIC ATOMIC THEORY

In this section we will consider the basic structure and components of atoms using the nuclear atom model. Later, the model will be refined with respect to the location of the electrons.

The English chemist John Dalton first formulated the modern atomic theory by consolidating three macroscopic laws that had been established by several scientists.

➤ The law of conservation of mass (or matter), which states that during a chemical reaction the total mass of the starting reactants equals the total mass of the products.
➤ The law of definite composition (or proportions), which states that a compound consists of two or more elements combined in a fixed ratio by mass.
➤ The law of multiple proportions, which states that if a pair of elements forms more than one compound, the combining masses of one of the elements with a fixed mass of the other element are in the ratio of small whole numbers.

Experiments with gases contributed to Dalton's theory. Dalton considered the data and concluded that the best explanation was that all matter is made of tiny, indivisible particles called atoms. The tenets of Dalton's atomic theory are summarized as follows:

➤ All matter is composed of tiny indivisible particles called atoms.
➤ Atoms of a given element are identical in all properties, and atoms of differing elements are different in some properties.
➤ Compounds are atoms combined together in a fixed ratio of individual atoms.
➤ Chemical reactions are the rearrangement of atoms to form different compounds in new fixed ratios of atoms.

The law of conservation of mass follows from the indivisibility of atoms. The laws of definite composition and multiple proportions result from the fixed combining ratios of different atoms of differing masses, which are observed macroscopically as fixed ratios of masses of elements. Inaccuracies have been found in each of Dalton's four points, but Dalton's theory provided a framework for experimental investigations supporting atomic theory in the nineteenth century and led to modern atomic theory in the twentieth century.

THE MODERN THEORY OF THE ATOM

The modern theory of the atom was developed in the first 30 years of the twentieth century. The French physicist Antoine-Henri Becquerel discovered that some elements spontaneously emit rays that can expose a photographic plate. These rays are called alpha particles (particles with a +2 relative charge), beta particles (particles with a −1 relative charge), and gamma rays (energy with no charge). Together, these rays were called radioactivity, and this phenomenon hinted that atoms contained particles smaller than the whole atom.

The English physicist J. J. Thomson studied the rays generated from metal plates exposed to a current in an evacuated tube called a cathode ray tube. Thomson called the cathode rays electrons, and eventually it was shown that cathode rays and beta particles are identical. Thomson's experiment allowed the determination of the mass-to-charge ratio of the electron. The American physicist Robert Millikan determined the charge on the electron, and multiplying this charge by the mass-to-charge ratio yielded the mass of the electron, which is 9.100×10^{-28} g. If the negative electron is part of a neutral atom, then there must also be a positive part.

The atom is composed mostly of empty space with the positive charge concentrated at the center, or nucleus. This nuclear atom is the currently accepted model for the atom, though it has been greatly refined. The positive particles at the center are called protons. Later, the nucleus was found also to contain neutrons, particles with a mass similar to the proton, but with no charge. Subatomic particles are summarized in Table 10.1. Chemical processes do not affect the particles in the nucleus, but nuclear reactions or radioactivity can alter the number of nuclear particles.

Table 10.1 Subatomic Particles				
Name	**Symbol**	**Relative Charge**	**Relative Mass**	**Location**
Proton	p^+ or p	+1	≈ 1 amu	Nucleus
Neutron	n	0	≈ 1 amu	Nucleus
Electron	e^-	−1	$1/1{,}836$ amu	Circulating outside the nucleus

All atoms of the same element have the same number of protons. This number is called the element's atomic number (Z). Carbon atoms have six protons. Gold atoms have 79 protons. The number of neutrons in the nucleus may vary. Atoms with different numbers of neutrons but identical numbers of protons are called isotopes. These atoms have a different mass but are chemically almost identical. The total number of protons and neutrons in the nucleus is called the mass number (A). The much smaller electrons are insignificant in the mass of the atom. Each element has a corresponding one- or two-letter symbol. Carbon is C, nitrogen is N, gold is Au, and hydrogen is H. The atomic symbol of a particular isotope is written with the mass number (A) as a left superscript and the atomic number (Z) as a left subscript. For example, a carbon atom with 6 neutrons is $^{12}_{6}$C. The carbon isotope with eight neutrons is $^{14}_{6}$C. The atomic number, Z, is redundant and is often omitted. The number of neutrons is A − Z. For ^{238}U, Z = 92 (92 p^+) and A = 238, so $238 - 92 = 146$ neutrons.

Each naturally occurring isotope makes up a specific fraction of the total atoms of that element called the relative abundance, usually given as a percentage. To convert a percentage to a fractional part, divide by 100. For boron, the two main isotopes are ^{11}B with a relative abundance of 80.09 percent and ^{10}B with a relative abundance of 19.91 percent. It is convenient to introduce a new unit that better matches the scale of atoms. The amu (atomic mass unit) is defined as $\dfrac{1}{12}$ of the mass of an atom of ^{12}C. 1 amu is close to the mass of a proton or a neutron. To calculate the average atomic mass of an atom of a given element, use the following formula (frac. = fraction):

$$\text{Avg. atomic mass} = (\text{frac. of isotope 1}) \times (\text{mass of isotope 1})$$
$$- (\text{frac. of isotope 2}) \times (\text{mass of isotope 2}) + \ldots$$

The sum will have as many terms as there are isotopes of the atom. For boron:

Isotope	Relative Abundance	Mass (amu)
^{10}B	19.91%	10.012939
^{11}B	80.09%	11.009305

$$\text{Avg. atomic mass} = (0.1991 \times 10.012939) + (0.8009 \times 11.009305) \text{ amu} = 10.81 \text{ amu}$$

Because the relative abundance of ^{11}B is greater than ^{10}B, the heavier element contributes a greater amount to the weighted average, which is closer to the mass of ^{11}B than to that of ^{10}B. Average atomic masses have been calculated from experimental data for most of the elements.

DETAILED ATOMIC STRUCTURE

This section will describe the properties of matter, including the interaction between matter and electromagnetic radiation. Electromagnetic radiation is energy such as visible light, radio waves, x-rays, microwave radiation, and ultraviolet radiation. Electromagnetic radiation is characterized by oscillating periodic waves. The wavelength (λ) is the distance between successive crests or troughs in a wave. The units of wavelength are the units of length such as a meter. The frequency (ν) is the number of wavelengths passing a given point per second. The units of frequency are 1/s or equivalently Hertz (Hz).

All electromagnetic radiation travels at the speed of light, c, which is 2.998×10^8 m/s in a vacuum. The frequency and wavelength of light are related by the equation: $\nu\lambda = c$.

> **PROBLEM:** A radio station has a frequency of 880 kHz. What is its wavelength?

> **SOLUTION:** kHz means 10^3 Hz, so 880 kHz is 8.80×10^5/s.

$$\lambda = \frac{c}{\nu} = \frac{2.998 \times 10^8}{8.80 \times 10^5} \rightarrow \lambda = 341 \, \text{m}$$

Until about 1900, matter and energy were thought to have entirely different properties. Matter was believed to behave as discrete particles described by Newton's laws of motion, and energy was believed to behave as continuous waves. In the first 30 years of the twentieth century, modern science showed that matter and energy can both behave with particle-like and wavelike properties. German physicist Max Planck was able to explain the emission spectrum from a heated body by assuming that energy was not emitted in a continuous way but came in bundles of energy called quanta, dependent on the frequency.

$$E_q = h\nu$$

where E_q is the energy of the quantum, h is Planck's constant (6.626×10^{-34} J-s), and ν is the frequency of the light.

Albert Einstein used Planck's idea to explain the photoelectric effect. In the photoelectric effect, light shining on a metal electrode in a vacuum can eject electrons that travel through the vacuum to another electrode, completing an electrical circuit. Einstein proposed that particles of light called photons supplied the energy to eject the electrons. Einstein's work showed the dual nature of light.

During the 1800s, scientists studied emissions from gas-filled tubes that were subjected to an electrical discharge, such as a neon bulb. Unlike the emissions from heated objects, which give continuous spectra of all wavelengths, the emissions from the gas-filled tubes gave only a few lines, which were a function of the gas in the tube. These spectra are called line emission spectra. For hydrogen, in the region of visible light, the line spectrum contains only four prominent lines, at 656, 486, 434, and 410 nm (1 nm = 1 × 10⁻⁹ m). Because the spectra are a function of the material in the tube, scientists believed the spectra reflected something about the energy and structure of the atoms of the gas in the tube. A formula was derived by the Swedish physicist Johannes Rydberg for the reciprocal of the wavelength of the lines in the emission spectrum of hydrogen:

$$\frac{1}{\lambda} = 10{,}967{,}758 \text{ m}^{-1}\left(\frac{1}{n_1^2} - \frac{1}{n_2^2}\right)$$

where n_1 and n_2 are integers with $n_1 < n_2$.

Bohr Model

The Bohr model of the hydrogen atom was the first explanation for the line spectra. The Danish physicist Niels Bohr assumed that in hydrogen, the electron travels around the hydrogen nucleus, a proton, in circular orbits similar to the solar system. Bohr assumed that the energy of the electron in an orbit was quantized, or restricted to specific energy levels labeled with quantum numbers, n. The values for n are integers beginning with 1. The lowest energy level, n = 1, has the smallest radius. The radius of the orbit for the next higher energy level, n = 2, is larger.

Bohr calculated that the energy of a given level in the hydrogen atom is: $E_n = -2.179 \times 10^{-18} \text{ J}\left(\frac{1}{n^2}\right)$. The energy is negative because the energy of a completely separated proton and electron was defined by Bohr to be zero. The energy of the transition between orbits is easily calculated. If the initial orbital is labeled n_i and the final orbit n_f, the energy of the transition between levels is shown in Figure 10.1.

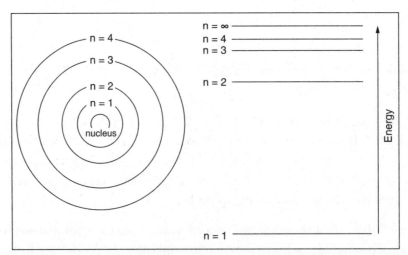

FIGURE 10.1 The Bohr model of the atom.

For the transition between $n_i = 4$ to $n_f = 2$:

$$\Delta E = -2.179 \times 10^{-18} \left(\frac{1}{n_1^2} - \frac{1}{n_2^2} \right)$$

$$\Delta E = -2.179 \times 10^{-18} \left(\frac{1}{4} - \frac{1}{16} \right)$$

$$\Delta E = -2.179 \times 10^{-18} (0.1875) = -4.086 \times 10^{-19} \, J$$

The negative sign indicates that energy is leaving the atom; that is, the process is exothermic. Bohr postulated that this photon is emitted by the atom with an energy equivalent to the energy difference of the two orbits. If the transition were reversed, the ΔE would be positive, indicating an endothermic process in which a photon is absorbed by the atom.

The frequency of the photon associated with this transition may be calculated from $\Delta E = h\nu$ or $\nu = \frac{E}{h}$. (The negative sign in the energy is ignored because it simply gives the direction of energy flow. A frequency is a positive number.)

$$\frac{4.086 \times 10^{-19} \, J}{6.626 \times 10^{-34} \, J \cdot s} = \frac{6.1667 \times 10^{14}}{s}$$

The wavelength of light is determined using the relation $\nu\lambda = c$ in the form $\lambda = \frac{c}{\nu}$.

$$\lambda = \frac{2.999 \times 10^8 \, m/s}{6.1667 \times 10^{14}} = 4.86 \times 10^{-7} \, m \text{ or } 486 \text{ nm}.$$

Note that this calculated value corresponds to one of the wavelengths in the line emission spectra of hydrogen. Through theoretical means, Bohr had derived the experimental value for this wavelength and other wavelengths from the emission spectrum of hydrogen. Bohr attempted to extend his model to atoms with more than one proton. The model did not work for any other atoms. Attempts to refine the model did not work. The energies were correct, but there was something fundamentally wrong with Bohr's model.

The Quantum Atom

The problem with Bohr's model was that it did not account for a fundamental property of the electron. In 1924, after Bohr's model was established, French physicist Louis de Broglie thought that if light can behave both as a particle and as a wave, then matter might behave both as a particle and as a wave with a de Broglie wavelength given by:
$\lambda = \frac{h}{mv}$ where m is the mass of the particle and v is the particle's velocity.

The de Broglie wavelength is negligible for everyday objects such as baseballs and trucks, but the size of the de Broglie wavelength of an electron is close to the size of an atom.

The wavelength of matter was confirmed experimentally by the diffraction of electrons by aluminum foil. The quantum mechanical model of the atom replaced Bohr's model. It was developed separately by German physicist Werner Heisenberg and the Austrian physicist Erwin Schrödinger. Schrödinger developed an equation based on de Broglie's wavelength and the basic wave equation from physics. The solutions to his equation are called wave functions or orbitals, to distinguish them from Bohr's orbits. Electrons are described by the probability of finding the electron at a point in space called electron density by chemists. Regions with high probabilities of finding an electron have larger electron densities.

Heisenberg also added to the quantum mechanical model of the atom by introducing the uncertainty principle. When this concept is applied to electrons (because of their very low mass), the Heisenberg uncertainty principle states that it is impossible to determine both the momentum and location of an electron at any one time. Instead, we can only look at the probability of finding an electron in a certain region about the atom's nucleus.

Quantum Numbers

Each solution to Schrödinger's equation is labeled by three integers. These integers are called quantum numbers—n, l, and m_l. Schrödinger's equation restricts the values of these quantum numbers. A fourth quantum number, m_s, is due to the spin of the electron. The principal quantum number, n, is restricted to positive integer values starting with 1. In other words, its possible values are 1, 2, 3, 4, 5, 6, and so on. The value of n primarily determines the energy of the electron. The lower the value of n, the lower the energy and the closer the electron is to the nucleus.

The azimuthal quantum number (or angular momentum quantum number), l, is restricted by the value of n to values from 0 and increases by one until $n - 1$ is reached.

Principal	Possible l Values
1	0
2	0, 1
3	0, 1, 2
4	0, 1, 2, 3
5	0, 1, 2, 3, 4

The azimuthal quantum number determines the shape of the orbital. Each number corresponds to a letter that names an orbital.

l value	0	1	2	3	4	5
Name	s	p	d	f	g	h

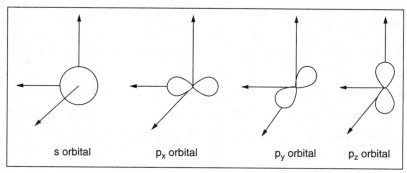

FIGURE 10.2 Shapes of s and p orbitals.

The magnetic quantum number, m, is restricted by the value of l to integers beginning at $-l$ and increasing by 1 until $+l$ is reached, and ml determines an orbital's orientation in space.

l Value		Possible ml Values
0	s	0
1	p	$-1, 0, 1$
2	d	$-2, -1, 0, 1, 2$
3	f	$-3, -2, -1, 0, 1, 2, 3$

From the preceding table, you can see that for any given value of n, there is one n_s orbital, three n_p orbitals, five n_d orbitals, seven n_f orbitals, etc. The spin quantum number, m_s, is restricted to values of $+\frac{1}{2}$ and $-\frac{1}{2}$.

The orbitals have shapes that are determined by the quantum number l. All s orbitals are spherical and centered on the nucleus. As n increases, the size of the sphere increases (1s < 2s < 3s < 4s < 5s, etc.). All p orbitals are dumbbell-shaped, and on each n level the three p orbitals are oriented in three mutually perpendicular directions along the x, y, and z axes respectively. As with the s orbital, size increases with increasing n value. Four of the d orbitals have a similar shape, usually described as a cloverleaf; one has a different shape. Representations of the shapes of s and p orbitals are shown in Figure 10.2.

ELECTRON CONFIGURATIONS

The atoms of the elements in the periodic table may be built up one by one by placing electrons in the lowest available orbital. Several rules must be followed.

➤ The **Pauli exclusion principle** states that no two electrons in an atom may have all four quantum numbers of identical value. If the first three quantum numbers are identical, the only possibilities for the fourth quantum number, ms, are $+\frac{1}{2}$ or $-\frac{1}{2}$. This means that an orbital can have at most two electrons, and if there are two electrons in an orbital, the electrons must have opposite values for ms. When two electrons occupy one orbital with ms values of $+\dfrac{1}{2}$ and $-\dfrac{1}{2}$, the spins are said to be paired. If two electrons are in separate orbitals with the same value for ms, the spins are said to be parallel.

➤ **Hund's rule** states that if a set of orbitals with equivalent energy is not completely filled, electrons will fill the orbitals to give a maximum number of half-filled orbitals with parallel spins. For example, if electrons are added to an unfilled 3p level (three orbitals), an electron will be placed in each orbital with parallel spins before any electron is paired up.

The energies of the orbitals are a function of both n and l. For a given value of n, the energies of the orbitals in a multielectron atom are in the order ns < np < nd < nf < etc. For lower values of n, the orbitals are well separated in energy. As n increases, the orbitals from different values of n begin to overlap.

The resulting order 1s → 2s → 2p → 3s → 3p → 4s → 3d → 4p → 5s → 4d → 5p → 6s → 4f → 5d → 6p → 7s → 5f → 6d → 7p will be adequate for most atoms, with a few exceptions. The periodic table itself may also be used to determine the filling order. The electron configuration for an element lists the orbitals that contain electrons and the number of electrons in each orbital. There are several ways to represent the electron configuration. Line diagrams use lines to represent the orbitals and arrows to represent the electron spin. An up arrow corresponds to $m_s = +\dfrac{1}{2}$ and a down arrow corresponds to $m_s = -\dfrac{1}{2}$. The *aufbau* (German for "to build up") approach is generally used. Hydrogen is first with one electron and one proton. Successive elements are "created" by adding one proton to the nucleus and one electron to the next lowest available orbital, following Hund's rule when necessary. The number in parentheses is the atomic number, which equals the number of electrons. In Figure 10.3 we see the line diagrams for the first 10 elements.

Line diagrams become cumbersome as the number of electrons increases. Orbitals may be represented as a number-letter combination. The number of electrons in an orbital is represented as a superscript. The first 10 electronic configurations may be rewritten as:

H	$1s^1$ (Pronounced "one s one")
He	$1s^2$
Li	$1s^2 2s^1$
Be	$1s^2 2s^2$
B	$1s^2 2s^2 2p^1$
C	$1s^2 2s^2 2p^2$
N	$1s^2 2s^2 2p^3$
O	$1s^2 2s^2 2p^4$
F	$1s^2 2s^2 2p^5$
Ne	$1s^2 2s^2 2p^6 = [Ne]$

H	↑				
	1s				
He	↑↓				
	1s				
Li	↑↓	↑			
	1s	2s			
Be	↑↓	↑↓			
	1s	2s			
B	↑↓	↑↓	↑		
	1s	2s	2p		
C	↑↓	↑↓	↑	↑	
	1s	2s	2p		
N	↑↓	↑↓	↑	↑	↑
	1s	2s	2p		
O	↑↓	↑↓	↑↓	↑	↑
	1s	2s	2p		
F	↑↓	↑↓	↑↓	↑↓	↑
	1s	2s	2p		
Ne	↑↓	↑↓	↑↓	↑↓	↑↓
	1s	2s	2p		

FIGURE 10.3 Line diagrams for the first 10 elements.

Because the electrons in neon will also be present in all following atoms, the electron configurations for each noble gas may be abbreviated as shown previously. This abbreviation will also be used in the following electron configurations for the next eight elements.

Na   [Ne] $3s^1$

Mg   [Ne] $3s^2$

Al   [Ne] $3s^2 3p^1$

Si   [Ne] $3s^2 3p^2$

P   [Ne] $3s^2 3p^3$

S   [Ne] $3s^2 3p^4$

Cl   [Ne] $3s^2 3p^5$

Ar   [Ne] $3s^2 3p^6$ = [Ar]

The next 18 elements will fill the 4s(2e−), 3d(10e−), and 4p(6e−) orbitals. A more common problem is to write the electron configuration of a given element.

PROBLEM: What is the electron configuration of Pt?

SOLUTION: Pt has 78 electrons. Fill the orbitals in order until 78 electrons are placed in orbitals.

Pt $\quad 1s^2 2s^2 2p^6 3s^2 3p^6 4s^2 3d^{10} 4p^6 5s^2 4d^{10} 5p^6 6s^2\, 4f^{14} 5d^8$

When the Russian chemist Dmitry Mendeleyev prepared the original periodic table, he placed elements in groups by their chemical properties before the electron had ever been discovered. The modern view of the periodic table recognizes that the elements are in groups because they have similar electron configurations. The shape of the periodic table can now be understood:

➤ The first two columns (groups 1 and 2) are where the s orbitals are being filled.
➤ The last six columns (groups 13 through 18) are where the p orbitals are being filled.
➤ The 10 columns in the middle (groups 3 through 12) are where the d orbitals are being filled.
➤ The two rows at the bottom of the table (the lanthanide and actinide series) are elements where the f orbitals are being filled.

The electron configurations of the alkali metals are generalized as $[NG]ns^1$ where $[NG]$ is the electron configuration of the preceding noble gas. The electron configurations of the alkali metal cations are those of each immediately preceding noble gas, for example, $Na^+ = [Ne]$. Electron configurations of the noble gases are called core electrons. These electrons are especially stable and do not normally take part in chemical reactions. A filled set of d electrons is unreactive and considered part of the core. Electrons that are not contained in the core electrons are called valence electrons. Valence electrons are the chemically reactive electrons. Each alkali metal has one valence electron (the ns^1 electron). The valence electron configuration is a function of the group in the periodic table. The valence electron configurations for each of the main group elements are:

Group	1	2	13	14	15	16	17	18
Number of valence electrons	1	2	3	4	5	6	7	8

Electron Configuration of Ions

Main group elements gain or lose electrons to achieve the electron configuration of the closest noble gas. For the third period of the periodic table:

Atom	Ion
Na $[Ne]3s^1$	Na^+ $[Ne]$
Mg $[Ne]3s^2$	Mg^{2+} $[Ne]$
Al $[Ne]3s^2 3p^1$	Al^{3+} $[Ne]$
Si $[Ne]3s^2 3p^2$ usually forms covalent compounds	

Atom	Ion
P [Ne]$3s^2 3p^3$	P^{3-} [Ne]$3s^2 3p^6$ = [Ar]
S [Ne]$3s^2 3p^4$	S^{2-} [Ne]$3s^2 3p^6$ = [Ar]
Cl [Ne]$3s^2 3p^5$	Cl^- [Ne]$3s^2 3p^6$ = [Ar]

Transition metal cations are different. The last electron that goes into a transition metal is a d electron. When ions form, the energy levels change in such a way that the (n + 1) s electrons are lost before the nd electrons. In the case of Fe^{3+}:

Fe [Ar]$4s^2 3d^6$ Fe^{3+} [Ar]$3d^5$

First the two 4s electrons are lost. Next one 3d electron is removed. For most of the transition metal cations, the electron configuration will be [NG]nd^x.

Each electron has a spin and functions as a tiny magnet. When two electrons are paired in an orbital, the two spins cancel each other out.

➤ Species with all electrons paired are diamagnetic and are repelled by a magnetic field.
➤ Species with unpaired electrons are paramagnetic and are attracted to a magnetic field.

PROBLEM: Which of the following atoms or ions are paramagnetic? Note: all the electrons in a noble gas configuration are paired.

N   Fe   Be S^{2-}

SOLUTION: The appropriate electron configurations are:

N	[He]↑↓ 2s	↑ ↑ ↑ 2p				three unpaired electrons paramagnetic 2s 2p
Fe	[Ar]↑↓ 4s	↑↓ ↑ ↑ ↑ ↑ 3d				four unpaired electrons paramagnetic 4s 3d
Be	[He]↑↓ 2s					zero unpaired electrons diamagnetic 2s
S^{2-}	[Ar]					zero unpaired electrons diamagnetic

All the electron configurations discussed previously are the most stable or ground state configurations for each atom or ion. If the correct amount of energy is supplied, an atom may enter an excited state with electrons in higher energy orbitals than the ground state. For example, the ground state and two excited states for an Fe atom are:

Fe [Ar]$4s^2 3d^6$ (ground state)
Fe [Ar]$4s^2 3d^5 4p^1$ (excited state)
Fe [Ar]$4s^0 3d^6 4p^2$ (excited state)

Atoms in excited states are not stable and will return to the ground state with a release of energy in the form of heat or light.

CHAPTER 11

The Periodic Table and Periodic Trends

Read This Chapter to Learn About

➤ The Periodic Table
➤ Atomic Radius
➤ Ionization Energy
➤ Electron Affinity
➤ Electronegativity

THE PERIODIC TABLE

The periodic table of the elements, first formulated by the Russian chemist Dmitry Mendeleyev, is a powerful and useful tool that organizes a large amount of information in a compact document. With increasing atomic number, certain properties of the elements repeat in a periodic pattern. The patterns are not as exact as a sine wave or the phases of the moon, to take two examples, but patterns are clearly seen. Chemistry students must be familiar with the parts of the periodic table (Figure 11.1). Periodic tables generally display the atomic number, the elemental symbol, and the average atomic mass for each element. The following figure shows the periodic table information for magnesium:

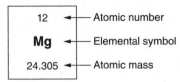

The shape and numbering scheme for a modern periodic table are shown in Figure 11.1. The rows of the table are called periods and are numbered from 1 to 7 from the top down. Columns in the table are called groups or families and are numbered from 1 to 18.

A line on the table under the boxes for B, Si, As, Te, and At separates the metals (to the left) from the nonmetals (to the right). The majority of the elements are metals. Metals form cations (positively charged ions), are good conductors of heat and electricity, tend to be shiny, and can be drawn into wires. Nonmetals tend to be dull, poor conductors, and brittle. Several elements have properties that are borderline between metallic and nonmetallic. These elements (B, Si, Ge, As, Sb, and Te) are called metalloids or semimetals. Note that these elements straddle the line that separates metals from nonmetals.

Periodic Table of the Elements

	1	2	3	4	5	6	7	8	9	10	11	12	13	14	15	16	17	18
1	1 **H** 1.0079																	2 **He** 4.0026
2	3 **Li** 6.941	4 **Be** 9.0122											5 **B** 10.81	6 **C** 12.011	7 **N** 14.007	8 **O** 15.999	9 **F** 18.998	10 **Ne** 20.179
3	11 **Na** 22.989	12 **Mg** 24.305											13 **Al** 26.981	14 **Si** 28.086	15 **P** 30.974	16 **S** 32.06	17 **Cl** 35.453	18 **Ar** 39.948
4	19 **K** 39.098	20 **Ca** 40.08	21 **Sc** 44.956	22 **Ti** 47.88	23 **V** 50.941	24 **Cr** 51.996	25 **Mn** 54.938	26 **Fe** 55.847	27 **Co** 55.933	28 **Ni** 58.69	29 **Cu** 63.546	30 **Zn** 65.38	31 **Ga** 59.72	32 **Ge** 72.59	33 **As** 74.922	34 **Se** 78.96	35 **Br** 79.904	36 **Kr** 83.80
5	37 **Rb** 85.468	38 **Sr** 87.62	39 **Y** 88.906	40 **Zr** 91.22	41 **Nb** 92.905	42 **Mo** 95.94	43 **Tc** (98)	44 **Ru** 101.07	45 **Rh** 102.91	46 **Pd** 106.42	47 **Ag** 107.87	48 **Cd** 112.41	49 **In** 114.82	50 **Sn** 118.69	51 **Sb** 121.75	52 **Te** 127.60	53 **I** 126.90	54 **Xe** 131.29
6	55 **Cs** 132.91	56 **Ba** 137.33	57 ***La** 138.90	72 **Hf** 178.49	73 **Ta** 180.95	74 **W** 183.85	75 **Re** 186.21	76 **Os** 190.2	77 **Ir** 192.22	78 **Pt** 195.08	79 **Au** 196.97	80 **Hg** 200.59	81 **Tl** 204.38	82 **Pb** 207.2	83 **Bi** 208.98	84 **Po** 209	85 **At** 210	86 **Rn** 222
7	87 **Fr** (223)	88 **Ra** 226.0	89 **#Ac** 227.03	104 **Rf** (261)	105 **Db** (262)	106 **Sg** (263)	107 **Bh** (262)	108 **Hs** (265)	109 **Mt** (266)	110 **Uun** (269)	111 **Uuu** (272)	112 **Unb** (277)						

* Lanthanides	58 **Ce** 140.12	59 **Pr** 140.91	60 **Nd** 144.24	61 **Pm** (145)	62 **Sm** 150.36	63 **Eu** 151.96	64 **Gd** 157.25	65 **Tb** 158.92	66 **Dy** 162.50	67 **Ho** 164.93	68 **Er** 167.26	69 **Tm** 168.93	70 **Yb** 173.04	71 **Lu** 174.97
# Actinides	90 **Th** 232.03	91 **Pa** 231.03	92 **U** 238.03	93 **Np** 237.05	94 **Pu** (244)	95 **Am** (243)	96 **Cm** (247)	97 **Bk** (247)	98 **Cf** (251)	99 **Es** (254)	100 **Fm** (257)	101 **Md** (257)	102 **No** (255)	103 **Lr** (256)

FIGURE 11.1 Periodic table.

The first two columns and the last six columns of the periodic table include what are called the main group elements. Columns 3 through 12 are called the transition metals. These metals are known for their multiple oxidation states and colored salts and solutions. The two rows separated from the main table beginning with Ce and Th are called the lanthanides and the actinides, respectively.

In addition to the divisions discussed previously, there are four groups whose names you should know:

- Group 1, the alkali metals, includes the common metals sodium and potassium.
- Group 2, the alkaline earth metals, includes magnesium and calcium.

➤ Group 17, the halogens, includes fluorine, chlorine, and bromine.
➤ Group 18, the noble gases, includes neon and argon.

Certain physical properties show periodic behavior when plotted against the atomic number; in other words, there is a repeating rise and fall in the values. The periodicity is not exact like a sine wave, but the trends are relatively clear and useful for predicting some chemical and physical behaviors of the elements.

ATOMIC RADIUS

Atomic radius is a measure of the size of an atom. The atomic radius is usually defined as one-half the distance between two atomic nuclei, which assumes that the atoms are spherical and are in physical contact with each other. The trend in atomic radii for main group elements is that the radii increase in size going down a column and the radii decrease in size going across a period from left to right. The increase as you go down a period is easily explained because the outermost electron is in an orbital with a larger value of n, meaning a bigger orbital. Li < Na < K < Rb < Cs because 2s < 3s < 4s < 5s < 6s.

There is a large jump in radius between a noble gas and the following alkali metal because the alkali metal introduces a new principal quantum number. For example, Ar [Ne]$3s^23p^6$ has a radius of 98 pm (1 pm = 10^{-12} m). K [Ar]$4s^1$ has a radius that is over twice this big, 227 pm, because the last electron added to K is in the 4s orbital.

For ions, the radii of cations of the same charge show a regular increase when going down a column. The same is true of anions of the same charge when going down a column. Both of these effects are due to the increasing size of the orbitals.

Li$^+$ (90 pm) < Na$^+$ (116 pm) < K$^+$ (153 pm) < Rb$^+$ (166 pm) < Cs$^+$ (181 pm)
F$^-$ (119 pm) < Cl$^-$ (167 pm) < Br$^-$ (182 pm) < I$^-$ (206 pm)

If you compare the radius of an ion to the radius of the atom from which that ion is derived, the cations are smaller than the parent atom because there is an excess of protons in the cation that can pull the electrons closer. Anions are larger than the parent atom because there is an excess of electrons over protons.

Na$^+$ (116 pm) < Na (186 pm)		Cl$^-$ (167 pm) > Cl (100 pm)	
11 p$^+$	11 p$^+$	17 p$^+$	17 p$^+$
10 e$^-$	11 e$^-$	18 e$^-$	17 e$^-$
[Ne]	[Ne]$3s^1$	[Ar]	[Ne]$3s^23p^5$

These effects are most prominent in highly charged ions. For example, B^{3+} (25 pm) is less than one-third the size of a B atom (85 pm).

Comparisons across a period are not valid because in a given period, both cations and anions are formed. A more apt comparison is that of isoelectronic ions, which are ions with the same number of electrons. For example, consider these ions, which all have the electron configuration of [Ne]:

Ion	Al^{3+} <	Mg^{2+} <	Na^+ <	F^- <	O^{2-} <	N^{3-}
p^+	13	12	11	9	8	7
e^-	10	10	10	10	10	10
Radius (pm)	68	86	116	119	126	132

If an element forms more than one cation, the cation with the higher charge will be smaller. Lead can form either a 2^+ or a 4^+ cation.

$$Pb^{4+} \ (92 \text{ pm}) < Pb^{2+} \ (133 \text{ pm})$$
$$82 \text{ p}^+ \qquad\qquad 82 \text{ p}^+$$
$$78 \text{ e}^- \qquad\qquad 80 \text{ e}^-$$

IONIZATION ENERGY

Ionization energy (IE) is defined as the energy required to remove an electron from an atom in the gas phase. Removing the first electron is the first ionization energy. Removing a second electron is the second ionization energy, and so on as long as there are electrons to remove.

$$Mg(g) \rightarrow Mg^+(g) + e^- \ \Delta E = \text{first ionization energy} = 737 \text{ kJ/mol}$$
$$Mg^+(g) \rightarrow Mg^{2+}(g) + e^- \ \Delta E = \text{second ionization energy} = 1451 \text{ kJ/mol}$$
$$Mg^{2+}(g) \rightarrow Mg^{3+}(g) + e^- \ \Delta E = \text{third ionization energy} = 7,732 \text{ kJ/mol}$$

The ionization energies increase in value as electrons are removed because as the positive charge increases, it becomes harder to remove a negatively charged electron. If a core electron is removed, there will be a large increase in the ionization energy. This is demonstrated for Mg. The second ionization energy is approximately double the first, but the third ionization energy is over five times as large as the second. Mg^{2+} has the electron configuration [Ne]. The third electron is removed from the neon core electrons.

In going down a group of the periodic table, the trend is that the first ionization energy decreases. This makes sense because the outer electrons are farther away from the nucleus in the elements lower in the table, and those electrons would be expected to be relatively easy to remove. As you go across the table from left to right, the general trend is for the first ionization energy to increase. There are some exceptions to this general trend that can be explained by considering the electron configuration of the elements.

ELECTRON AFFINITY

Electron affinity is defined as the energy change when an electron is added to an atom in the gas phase.

$$Cl(g) + e^- \rightarrow Cl^-(g) \ \Delta E = \text{Electron affinity} = -349 \text{ kJ/mol}$$

The electron affinity for Cl has a large negative value due to the fact that adding an electron is a favorable process because a noble gas configuration is formed. The halogens each form a noble gas electron configuration upon adding an electron, so atoms of each of these elements have large negative electron affinities. The trends in electron affinities are not as regular as those for atomic radii or first ionization energy. The electron affinities for noble gases are positive (+) because when an electron is added, the stable noble gas configuration is broken, an unfavorable process.

ELECTRONEGATIVITY

Electronegativity is an important periodic property that is used to understand bonding. Electronegativity is defined as the power of an atom in a compound to draw electrons to itself. Electronegativity tends to increase as you go up a group and as you cross a period from left to right. Electronegativity will be used extensively in the discussion of chemical bonding in the next chapter.

CHAPTER 12

Bonding

> ### Read This Chapter to Learn About
>
> ➤ Compounds, Molecules, and Ions
> ➤ Naming Compounds
> ➤ Chemical Bonding
> ➤ Covalent Bonds and Lewis Structures
> ➤ Resonance
> ➤ Polarity of Molecules

COMPOUNDS, MOLECULES, AND IONS

In this section we look in more detail at the types of possible compounds. Compounds are divided into two broad categories depending on the components that make up the sample. The two major classes of compounds are covalent compounds, which are formed by sharing electrons between atoms, and ionic compounds, which are made by transferring electrons from one atom to another. The covalent compounds are made up of collections of two or more atoms joined together in a unit called a molecule. Ionic compounds are made up of ions, which are charged particles.

In the chemical formula for a compound, the number of each type of atom present is shown by a subscript. If only one atom of a given element is present, the number 1 is omitted. Sometimes a group is placed in parentheses and given a subscript, for example, iron (II) nitrate, $Fe(NO_3)_2$, contains 1 Fe, 2 N, and 6 O.

You can determine whether a compound is covalent or ionic by looking at the formula.

Binary Compounds (Made of Two Elements)

➤ Two nonmetals: covalent; molecules—H_2O, SO_2, NCl_3, PF_3, P_4S_3, and SBr_2
➤ A metal and a nonmetal: ionic; ions—MgO, NaBr, CaF_2, $FeCl_3$, and Na_2S
➤ A metal and metal: metallic bonding

Compounds Containing More Than Two Elements

➤ Polyatomic ion present: ionic; ions—$Ca(NO_3)$, NH_4Cl, $Fe_3(PO4)_2$, and K_2CO_3

➤ All nonmetal: may be a molecular organic compound, which must contain carbon and may contain hydrogen and other elements.

NAMING COMPOUNDS

A number of conventions are used in naming binary covalent and ionic compounds. These conventions enable consistency in the naming of complex compounds.

Binary Covalent Compounds

In naming binary covalent compounds, the leftmost element in the periodic table is named first and the rightmost element last. If the two elements are in the same group, the lower element is named first. The format for the name is:

prefix + first element name + prefix + second element root + -*ide*

The prefix indicates the number of atoms in the molecule. If there is only one atom of the first element, the prefix (*mono-*) is excluded.

Prefix	mono-	di-	tri-	tetra-	penta-	hexa-
Number of atoms	1	2	3	4	5	6
Examples	CO	N_2O_4	NO_2	P_4S_3	CF_4	SF_6
Name	Carbon monoxide	Dinitrogen tetraoxide	Nitrogen dioxide	Tetraphosphorus trisulfide	Carbon tetrafluoride	Sulfur hexafluoride

Several compounds do not adhere to this system and have longstanding common names. Some of these include H_2O (water), NH_3 (ammonia), and NO (nitric oxide).

Ionic Compounds

In the process of forming a compound, if an atom gains one or more electrons, a negative ion or anion is formed. If an atom loses one or more electrons, a positive ion or cation is formed. Cations and anions are attracted to one another due to the opposite charges. The total number of cation positive charges must equal the total number of anion negative charges to make a neutral compound. The ions in an ionic crystal are arranged in a pattern like a three-dimensional checkerboard. A portion of the structure of sodium chloride is shown in the following figure (+ indicates cations, − indicates anions). Ions continue in the crystal up and down, right and left, and in front of and behind the page.

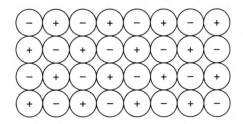

There is no molecule of sodium chloride in the structure. For ionic crystals, the smallest unit of the crystal that has the simplest whole number ratio of the ions is called the formula unit. Thus for sodium chloride, the formula unit consists of one sodium cation and one chloride anion.

For most of the main group elements, the charge formed by a monoatomic ion is related to the atom's position in the periodic table. Third-period elements are shown in the following table.

1	2	13	14	15	16	17	18
Na^+	Ca^{2+}	Al^{3+}	–	P^{3-}	O^{2-}	Cl^-	–

For the anions, the absolute value of the charge is the number of columns the element is to the left of the noble gases, Group 18. Group 14 elements tend to form covalent compounds instead of ionic compounds. (Sn and Pb may form ionic compounds with +2 or +4 charges.) Group 18, the noble gases, are not very reactive and do not form ions. The ions formed by transition metals are not so easily predicted, and some transition metals form ions of more than one charge (Fe^{2+} and Fe^{3+}). Most of the more common polyatomic ions are anions, with the main exception being the ammonium ion, NH^{4+}. Some of the more common polyatomic anions are NO_3^- (nitrate), SO_4^{2-} (sulfate), PO_4^{3-} (phosphate), OH^- (hydroxide), CO_3^{2-} (carbonate), and HCO_3^- (hydrogen carbonate).

Ionic compounds are made up of ions, and the compound must have no overall charge. The total positive charges are equal to the total negative charges. Examples are shown in the following table.

Cation	Anion	Ion	Ion	Formula
Calcium	Oxygen	Ca^{2+}	O^{2-}	CaO
Barium	Chlorine	Ba^{2+}	Cl^-	$BaCl_2$
Calcium	Nitrogen	Ca^{2+}	N^{3-}	Ca_3N_2
Iron (2+)	Chlorine	Fe^{2+}	Cl^-	$FeCl_2$
Iron (3+)	Chlorine	Fe^{3+}	Cl^-	$FeCl_3$
Calcium	Phosphate	Ca^{2+}	PO_4^{3-}	$Ca_3(PO_4)_2$
Ammonium	Nitrate	NH_4^+	NO_3^-	NH_4NO^3
Cobalt (2+)	Perchlorate	Co^{2+}	ClO_4^-	$Co(ClO_4)_2$

One way of obtaining the formula is to make the cation charge equal to the subscript on the anion and make the subscript on the cation equal to the charge on the anion, ignoring the negative sign. For ionic compounds, if a formula has a common factor in the subscripts, the common factor is divided out. Consider Ti^{4+} and O^{2-}. Crossing the charges gives Ti_2O_4. Dividing out the common factor of 2 gives TiO_2.

Ionic compounds are named simply by cation name plus anion name. The name of monoatomic cations is the element name. The sodium atom, Na, and sodium cation, Na^+, are both called sodium. Anions are named by a combination of the root of the element name plus the suffix *-ide*. Sulfur, S, becomes S^{2-}, sulfide; oxygen, O, becomes O^{2-}, oxide; nitrogen, N, becomes N^{3-}, nitride; and chlorine, Cl, becomes Cl^-, chloride.

Formula	Name
NaCl	Sodium chloride
$CaCl_2$	Calcium chloride
K_2O	Potassium oxide
Na_3N	Sodium nitride
$AlBr_3$	Aluminum bromide

A Roman numeral in parentheses is used for cations with more than one possible charge.

Formula	Ions Present	Name
$FeCl_2$	Two Cl^- ions are balanced by one Fe^{2+} ion	Iron (II) chloride
CoS	One S^{2-} ion is balanced by one Co^{2+} ion	Cobalt (II) sulfide
Cr_2O_3	Three O^{2-} ions are balanced by two Cr^{3+} ions	Chromium (III) oxide

With polyatomic ions, simply substitute the name of the polyatomic ion.

Formula	Name
$Ca(ClO_4)_2$	Calcium perchlorate
$Mg_3(PO_4)_2$	Magnesium phosphate
Rb_2SO_4	Rubidium sulfate
$(NH_4)_2C_2O_4$	Ammonium oxalate
$K_2Cr_2O_7$	Potassium dichromate
$Fe(NO_3)_3$	Iron (III) nitrate (Fe^{3+} balances three NO_3^- ions)
$CoSO_4$	Cobalt (II) sulfate (Co^{2+} balances one SO_4^{2-})
NH_4NO_2	Ammonium nitrite

CHEMICAL BONDING

There are three main types of chemical bonding:

➤ Ionic bonding occurs when electrons are transferred between atoms.
➤ Covalent bonding occurs when atoms share electrons between bonded atoms.
➤ In metallic bonding, fixed metal cations are surrounded by freely moving electrons.

Metallic bonding is important only for metals and a few compounds. Metals conduct electricity. Conduction occurs when charged particles can move through a continuous circuit. In the case of metals, the current is carried by freely moving electrons. Bonding in metals is described as metal cations in fixed positions surrounded by electrons that can move freely through the solid. Some chemists describe this as cations in a sea of electrons. This bonding explains many of the properties of metals discussed later.

Classifying Bond Types Based on Formulas

You can classify the type of bonding in different substances by considering the chemical formula of the substance:

Single Element in the Formula

➤ Metal element—metallic bonding
➤ Nonmetal element—covalent bonding (except noble gases = no bonding)
➤ Metalloid element—covalent or metallic bonding depending on the element and structure

Two Elements in the Formula (Binary Compound)

➤ Metal and metal—metallic bonding
➤ Metal and nonmetal—ionic bonding
➤ Nonmetal and nonmetal—covalent bonding

More Than Two Elements in the Formula

➤ Polyatomic ion present—ionic bonding
➤ All nonmetals, no polyatomic ion—covalent bonding

Most nonmetal elements exist as covalently bonded discrete molecules such as O_2, N_2, P_4, S_8, C_{60}, and Cl_2. Some nonmetals exist as network solids. These substances can be best described as giant molecules that are covalently bonded, forming one-, two-, or three-dimensional continuous networks. Examples of nonmetal elements that exist as network solids are Si, C (diamond), C (graphite), and As.

Polyatomic ions are covalently bonded within the ion, but they form ionic compounds with ions of opposite charge. Examples:

Formula	Type of Element(s)	Bonding
Fe	One metal	Metallic
Si	One metalloid	Covalent
Br_2	One nonmetal	Covalent
Ne	Nonmetal (noble gas)	No covalent bonding
KBr	Metal + nonmetal	Ionic

Formula	Type of Element(s)	Bonding
CO_2	Nonmetal + nonmetal	Covalent
$MgBr_2$	Metal + nonmetal	Ionic
$NaNO_3$	Polyatomic ion (NO_3^-)	Ionic
NH_4NO_3	Polyatomic ion(s) (NH_4^+, NO_3^-)	Ionic
NH_4Cl	Polyatomic ion (NH_4^+)	Ionic
$C_6H_{12}O_6$	Nonmetals (no polyatomic ions)	Covalent

Ionic Bonding

Ionic bonding is the electrical attraction between the positively charged cations and the negatively charged anions. The strength of an ionic bond is measured by the lattice energy, which is the energy released when gaseous ions condense into the ionic solid. The strength of an ionic bond depends on two main factors:

➤ Higher-charged ions form stronger ionic bonds.
➤ Smaller ions form stronger bonds due to the closer approach of the ions.

For example, magnesium oxide, MgO, has a lattice energy more than four times greater than that of NaF because the ions in MgO are 2+ and 2− and the ions in NaF are 1+ and 1−. MgO has a shorter interionic distance, allowing closer interaction of the ions. Both factors strengthen the electrical attraction between ions in MgO, as compared to NaF.

COVALENT BONDS AND LEWIS STRUCTURES

The American physicist Gilbert Newton Lewis first postulated that atoms share electrons so as to achieve a noble gas configuration, and that the electrons in molecules arrange into pairs of electrons. These pairs may be shared between two atoms (a bond pair) or belong to a single atom (a lone pair). Simple electron dot structures to indicate the distribution of electrons are called Lewis structures to honor Lewis's theory.

A simple Lewis structure for hydrogen shows a pair of shared electrons between two hydrogen atoms, H:H. These shared pairs of electrons are generally represented by a line standing for the two electrons forming the bond, H-H. Each hydrogen atom achieves the noble gas configuration of [He] by allowing the shared pair to count for both atoms.

A more complicated example is the Lewis structure of F_2. F has seven valence electrons. Two F atoms can contribute one electron each to the bond pair between the atoms. This gives both F atoms an octet or [Ne] configuration, as shown in the following figure.

$$:\ddot{F}\cdot \ + \ \cdot\ddot{F}: \ \longrightarrow \ :\ddot{F} \ — \ \ddot{F}:$$

Lewis Structures

1. Sum up the number of valence electrons contributed by each atom in the molecule or ion. The group number is equivalent to the number of valence electrons or the number of valence electrons plus 10. For anions, add an electron for each negative charge. For cations, subtract an electron for each positive charge.
2. Write the skeletal structure of the molecule or ion. Most structures have a single atom in the middle, which will be the least electronegative atom.
3. Using two valence electrons, form a bond from the central to the outer atoms.
4. Hydrogen is satisfied with two electrons, giving it a [He] electron configuration. For other elements, the octet rule applies. The octet rule states that an atom is most stable if there are eight electrons from the lone pairs and bond pairs surrounding the atom. Put lone pairs on the outer atoms first, and if electrons are left over, place lone pairs on the central atom. Do not use more electrons than the initial total.
5. Check that each nonhydrogen atom obeys the octet rule. If an atom has less than an octet, it may be necessary to convert a lone pair on an adjacent atom into a bond pair. This creates a four-electron double bond. Triple bonds are also possible.

Additional Rules

➤ Do not violate the octet rule for C, N, O, and F. (There are a few exceptions to this rule. For example, NO_2 has an odd number of electrons, and N will only have seven electrons around it.)

➤ Be and B may have less than an octet because they are not very electronegative. There are structures of Be and B that follow the octet rule, but do not move an electron from a very electronegative atom to Be or B just to meet the octet rule.

➤ Elements in the third period of the periodic table or below (such as P, S, Cl, and Br) may exceed the octet rule. Only exceed the octet rule if necessary or if a more reasonable formal charge results. (Formal charge is described later.)

➤ Some structures have more than one "central" atom. In these cases, apply the preceding rules to each atomic center.

Examples: All of the structures shown in the following figure follow the octet rule. The initial structures for SO_4^{2-} and ClO_2^- will be modified later to give more reasonable formal charges.

CH_4	NH_3	SO_4^{2-}	NH_4^+	ClO_2^-
1C = 4e⁻	1N = 5e⁻	1S = 6e⁻	1N = 5e⁻	1Cl = 7e⁻
4H = 4e⁻	3H = 3e⁻	4O = 24e⁻	4H = 4e⁻	2O = 12e⁻
		2- = 2e⁻	1+ = -1e⁻	1- = 1e⁻
8e⁻	8e⁻	32e⁻	8e⁻	20e⁻

The three examples in the following figure require formation of multiple bonds.

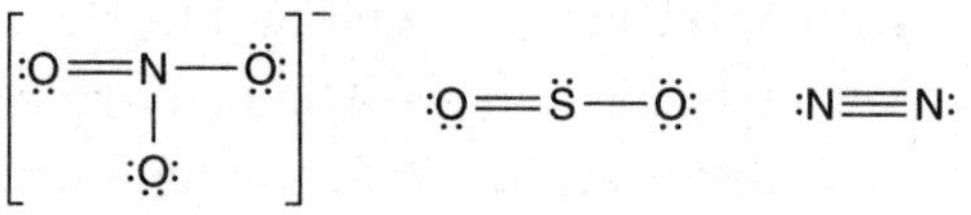

$$\left[:\ddot{O}=N-\ddot{O}: \atop \quad\;\; :\ddot{O}: \right]^{-} \qquad :\ddot{O}=\ddot{S}-\ddot{O}: \qquad :N\equiv N:$$

NO_3	SO_2	N_2
1N = 5e⁻	1S = 6e⁻	2N = 10e⁻
3O = 18e⁻	2O = 12e⁻	
1- = 1e⁻		
24e⁻	18e⁻	10e⁻

RESONANCE

In NO_3^- there are three choices for the oxygen atom to which the double bond is drawn. In SO_2 there are two choices. This choice is arbitrary. The three possible structures for a nitrate ion are shown in the following figure.

$$\left[\ddot{O}=N-\ddot{O}: \atop \quad\;\; :\ddot{O}: \right]^{-} \longleftrightarrow \left[:\ddot{O}-N-\ddot{O}: \atop \quad\;\; :\ddot{O}: \right]^{-} \longleftrightarrow \left[:\ddot{O}-N=\ddot{O} \atop \quad\;\; :\ddot{O}: \right]^{-}$$

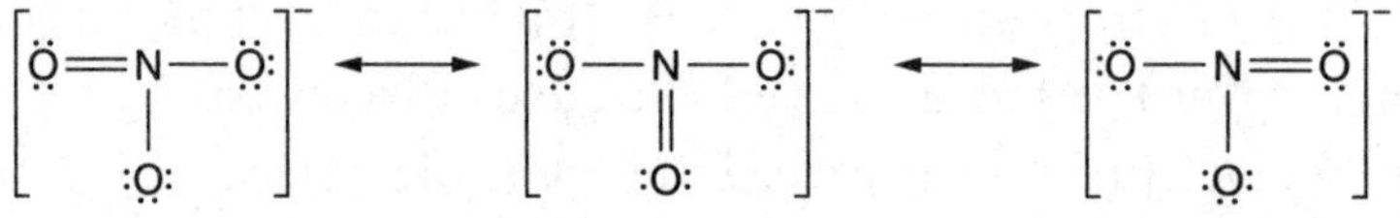

Each structure has two single bonds to O and one double bond to O. Structures such as these, which differ only by the distribution of electrons, are called resonance structures. The double-bond electrons are said to be delocalized over three atoms. A quantum chemical effect of delocalizing electrons throughout the molecule is that the structure is more stable than similar structures without resonance. The actual structure of NO_3^- is an average of all three structures called a resonance hybrid. Resonance "smears" the two electrons of the double bond throughout the molecule, making each N-O bond equivalent and effectively one and one-thirds bonds. The structure shown in the following figure attempts to represent the delocalization.

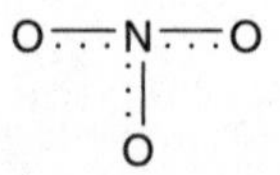

$$O\cdots N\cdots O \atop \quad\; O$$

Structures That Violate the Octet Rule

Some examples of Be and B compounds are shown in the following figure. The first two on the left have less than an octet, but the two on the right have an octet for Be or B.

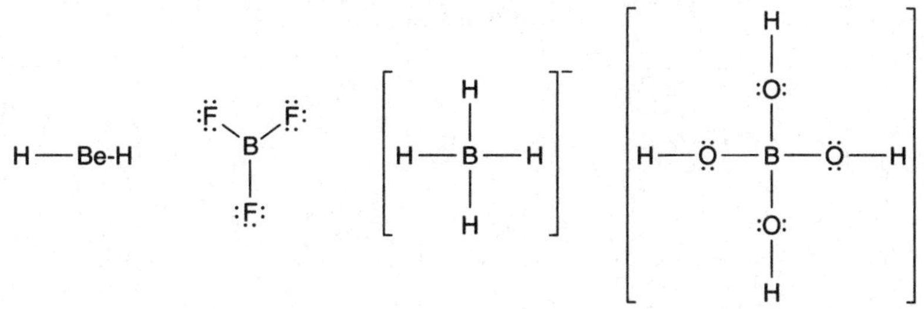

Some examples of hypervalent species (having more than an octet) are SF_4, PCl_5, XeF_4, and $BrCl_3$, shown in the following figure. The Lewis structures of these species can be constructed following the rules outlined previously. Xenon tetrafluoride is an example of a noble gas compound. The heavier noble gases Kr and Xe can form compounds with more reactive elements like oxygen and fluorine. The three lone pairs on each F and Cl have been omitted for clarity.

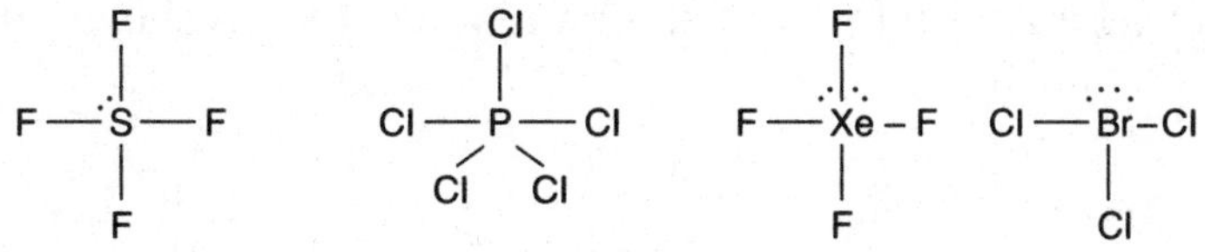

Formal Charge

There are three equivalent resonance structures for a nitrate ion. The energies of these three structures are equivalent and contribute equally to the total structure of the molecule. Some species such as the cyanate ion, OCN^-, have nonequivalent resonance structures. Three resonance structures for cyanate are shown in the following figure.

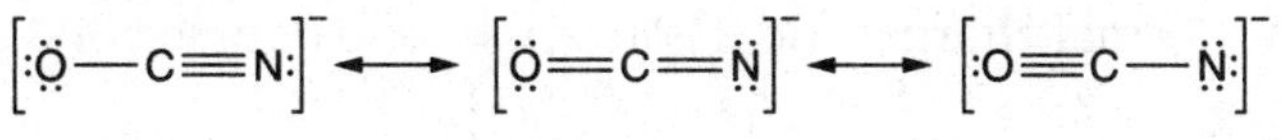

The energies of these three structures are different. Assigning formal charges is a way of measuring the number of electrons associated with a given atom in a compound relative to the number of valence electrons in the uncombined atom. Lone pair electrons belong to the atom on which they reside. Bond pair atoms are split equally between the two atoms sharing the bond.

Rules for Assigning Formal Charge

➤ Formal charge = valence electrons – [lone pair electrons + $\frac{1}{2}$ (bond pair electrons)]

➤ The sum of the formal charges must equal the overall charge. For neutral molecules the overall charge is zero.

➤ If several structures exist, the best structures are those with the fewest formal charges and with any negative charges on the more electronegative atoms. Charges of 2+ or higher on a single atom or 2− or lower on a single atom are unreasonable if there are resonance structures with charges closer to zero.

Look at the sulfate structure in the following figure.

The formal charges are:

$$S = 6 - \left[0 + \frac{1}{2}(8)\right] = +2$$

$$O = 6 - \left[6 + \frac{1}{2}(2)\right] = -1$$

Formal charges are indicated on structures with the formal charge next to the atom. The sum of the formal charges equals −2, the overall charge. In this structure, every atom has a formal charge. S has a 2+ charge. A better structure is obtained if a double bond is made between the sulfur atom and an oxygen atom as shown in the following figure.

$$S = 6 - \left[0 + \frac{1}{2}(10)\right] = +1$$

$$O(A) = 6 - \left[4 + \frac{1}{2}(4)\right] = 0$$

$$O(B) = 6 - \left[6 + \frac{1}{2}(2)\right] = -1$$

One less atom has a formal charge, and S is +1. A second double bond gives:

$$S = 6 - \left[0 + \frac{1}{2}(12)\right] = 0$$

$$O(A) = 6 - \left[4 + \frac{1}{2}(4)\right] = 0$$

$$O(B) = 6 - \left[6 + \frac{1}{2}(2)\right] = -1$$

For a −2 ion, as shown in the following figure, two atoms each with a −1 charge is the best possible structure you can draw. The addition of double bonds also allows for resonance structures, which add stability that more than makes up for violating the octet rule.

PROBLEM: Assign formal charges to the cyanate ion to determine the best structure (see the following figure):

$$:\ddot{O}-C\equiv N: \quad \longleftrightarrow \quad \ddot{O}=C=\ddot{N} \quad \longleftrightarrow \quad :O\equiv C-\ddot{N}:$$
$$\ominus \qquad\qquad\qquad \ominus \qquad\qquad \oplus \qquad ②-$$

SOLUTION:

$$O = 6 - \left[6 + \frac{1}{2}(2)\right] = -1 \qquad O = 6 - \left[4 + \frac{1}{2}(4)\right] = 0 \qquad O = 6 - \left[2 + \frac{1}{2}(6)\right] = +1$$

$$C = 4 - \left[0 + \frac{1}{2}(8)\right] = 0 \qquad C = 4 - \left[0 + \frac{1}{2}(8)\right] = 0 \qquad C = 4 - \left[0 + \frac{1}{2}(8)\right] = 0$$

$$N = 5 - \left[2 + \frac{1}{2}(6)\right] = 0 \qquad N = 5 - [4 + (4)] = -1 \qquad N = 5 - \left[6 + \frac{1}{2}(2)\right] = -2$$

The right structure is least stable because it has two atoms with formal charge, one of which is 2–. The center and left structures differ in that the –1 charge is either on N or O. The O atom is more electronegative than N, so the best structure is the one on the left.

Valence Shell Electron Pair Repulsion (VSEPR) and Molecular Shape

A Lewis structure simply gives the correct distribution of electrons and bonded atoms but does not describe the molecular geometry. A simple way to determine the shape is the valence shell electron pair repulsion (VSEPR) model, in which electrons are distributed to minimize repulsions between pairs of electrons on the center atom. To assign a VSEPR shape:

1. Obtain a valid Lewis structure.
2. Assign effective electron pairs to the bonds and lone pairs about the central atom. An effective pair of electrons is defined as either:
    ➤ A lone pair (2 electrons)
    ➤ A single bond pair (2 electrons)
    ➤ A double bond (4 electrons)
    ➤ A triple bond (6 electrons)
    Another possible name used for an effective electron pair is the steric number. Electrons in multiple bonds occupy the same region in space, so these electrons (for VSEPR purposes) are counted as effectively a single electron pair.
3. Count the number of effective electron pairs about an atom. These electrons will be arranged in geometries according to the table in Figure 12.1. The central atom is A and the attached atoms are B in the molecular structures. Atoms in the plane of the page are shown with a regular line. Atoms above the plane of the page are shown with a wedged line. Atoms that are behind the plane of the page are shown with a dashed wedge.

Effective electron pairs	Geometry	Structure	Angles	Examples
2	Linear	B—A—B	180°	CO_2, OCN^-
3	Trigonal planar	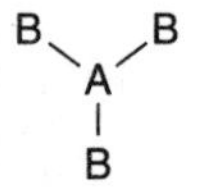 B, B / A / B	120°	NO_3^-, BF_3, SO_3
4	Tetrahedral	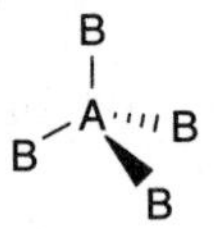 B / A / B B B	109.5°	CH_4, SO_4^{2-}, XeO_4
5	Trigonal bipyramidal	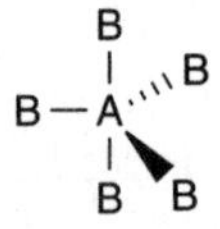 B / B—A—B / B B	120°, 180°, 90°	PF_5, SF_5^+
6	Octahedral	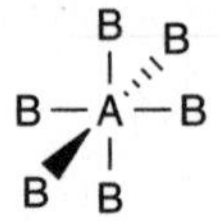 B B / B—A—B / B B	180°, 90°	SF_6, BrF_6^-

FIGURE 12.1 Important molecular geometries.

The effect of lone pairs can be seen in the structures of CH_4, NH_3, and H_2O, which have a tetrahedral arrangement of effective electron pairs. Removing the lone pairs yields the molecular shape. The bond angle is reduced because the relative sizes of the effective electron pairs about the central atom are lone pair > triple bond > double bond > single bond. Figure 12.1 summarizes what is important to know regarding molecular geometries.

The following figures show some common molecular shapes:

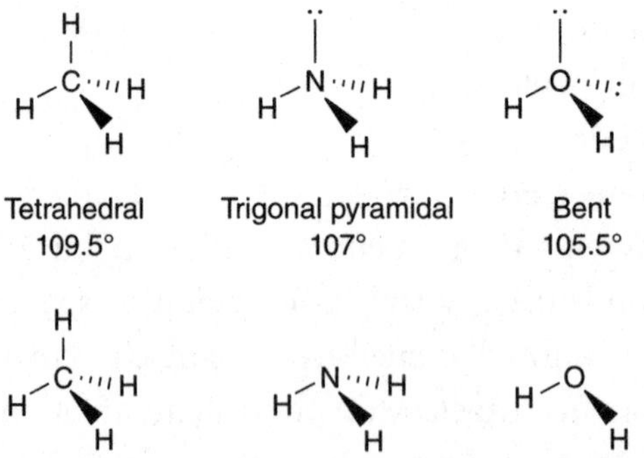

Tetrahedral 109.5°	Trigonal pyramidal 107°	Bent 105.5°

The most common shapes encountered when applying the VSEPR method are shown in Figure 12.2.

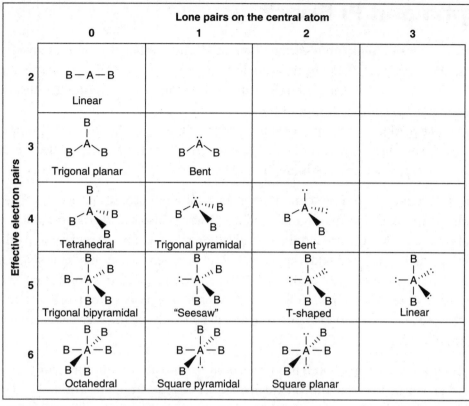

FIGURE 12.2 Common shapes encountered using VSEPR method.

The following figures show a few examples of Lewis structures and the predicted molecular shapes. The three lone pairs on each external F and Cl have been omitted for clarity. Note that the Lewis structures may not necessarily be a good indicator of the actual shape.

Effective electron pairs	6	3	3
Lone pairs	2	0	1
Shape	Square planar	Trigonal planar	Bent

Effective electron pairs	5	5	4
Lone pairs	2	0	0
Shape	T-shape	Trigonal pyramidal	Tetrahedral

Sigma and Pi Bonds

One more topic of discussion regarding bonding is the overlap of orbitals. Consider the bonding in a molecule of H_2. In this simple example we have both $1s^1$ electrons being shared. In order to do so, the s orbitals of the two H atoms must overlap. This overlap is called a sigma (σ) bond. This type of bond is not limited to just s orbitals, as the overlap of an s and a p orbital, or p and p orbitals, will yield the same sigma bond. Examples of these are the overlap of an s orbital and p orbital in HBr or the overlap of two p orbitals between the carbon atoms in ethane, H_3C-CH_3.

The hybridization of an atom can arrange for additional orbitals to overlap. The first orbitals to overlap will form a sigma bond. But there is also the overlap of additional p orbitals that were not involved in the hybridization process. The second set of p orbitals to overlap will create a pi bond, the second bond between two atoms. This stems from the sp^2 hybridization of the carbon atom (one s and two p orbitals combine to form a trigonal planar set of orbitals). However, there is still one more set of p orbitals that did not hybridize and can overlap to form the first pi bond. This is the case between the carbon atoms in ethene, H_2C=CH_2.

Should a third bond (triple bond) be formed between two atoms, another pair of p orbitals need to overlap to create the second pi bond. This stems from one s orbital and one p orbital hybridizing to form an sp hybridized carbon atom. There are still two untouched p orbitals about the carbon atoms that will form the two pi bonds between the atoms. This is the case between the two carbon atoms in ethyne, HC≡CH. More of this topic will be covered in Chapter 19.

POLARITY OF MOLECULES

Once the shape of a molecule is known, the polarity of the molecule may be determined. A molecule is polar if there is a separation between the center of the positive charge and the center of the negative charge. Polar molecules have a permanent dipole, which points in the direction from the center of positive charge toward the center of negative charge. The polarity can be determined by considering the sum of the bond polarities.

The polarity of the bond is determined by the difference in electronegativities of the atoms in the bond:

➤ A difference of 0.0 to 0.4 is considered a nonpolar covalent bond.
➤ A difference of 0.5 to 1.7 is considered a polar covalent bond.
➤ A difference of 1.8 or greater is considered an ionic bond.

These numbers are estimates for the boundary between the bond types.

Bond polarity is due to unequal sharing of electrons. The more electronegative atom develops less than a full negative charge, indicated by a δ^-. The less electronegative atom develops less than a full positive charge, indicated by a δ^+. The bond polarity can be represented by a bond vector from the less electronegative to the more electronegative atom that is proportional to the difference in electronegativity. Bond polarity should not be confused with molecular polarity, which applies to the entire molecule. The bond vector for HF is shown in the following figure. With only one bond, the bond vector is also the dipole.

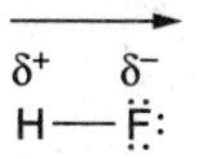

$$\overrightarrow{\underset{H-\ddot{F}:}{\underset{\delta^+ \quad \delta^-}{}}}$$

The electronegativities of selected elements are given in the following table for use in determining bond polarity and molecular polarity. When considering the difference in electronegativity, the absolute value of the difference is used.

$H = 2.1$	$C = 2.5$	$N = 3.0$	$O = 3.5$	$F = 4.0$
$Li = 0.9$	$Si = 1.8$	$P = 2.1$	$S = 2.5$	$Cl = 3.0$

PROBLEM: Classify the bond polarity of the following bonds: Li-F, C-H, C-O, P-S, C-F, O-H, and N-Cl.

SOLUTION:

Elements	First	Second	Difference	Type
Li-F	0.9	4.0	3.1	Ionic
C-H	2.5	2.1	0.4	Nonpolar covalent
C-O	2.5	3.5	1.0	Polar covalent
P-S	2.1	2.5	0.4	Nonpolar covalent
C-F	2.5	4.0	1.5	Polar covalent
O-H	3.5	2.1	1.4	Polar covalent
N-Cl	3.0	3.0	0.0	Nonpolar covalent

To determine whether a molecule is polar, obtain a valid VSEPR structure. Draw bond vectors in space along the bonds for each polar bond in the molecule.

➤ If there are no vectors because all the bonds are nonpolar, the molecule is nonpolar.
➤ If there are polar bonds, add the vectors in space. If the vectors cancel out, the molecule is nonpolar. If the vectors do not cancel out, the molecule is polar and the dipole is in the direction of the vector sum.
➤ There are a limited number of ways that bond vectors can interact. The following vector combinations will cancel out:
  ➤ Two equivalent vectors at 180°, such as in CO_2
  ➤ Three equivalent vectors at 120°, such as in SO_3
  ➤ Four equivalent vectors at 109.5°, such as in CH_4

The molecular shape and partial charges are shown on the left in the following figures (lone pair electrons except those on the central atom are omitted), and the bond vectors are shown on the right for some nonpolar molecules. XeF_4, shown in the following figure, is square planar, and the two pairs of Xe-F bonds at 180° cancel out in pairs.

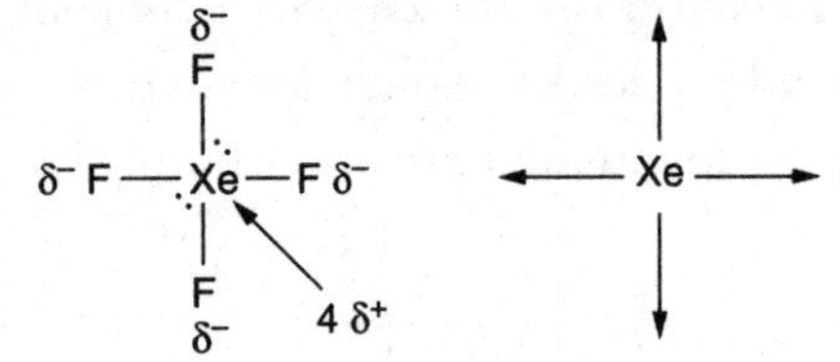

PF_5, shown in the following figure, has two P-F bond vectors at 180° that cancel each other out. There are also three bond vectors at 120° that cancel out.

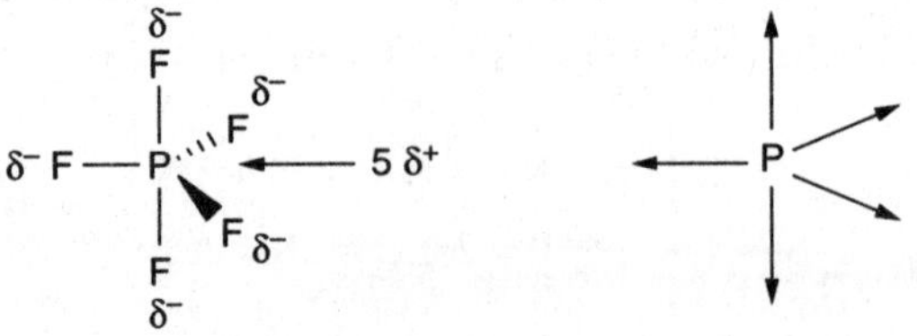

The following figure shows some examples of polar molecules. Lone pairs except those on the central atom have been omitted. NH_3 is trigonal pyramidal because of the lone pair on nitrogen. The bond vectors point towards the nitrogen. The net result of the three N-H bonds is a dipole pointing away from the nitrogen, on the side opposite the hydrogens. This molecule is polar.

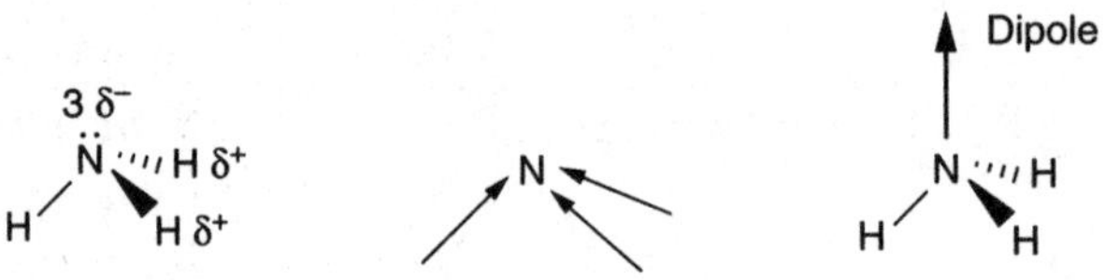

SF_4, shown in the following figure, has a seesaw shape. The two S-F vectors at 180° (A and B) cancel each other out, but the two at 120° (C and D) are not canceled, and the molecule is polar.

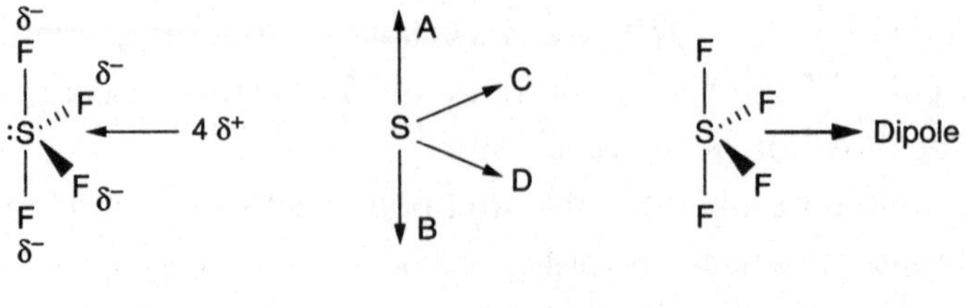

In conclusion, after achieving the correct electron pair geometry, it is important to achieve the correct molecular geometry so that the overall dipole moment can be determined.

CHAPTER 13

Gases, Liquids, and Solids

Read This Chapter to Learn About
➤ Matter and Change
➤ Gases
➤ Kinetic Molecular Theory
➤ Intermolecular Forces of Solids and Liquids
➤ Liquids
➤ Solids

MATTER AND CHANGE

Chemistry is defined as the science of matter. Matter is defined as anything that has mass and occupies space. The concept of matter may easily be visualized by considering the three states of matter: solid, liquid, and gas. You will be familiar with these states, and you can conclude that all the material that makes up our universe is matter, including air, steel, bricks, our bodies, dirt, wood, copper, gold, aluminum, water, and so on. Chemistry is concerned primarily with three aspects of matter:

➤ The physical and chemical properties of matter
➤ The physical and chemical changes that matter undergoes
➤ The energy transfer associated with these changes

Properties of matter are divided into physical properties, such as color, electrical conductivity, shape, hardness, density, melting point, and ductility. These properties are further divided into quantitative (those with an associated number), such as a boiling point of 78.5°C or a density of 2.70 g/mL, and qualitative (having no associated number), such as color or ductility (that is, the ability to be drawn into a wire). Chemical properties are the possible chemical reactions that a substance undergoes, such as flammability or the ability of a metal to react with an acid to produce hydrogen gas.

Associated with physical and chemical properties are physical and chemical changes. Physical changes are changes in matter in which only the form changes while the chemical makeup remains intact. Changes of state such as boiling, freezing, melting, sublimation, and condensation are examples. In contrast, a chemical change (or chemical reaction) requires a change in chemical composition. An example of a chemical reaction is the combination of hydrogen gas and oxygen gas to form liquid water.

Chemistry involves three levels of description of matter:

➤ **Macroscopic:** processes that can be seen by the normal senses
➤ **Microscopic:** explanations of macroscopic observations in terms of atoms, molecules, and ions
➤ **Symbolic:** representing atoms, molecules, and ions with chemical symbols

PROBLEM: Give macroscopic, microscopic, and symbolic descriptions for the formation of water.

SOLUTION:

➤ Macroscopic: Clear, colorless hydrogen and oxygen gases combine to form colorless liquid water.
➤ Microscopic: Diatomic hydrogen molecules combine with diatomic oxygen molecules in a ratio of 2:1 (hydrogen:oxygen) to produce triatomic water molecules.
➤ Symbolic (chemical symbols): $2H_2(g) + O_2(g) \rightarrow 2H_2O(l)$

The path from macroscopic observations to microscopic explanations aided by symbolic representation mirrors the steps of the scientific method. To have a good grasp of chemistry, you must be able to think on all three levels (macroscopic, microscopic, and symbolic) and be able to convert between the three representations.

Matter may be classified by the chemical composition of a sample. A broad division is between matter that has a fixed composition (pure substances) and matter that may have a variation in composition (mixtures). Mixtures may be either heterogeneous (clear phases can be seen by the eye or a microscope) or homogeneous (the matter consists of one continuous phase). Homogeneous mixtures are also called solutions. Heterogeneous mixtures may be separated into homogeneous mixtures by physical methods. A homogeneous mixture may be further separated into the pure substances that it is composed of by physical means. Pure substances come in two forms: elements and compounds. Elements cannot be broken down into simpler substances by chemical means. Elements consist of only one type of atom. Compounds are pure substances that can be separated into elements by chemical methods. Compounds contain two or more atoms combined in a fixed ratio. Figure 13.1 illustrates the relationships between the various classifications of matter.

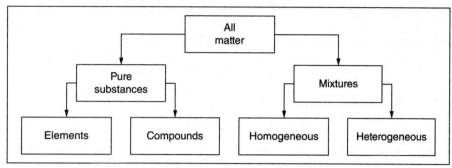

FIGURE 13.1 Classification of matter.

GASES

Gases are easier to study than solids or liquids because the molecules of gases are well separated from one another. In solids and liquids, the molecules are in contact. The equations that describe the behavior of gases are similar for all gases as long as the temperature is not too low or the pressure is not too high. Gases under these conditions are described as ideal gases.

One variable used in describing the state of a gas is pressure, which is defined as the force exerted per unit area. The most common unit of pressure is the atmosphere (atm), equivalent to the average pressure of the earth's atmosphere at sea level. Pressure is also measured by the length of a column of mercury that can be supported by the atmosphere in an inverted tube. A pressure of 1 atm can support a column of 760 mm mercury. A pressure of 1 mm of mercury is also called a torr. The equation 1 atm = 760 torr = 760mm Hg is used often in working problems with gases. The official unit for pressure in the SI system is the Pascal: $Pa = N/m^2$. The conversion factor from atm to kPa is 1 atm = 101.325 kPa. Temperature for gases must usually be given in Kelvin. The conversion from Celsius to Kelvin is K = °C + 273.15. For most purposes, °C + 273 is adequate.

The variables in the state of a gas—volume, pressure, and so on—are related in ways that are either direct variations or inverse variations or proportions.

➤ In a direct variation, an increase in one variable results in an increase in the other. If y varies directly with x, then, $y = ax$, where a is a constant.
➤ In an inverse variation, an increase in one variable results in a decrease in the other. If y varies inversely with x, then, $y = \dfrac{b}{x}$, where b is a constant. An inverse variation can also represented as $xy = b$.

The graph of a direct variation is shown on the left, and the graph of an inverse variation is shown on the right in the following figure.

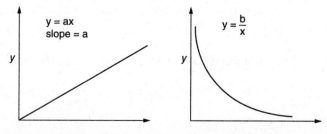

Three relationships discovered early in the study of gases are:

➤ **Boyle's law.** Volume (V) varies inversely with pressure (P).

$$V = \frac{constant}{P} \text{ or } PV = constant$$

➤ **Charles's law.** Volume varies directly with absolute (Kelvin) temperature (T).

$$V = constant \times T$$

➤ **Avogadro's law.** Volume varies directly with moles (n) of gas.

$$V = constant \times n$$

In each of these laws, variables not given in the equation are constant. For example, when using Boyle's law, the temperature and number of moles of gas are constant. You can rewrite these laws in a more convenient form by eliminating the constant of proportionality. For Boyle's law, consider two states of a gas:

$$P_1 V_1 = constant \text{ and } P_2 V_2 = constant, \text{ so } P_1 V_1 = P_2 V_2$$

In a similar way, Charles's law can be written as follows:

$$\frac{V_1}{T_1} = \frac{V_2}{T_2}$$

and Avogadro's law becomes:

$$\frac{V_1}{n_1} = \frac{V_2}{n_2}$$

These relationships can be used to evaluate the effect on one variable when another changes.

> **PROBLEM:** A sample of 34.0 L of helium at 0°C is heated to 75°C. If the pressure and number of moles of helium are fixed, what is the new volume?

> **SOLUTION:**

$$V_2 = ?$$
$$T_1 = 0 + 273 = 273 \text{ K}$$
$$T_2 = 75 + 273 = 348 \text{ K}$$
$$\frac{V_1}{T_1} = \frac{V_2}{T_2}$$
$$\frac{34.0 \text{ liters}}{273 \text{ K}} = \frac{x}{348 \text{ K}} = 43.3 \text{ liters}$$

The next thing is to ask if this answer makes sense. If the temperature increased, so should the volume. Sure enough, the volume increased from 34.0 L to 43.3 L.

These three laws can be combined into one general law called the ideal gas law:

$$PV = nRT$$

The quantity R is known as the ideal gas constant. $R = 0.08206 \, L \times atm/mol \times K$. When using this value of the ideal gas constant, volume must be in L, pressure in atm, and temperature in K.

PROBLEM: A 10.00 L flask contains 1.00 mol of neon. What is the pressure of the gas at 25°C? (25°C = 298 K)

SOLUTION:

$$P = \frac{nRT}{V}$$

$$P = \frac{(1.00 \, \text{mol})(0.08206 \, L \times atm/mol \times K)(298K)}{(10.00L)} = 2.45 \, atm$$

The ideal gas law contains moles, so stoichiometry problems with gases are possible.

PROBLEM: If 2.00 g of Mg (molar mass 24.305 g/mol) is reacted with excess hydrochloric acid, what volume of hydrogen gas is produced at 40°C at a pressure of 700 torr?

SOLUTION:

$$700 \, torr \times \frac{1 \, atm}{760 \, torr} = 0.921 \, atm$$

$$40°C + 273 = 313K$$

$Mg(s) + 2HCl(g) \rightarrow MgCl_2(aq) + H_2(g)$, so g of Mg → mol of Mg → mol of H_2 → V of H_2

$$2.00g \, Mg \times \frac{1 \, mol \, mg}{24.305 \, g \, Mg} \times \frac{1 \, mol \, H_2}{1 \, mol \, Mg} = 0.0823 \, mol \, H_2$$

$$PV = nRT$$

$$V = \frac{nRT}{P}$$

$$P = \frac{(0.0823 \, mol)(0.08206 \, L \times atm/mol \times K)(313 \, K)}{(0.921 \, atm)} = 2.30 \, L$$

Gases and Molar Masses

The number of moles of a substance is determined by dividing the mass of the substance, m, by the molar mass, M (a script M is used to prevent confusion with molarity). Substituting m/M for the number of mol, n, in the ideal gas law gives $PV = (m/M)(RT)$, which can be rearranged to: $PM = (m/V)RT$. The quantity m/V is simply the density, so the previous equation becomes $PM = dRT$. This equation may be used to determine the molar mass of a gas.

Dalton's Law of Partial Pressures

In a mixture of gases, the gas molecules are well separated, ideally. There is little interaction between the molecules of the different gases. Because of this lack of interaction, each gas behaves as if it were in the container by itself. For each gas in a mixture, the partial pressure, P_{total}, of the gas is calculated as if the gas were the only gas present. Dalton's law of partial pressures states that the total pressure of a mixture of gases is the sum of the partial pressures of all the gases in the mixture. This can be simply seen in the equation: $P_{total} = P_{gas1} + P_{gas2} + P_{gas3} \ldots$ Consider a container that has a mixture of hydrogen and helium gas, the two most ideal gases. If the pressure of the helium gas is 500 torr and the pressure of the hydrogen gas is 250 torr, what would the total pressure be? Using Dalton's law of partial pressures, the total pressure would be the sum of these individual pressures, 750 torr. The concept can also be used to find the partial pressure of an individual gas.

> **PROBLEM:** Write an equation for the partial pressures of a mixture of argon and fluorine gas. If the total pressure in the container is 900 torr and the partial pressure of the fluorine gas is 560 torr, what is the partial pressure of the argon gas?

> **SOLUTION:** The equation is $P_{total} = P_{F2} + P_{Ar}$. The total pressure of 900 torr minus the partial pressure of the fluorine gas, 560 torr, gives the pressure of the argon gas, 340 torr.

> **PROBLEM:** A container is 18% filled with oxygen gas, 32% filled with neon gas, and 50% filled with chlorine gas. If the total pressure inside the container is 760 torr, what is the partial pressure of each gas?

> **SOLUTION:**
>
> $(0.18)(760) = 136.8$ torr is the pressure of the oxygen gas.
> $(0.32)(760) = 243.2$ torr is the pressure of the neon gas.
> $(0.50)(760) = 380$ torr is the pressure of the chlorine gas.

KINETIC MOLECULAR THEORY

In the preceding discussion of gases, the macroscopic properties of gases such as pressure, temperature, and volume were described. The behavior of gases is explained on the molecular level by the kinetic molecular theory, which has the following postulates:

➤ Particles of gases are separated from one another by large distances when compared to the size of the particles.
➤ Particles of a gas are in constant and random motion.
➤ When the particles of a gas collide with other particles or the sides of the container, no energy is lost; the collisions are elastic.
➤ The particles exert neither repulsive nor attractive forces on one another.
➤ The average kinetic energy of gas particles is directly proportional to the absolute temperature in Kelvin.

The first four points are relatively clear and explain many of the properties of gases such as compressibility, pressure, and the similar behavior of different gases. The last point is important because it means that regardless of the gases involved, at the same temperature all gases have the same average kinetic energy. The last point can also be taken as a definition of temperature.

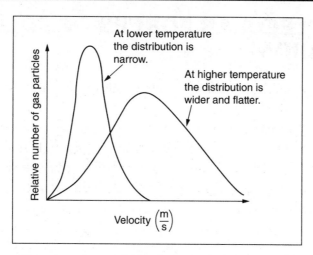

FIGURE 13.2 Distribution of velocities of gas molecules.

In a large sample of a gas such as oxygen there is a distribution of velocities. As the temperature increases, the speeds of the oxygen molecules shift to greater velocities and the distribution curve skews to higher velocities. A sample distribution of oxygen molecules at two temperatures is shown in Figure 13.2. At the higher temperature the distribution broadens and flattens.

The average kinetic energy of an individual molecule of a gas is given by $KE = \frac{1}{2}mu^2$, where u^2 is the average of the squares of the velocities of the molecules. The kinetic molecular theory states that the average kinetic energy is proportional to the temperature in Kelvin. The constant of proportionality for one mole of gas is $\frac{3}{2}RT$. With a little manipulation of the previous two equations, we can see that the root mean square velocity is:

$$u_{rms} = \sqrt{\frac{3RT}{M}}$$

In order to obtain the velocity in m/s, the gas constant must be R = 8.314 J/mol K and the molar mass must be given in kg/mol. (Simply divide the molar mass in g/mol by 1,000.) The quantity u is the root mean square velocity, which is an average velocity for a gas molecule. This quantity increases with temperature for a given gas. If two gases are compared at the same temperature, the velocity of the more massive gas will be smaller.

PROBLEM: Calculate the u_{rms} velocities of O_2 (molar mass = 32.00 g/mol) and Br_2 (molar mass = 159.8 g/mol) at 25°C.

SOLUTION:

$$U_{rms}O_2 = \sqrt{\frac{3 \cdot \dfrac{8.134\ J}{mol\ K}}{0.03200\ kg/mol}}$$

$$U_{rms}Br_2 = \sqrt{\frac{3 \cdot \dfrac{8.134\ J}{mol\ K}}{0.1598\ kg/mol}}$$

The Br_2 travels much more slowly than the lighter O_2 molecules.

INTERMOLECULAR FORCES OF SOLIDS AND LIQUIDS

All gases, if at low enough pressure and high enough temperature, behave in a similar fashion regardless of the composition of the gas. The much larger relative volumes of gases mean that gas particles (atoms or molecules) are well separated from one another. In solids and liquids, the particles are in contact. In liquids the particles can move freely about. In solids the particles vibrate about fixed positions. The behavior of solids and liquids depends upon the forces involved in the interactions of the particles. There are three types of intermolecular forces (interatomic for noble gases) present in solids and liquids:

➤ Nonpolar molecules and isolated atoms interact through London dispersion forces (also called van der Waals forces).
➤ Polar molecules interact through dipole-dipole forces.
➤ Certain molecules that contain hydrogen bound to the more electronegative elements (O, N, and F) interact with especially strong dipole-dipole interactions called hydrogen bonds.

London dispersion forces arise from a temporary asymmetric distribution of electrons in a molecule or atom. The random motion of electrons in a nonpolar species occasionally creates an instantaneous dipole, which is a temporary separation of positive and negative charge. Another instantaneous dipole will be induced in an adjacent molecule, creating a weak electrical attraction. London forces are the weakest intermolecular forces. The importance of London forces depends on how easily the electron cloud about the atom in a molecule can be deformed. This property is called polarizability. Polarizability increases as the total number of electrons and size of the atoms in the molecule increase. London forces increase with molar mass for molecules or atoms of similar structure and size. London forces are present in all matter, but they are important only if stronger interactions are not possible.

Polar molecules have permanent dipoles. Each molecule has a separation of positive charge from negative charge. In polar solids or liquids, the positive end of one molecule will interact through electrical attraction with the negative part of an adjacent molecule.

If hydrogen is bound to a highly electronegative atom such as nitrogen, oxygen, or fluorine, the hydrogen develops a slight positive charge. The positive hydrogen atom will be strongly attracted to the lone pair of highly electronegative atoms creating a hydrogen bond, which is an especially strong dipole-dipole interaction. Hydrogen-bonded compounds tend to have unusually high boiling points when compared to substances of similar molar masses that do not take part in hydrogen bonding. Hydrogen bonds are also important in water and in biological molecules such as proteins, DNA, and carbohydrates. Some examples of hydrogen bonds formed by water and urea are shown as dotted lines in the following figure.

The relative strengths of interparticle forces are as follows:

hydrogen bonds > dipole-dipole forces > London dispersion forces

LIQUIDS

Liquids can best be described as consisting of molecules in contact with one another but able to move randomly through the bulk of the liquid. Liquids have short-range order, but long-range disorder. Several physical properties are used to characterize liquids.

Viscosity is the resistance of a liquid to flow. Viscosity is high for substances with stronger intermolecular forces. The viscosity of gasoline is less than that of water, which is in turn less than that of honey due to the strong hydrogen bonding in water. The internal molecules of a liquid interact evenly in all directions with the other molecules of the liquid. Molecules on the surface interact with other molecules on the surface and within the liquid. Because there are no molecules above surface molecules, the uneven forces tend to draw surface molecules into the bulk of the liquid. The energy required to increase the surface area of a liquid is called the surface tension. The stronger the intermolecular forces, the higher the surface tension. Insects such as water bugs can be supported on the surface of water because of its high surface tension. In a small-diameter tube made of a substance to which a liquid is attracted (such as water in a thin glass tube), the liquid will tend to be drawn into the tube until the force of gravity stops the rise of the liquid. This tendency for water to rise in a thin tube is called capillary action. Capillary action is important in plants to draw water into the leaves against gravity.

Phase Changes

At any given temperature a fraction of the molecules will have sufficient energy to escape from the liquid phase to the gas phase. In an open container with a constant temperature the entire liquid will evaporate. In a closed container, at first molecules will leave the liquid faster than gaseous molecules return to the liquid. Over time the rate of molecules going from the liquid to the gas phase will equal the rate of gaseous molecules returning to the liquid. This is a dynamic equilibrium state. Both processes continue, but there will be no net change in the number of gas molecules above the liquid. The pressure of the vapor above the liquid is called the equilibrium vapor pressure.

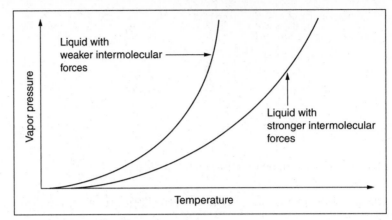

FIGURE 13.3 Sample vapor pressure curve.

The vapor pressure increases with temperature, but the increase is not linear. Vapor pressure decreases with increasing intermolecular forces. A sample vapor pressure curve versus temperature for two liquids is shown in Figure 13.3.

When the vapor pressure reaches the external atmospheric pressure, molecules form bubbles, the process called boiling. The temperature at which the boiling occurs at 1 atm pressure is called the normal boiling point.

Boiling is an example of a phase change in which a substance in one of the three states of matter converts to one of the other states of matter. Figure 13.4 shows all the types of phase changes, which include the following:

➤ For most substances, if you start with the substance in the solid state and increase the temperature, the substance will melt to a liquid.
➤ Then if you increase the temperature still further, the substance will boil or vaporize to a gas.
➤ If you cool down a gas, it will condense to a liquid.

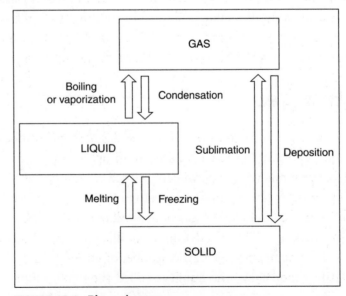

FIGURE 13.4 Phase changes.

➤ If you cool the liquid, it will freeze into a solid.

➤ Direct conversion from a solid to a gas is called sublimation, and its reverse is called deposition.

Each of these phase changes has enthalpy associated with the change. Phase change enthalpies for water are listed in the following table. For each reaction, the change assumes 1 mole of substance. If any of these processes are reversed, the enthalpy must be multiplied by –1.

$$H_2O(s) \rightarrow H_2O(l) \qquad \Delta H_{fusion}$$
$$H_2O(l) \rightarrow H_2O(g) \qquad \Delta H_{vaporization}$$
$$H_2O(s) \rightarrow H_2O(g) \qquad \Delta H_{sublimation}$$

All of the energy added during the phase change goes into the transition from one phase to another, so the temperature remains fixed during the phase change. The heat required to melt a substance is always less than the heat required to vaporize the substance. That is because melting simply breaks down the order of the solid without breaking the intermolecular forces, but boiling requires completely breaking the intermolecular forces to separate the molecules from one another.

Pure substances will show different boiling and melting points at different pressures. These data can be used to construct a phase diagram that shows what phase is stable for a given combination of pressure and temperature. A generic phase diagram is shown in Figure 13.5. The lines between the regions represent the combination of pressure and temperature where phase transitions occur. Phase transitions at 1 atm pressure are the normal melting point (solid to liquid), normal boiling point (liquid to gas), and normal sublimation point (solid to gas, not shown in this diagram). The point at which the three phases meet is called the triple point. This is the only combination of temperature and pressure where solid, liquid, and gas can be in equilibrium. The termination of the vapor-liquid line is called the critical point. At temperatures above the critical point, no amount of applied pressure can liquefy the gas. A substance in this region is called a supercritical fluid.

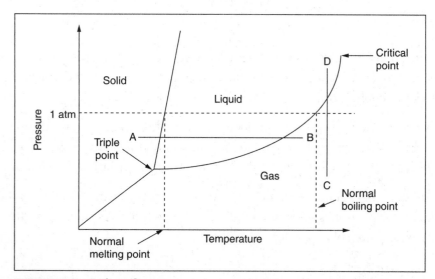

FIGURE 13.5 A phase diagram.

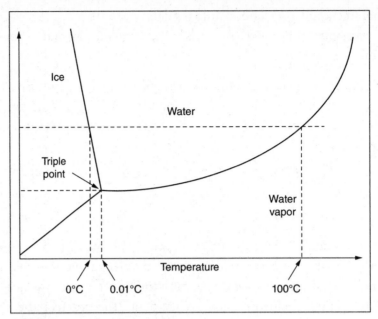

FIGURE 13.6 Phase diagram for water.

Referring to Figure 13.5, a horizontal line (AB) traces the changes that occur if the temperature changes at a fixed pressure. A substance beginning at A as a solid melts as the temperature reaches the solid-liquid line and boils when the temperature reaches the liquid-gas line.

A vertical line (CD) represents changes in temperature at a constant pressure. A substance that is a gas at C will convert to a liquid as the pressure is increased and the liquid-gas line is crossed. This phase diagram is typical of most substances that exist in only three phases. In most substances, the solid-liquid line has a positive slope. Water is unusual in that the solid phase is less dense than the liquid phase. This is why ice floats. A phase diagram for water is shown in Figure 13.6.

SOLIDS

Amorphous solids have no long-range order, but short-range order may be possible. Glass is an example of an amorphous solid. A good description of an amorphous solid is that it is a supercooled liquid.

Crystalline solids have long-range periodic order in three dimensions. Many common solids are crystalline. Examples are table salt, sugar, and most ionic solids. A crystalline solid is characterized by a unit cell that is the minimum translational repeat unit.

The interactions between the particles of a solid depend on the solid's composition. Properties of various solids are shown in the following table. All the entries are crystalline solids except amorphous solids.

Table 13.1 Properties of Various Solids				
Type	**Structural Units**	**Interparticle Forces**	**Example**	**Properties**
Ionic	Cations and anions	Ionic bonding	NaCl	Hard, brittle, high melting point, conduct electricity in liquid phase
Metallic	Metal cations surrounded by electrons	Metallic bonding	Fe	Malleable, ductile, conduct electricity, low to high melting and boiling points
Molecular	Covalently bonded discrete molecules	London dispersion dipole-dipole forces or hydrogen bonds	Ar CO H_2O	Soft, poor conductors of heat and electricity, low to moderate melting and boiling points
Network	Covalently bonded atoms in 1-, 2-, or 3-dimensional networks	Multidirectional covalent bonds	Si quartz	3-D networks, hard, lower dimensional species are softer, range of melting and boiling points
Amorphous	Covalent bonded species with no long-range order	Covalent bonds	Glass	Wide range of properties

The properties shown in Table 13.1, like many properties of matter in all phases, are largely the result of the type of bonds or forces that exist in each solid.

CHAPTER 14

Moles and Stoichiometry

Read This Chapter to Learn About

➤ The Mole Concept
➤ Chemical Reactions

THE MOLE CONCEPT

The amu is useful for individual atoms, but grams or kilograms are more practical units for a collection of atoms. A mole (abbreviated mol) is defined as the number of atoms in exactly 12 g of ^{12}C. This quantity is Avogadro's number (6.022×10^{23} particles/mol to four significant figures), and it should be memorized. One atom of ^{12}C has a mass of 12 amu. One mole of ^{12}C has a mass of exactly 12 g and contains 6.022×10^{23} 12-C atoms. The average atomic mass in amu is numerically equal to the mass in grams of one mole of a substance. Avogadro's number can be thought of as a conversion between the number of moles and the number of particles, which are usually atoms, ions, or molecules.

The mass in grams of one mole is called the molar mass (formerly called molecular weight). *Mass* is preferred because weight depends on gravity. The molar mass converts between grams of a substance and moles of a substance. An analogy is the way loose nails are normally sold in a hardware store. Nails are not counted individually but rather by weighing. If there are 1,000 nails in a pound, 5 pounds of nails contain 5,000 nails. Similarly, if there is 1 mole (6.022×10^{23} atoms) of carbon in 12.01 g of carbon, 5×12.01 g $= 60.06$ g of carbon would contain $5 \times 6.022 \times 10^{23}$ atoms of carbon. Here are some examples using molar mass:

PROBLEM: How many moles of gold are there in 200.0 g of gold (Au)?

SOLUTION: $200.0 \text{ g Au} \times \dfrac{1 \text{ mole Au}}{196.967 \text{ g Au}} = 1.015 \text{ mol Au}$

PROBLEM: How many g are needed to make 3.78 mol of sulfur?

SOLUTION: $3.78 \text{ mol S} \times \dfrac{32.07 \text{ g S}}{1 \text{ mol S}} = 121 \text{ g S}$

PROBLEM: How many individual copper atoms are in a piece of copper (Cu) with a mass of 0.00246 g?

SOLUTION: This calculation requires two steps:

$$\text{g Cu} \rightarrow \text{mol Cu} \rightarrow \text{Cu atoms}$$

$$0.00246 \text{ g Cu} \times \frac{1 \text{ mol Cu}}{63.546 \text{ g Cu}} \times \frac{6.022 \times 10^{23} \text{ Cu atoms}}{1 \text{ mol Cu}} = 2.33 \times 10^{19} \text{ Cu atoms}$$

Molar Mass

The sum of the molar masses of the atoms in a formula gives a compound's molar mass.

$$H_2O: (2 \times 1.008) + (1 \times 16.00) \text{ g} = 18.02 \text{ g/mol } H_2O$$
$$C_2H_6O: (2 \times 12.01) + (6 \times 1.008) + (1 \times 16.00) \text{ g} = 46.07 \text{ g/mol } C_2H_6O$$
$$K_2CO_3: (2 \times 39.10) + (1 \times 12.01) + (3 \times 16.00) \text{ g} = 138.21 \text{ g/mol } K_2CO_3$$
$$Ca(NO_3)_2: (1 \times 40.08) + (2 \times 14.01) + (6 \times 16.00) \text{ g} = 164.10 \text{ g/mol } Ca(NO_3)_2$$

The same calculation done with the molar mass of elements can be used for compounds.

PROBLEM: How many moles are there in 100.0 g of C_2H_6O?

SOLUTION: $100.0 \text{ g } C_2H_6O \times \dfrac{1 \text{ mol } C_2H_6O}{46.07 \text{ g } C_2H_6O} = 2.171 \text{ mol } C_2H_6O$

PROBLEM: How many grams of potassium carbonate are equivalent to 5.00 mol of K_2CO_3?

SOLUTION: $5.00 \text{ mol } K_2CO_3 \times \dfrac{138.21 \text{ g potassium carbonate}}{1 \text{ mole potassium carbonate}} = 691 \text{ g } K_2CO_3$

PROBLEM: How many oxygen atoms are there in 10.0 g of $Ca(NO_3)_2$?

SOLUTION: This is a three-step process:

$$\text{g Ca(NO}_3)_2 \rightarrow \text{mol Ca(NO}_3)_2 \rightarrow \text{formula units Ca(NO}_3)_2 \rightarrow \text{oxygen atoms}$$

$$10.0 \text{ g Ca(NO}_3)_2 \times \frac{1 \text{ mol Ca(NO}_3)_2}{164.10 \text{ g Ca(NO}_3)_2} \times \frac{6.022 \times 10^{23} \text{ formula units Ca(NO}_3)_2}{1 \text{ mol Ca(NO}_3)_2} =$$
$$3.67 \times 10^{22} \text{ formula units}$$

$$Ca(NO_3)_2 \times \frac{6 \text{ oxygen atoms}}{1 \text{ formula unit Ca(NO}_3)_2} = 2.20 \times 10^{23} \text{ O atoms}$$

Percent Composition and Determining Molecular Formulas

The percent composition is easily calculated from the formula of a compound. Ibuprofen, a common drug used in over-the-counter pain relievers, has the formula $C_{13}H_{18}O_2$. What is the percent composition by mass of each element in ibuprofen?

$$13 \times C = 13 \times 12.01 = \qquad 156.13 \text{ g C}$$
$$18 \times H = 18 \times 1.008 = \qquad 18.144 \text{ g H}$$
$$2 \times O = 2 \times 16.00 = \qquad \underline{32.00 \text{ g O}}$$
$$\qquad\qquad\qquad 206.27 \text{ g total in one mole of ibuprofen}$$

$$\%C = \frac{156.13 \text{ g C}}{206.27 \text{ g total}} \times 100 = \qquad 75.692 \text{ \% C}$$

$$\%H = \frac{18.444 \text{ g H}}{206.27 \text{ g total}} \times 100 = \qquad 8.942 \text{ \% H}$$

$$\%O = \frac{32.00 \text{ g O}}{206.27 \text{ g total}} \times 100 = \qquad \underline{15.51 \text{ \% O}}$$
$$\qquad\qquad\qquad\qquad 100.00\% \text{ total}$$

Given the percent composition of a substance, determining the molecular formula is more difficult. Before demonstrating this calculation, the empirical formula must be defined. The molecular formula of a compound occasionally contains a common factor in the subscripts. Dividing out this factor yields the empirical formula.

Molecular Formula	Empirical Formula
C_2H_6	CH_3
$B_3N_3Cl_6$	$BNCl_2$
C_6H_6	CH
C_2H_6O	C_2H_6O

Formulas obtained from the percent composition are always the empirical formula. This is because the molecular formula is a multiple of the empirical formula, the ratio of the mass of the elements is the same, and the percent composition will be the same.

PROBLEM: A compound was analyzed and the percent composition by mass was found to be 49.41 % K, 20.26 % S, and 30.33 % O. Determine the empirical formula. A convenient amount to use for this problem is 100.0 g because the percents are numerically equal to the number of grams of each element. From the grams of each element, you can determine the number of moles of each element. The ratio of the moles is directly related to the ratio of the atoms in the formula.

SOLUTION:

$$49.41 \text{ g K} \times \frac{1 \text{ mol K}}{39.10 \text{ g K}} = 1.264 \text{ mol K}$$

$$20.26 \text{ g S} \times \frac{1 \text{ mol S}}{32.00 \text{ g S}} = 0.6331 \text{ mol S}$$

$$30.33 \text{ g O} \times \frac{1 \text{ mol O}}{16.00 \text{ g O}} = 1.896 \text{ mol O}$$

These moles are in the correct ratio, but a fraction of an atom is not possible.

$$K_{1.264}S_{0.6331}O_{1.896}$$

Divide each number of moles by the smallest number of moles to get a whole number.

$$K_{\frac{1.264}{0.6331}} S_{\frac{0.6331}{0.6331}} O_{\frac{1.896}{0.6331}} = K_2SO_3$$

CHEMICAL REACTIONS

A chemical reaction is a chemical change in which a set of chemical substances called reactants are transformed into a new set of chemical substances called products. A chemical reaction is represented symbolically by a chemical equation. In chemical equations, (s) = solid, (l) = liquid, (g) = gas, and (aq) = aqueous solution.

PROBLEM: $CH_4(g) + 2O_2(g) \rightarrow 2H_2O(l) + CO_2(g)$

SOLUTION: The reactants are CH_4 and O_2, and the products are H_2O and CO_2. To make sure the equation is balanced, a number called a coefficient (in this case, 2) is placed in front of H_2O and O_2. That coefficient ensures that there is the same number of each type of atom in the reactants and in the products, as required by the law of conservation of mass.

Chemical reactions can be classified by the nature of the reactants and products.

➤ A **precipitation reaction** produces an insoluble compound called a precipitate. For example, the formation of a precipitate of barium sulfate:

$$Na_2SO_4(aq) + Ba(NO_3)_2(aq) \rightarrow 2NaNO_3(aq) + BaSO_4(s)$$

➤ A **neutralization reaction** is a reaction between a source of H^+, an acid, and a source of OH^-, a base, to form water and an ionic compound, a salt. For example, the reaction of HCl and NaOH:

$$HCl(aq) + NaOH(aq) \rightarrow H_2O(l) + NaCl(aq)$$

➤ An **oxidation-reduction reaction** is the transfer of electrons from one substance to another. For example, magnesium transfers electrons to oxygen, yielding magnesium oxide:

$$2Mg(s) + O_2(g) \rightarrow 2 MgO(s)$$

Balancing Chemical Equations

Most equations can be balanced by trial and error. Equations are balanced by changing the coefficients. Never change the subscripts because this will change the compound or produce a nonexistent compound.

PROBLEM: Balance the following equation:

$$Al(s) + Br_2(g) \rightarrow AlBr_3(s)$$

SOLUTION: Al is initially balanced. Balance Br atoms with a 3 in front of Br2 and a 2 in front of AlBr3. Rebalance the Al with a 2 in front of Al.

$$2Al(s) + 3Br_2(g) \rightarrow 2AlBr_3(s)$$

A common type of equation that is balanced is the combustion of an organic compound.

PROBLEM: Balance the following equation:

$$C_4H_{10}(g) + O_2(g) \rightarrow H_2O(l) + CO_2(g)$$

SOLUTION: Balance C with a 4 in front of CO_2. Balance H with a 5 in front of H_2O.

$$C_4H_{10}(g) + O_2(g) \rightarrow 5H_2O(l) + 4CO_2(g)$$

Balancing the oxygen is tricky because three compounds have oxygen. There is an odd number of O atoms on the product side, but O_2 from the reactant side will always give an even number of O atoms. A method to get around this problem is to use a fractional number of O_2 molecules in front of O_2 to balance the equation.

$$C_4H_{10}(g) + 6\frac{1}{2}O_2(g) \rightarrow 5H_2O(l) + 4CO_2(g)$$

In general, a balanced equation has all whole-number coefficients. Double all coefficients to remove the fraction. Check the final equation.

$$2\,C_4H_{10}\,(g) + 13O_2(g) \rightarrow 10H_2O(l) + 8CO_2(g)$$

Consider the combustion of methane:

$$CH_4(g) + 2O_2(g) \rightarrow 2H_2O(l) + CO_2(g)$$

The calculation of the relationships among the masses of reactants and products in a chemical reaction is called stoichiometry. Molar ratios are the ratios of the coefficients from the balanced equation. Examples of these molar ratios using the combustion of methane are:

$$1 \text{ mol } CH_4/2 \text{ mol } O_2 \text{ or } 2 \text{ mol } H_2O/2 \text{ mol } O_2 \text{ or } 1 \text{ mol } CH_4/2 \text{ mol } H_2O$$

The reciprocal of each ratio is also valid. A molar ratio is a conversion factor for the moles of one substance to an equivalent number of moles for another substance in a given chemical reaction. Putting together the molar ratios and the molar mass, a path from grams of a component of the reaction, A, to the grams of any other component, B, can be drawn.

$$g \text{ of } A \rightarrow \text{mol of } A \rightarrow \text{mol of } B \rightarrow g \text{ of } B$$

The first and last steps use the molar mass, and the middle step uses the molar ratio.

> **PROBLEM:** Given the reaction: $N_2(g) + 3H_2(g) \rightarrow 2NH_3(g)$, if 46.8 g of H_2 (molar mass = 2.016 g/mol) is completely reacted with N_2, how many g of NH_3 (molar mass = 17.03 g/mol) will be formed?

> **SOLUTION:**

$$g \text{ of } H_2 \rightarrow \text{mol of } H_2 \rightarrow \text{mol of } NH_3 \rightarrow g \text{ of } NH_3$$

$$46.8 \text{ g } H_2 \left(\frac{1 \text{ mol } H_2}{2.016 \text{ g } H_2} \right) \left(\frac{2 \text{ mol } NH_3}{3 \text{ mol } H_2} \right) \left(\frac{17.03 \text{ } NH_3}{1 \text{ mol } NH_3} \right) = 264 \text{ g } NH_3$$

This type of calculation can be carried out for any balanced equation.

Limiting Reactants

If there are two or more reactants in a chemical reaction, and the moles of the reactants are in the same ratio as the balanced equation, all the reactants will completely react. The other possibility is that one reactant is in limited supply, and there is not enough of that limiting reactant to completely consume the other reactants.

For the reaction: $4NH_3(g) + 5O_2(g) \rightarrow 4NO(g) + 6H_2O(l)$, a mixture of 4.0 mol of NH_3 can react completely with 5.0 mol of O_2 to produce products with no reactants left over. In this case, you would say the reactants are in a stoichiometric ratio. Consider the combination of 4.0 mol of NH_3 and 9.0 mol of O_2. In this case, the NH_3 would react with 5.0 mol of O_2 to form products, but after the 4.0 mol of NH_3 are reacted there is still $9.0 - 5.0 = 4.0$ mol of O_2 left over. The maximum amount of products formed is dependent on the limiting reactant, NH_3. The O_2 is in excess.

The maximum amount of product with a limiting reactant is determined by calculating the masses of products that are possible from the complete reaction of each reactant.

> **PROBLEM:** What is the maximum amount of H_2O formed from combustion of 25.0 g of C_3H_8 and 50.0 g of O_2 as per the reaction: $C_3H_8(g) + 5O_2(g) \rightarrow 3CO_2(g) + 4H_2O(l)$?

> **SOLUTION:** First, calculate the maximum amount of water formed from complete reaction of C_3H_8.

$$g \text{ of } C_3H_8 \rightarrow \text{mol of } C_3H_8 \rightarrow \text{mol of } H_2O \rightarrow g \text{ of } H_2O$$

$$25.0 \text{ g of } C_3H_8 \left(\frac{1 \text{ mol of } C_3H_8}{44.09 \text{ g } C_3H_8} \right) \left(\frac{4 \text{ mol of } H_2O}{1 \text{ mol of } C_3H_8} \right) \left(\frac{18.02 \text{ g of } H_2O}{1 \text{ mol of } H_2O} \right) = 40.9 \text{ g } H_2O$$

Assuming all the O_2 reacts, the calculation is as follows:

$$g \text{ of } O_2 \rightarrow \text{mol of } O_2 \rightarrow \text{mol of } H_2O \rightarrow g \text{ of } H_2O$$

$$50.0 \text{ g of } O_2 \left(\frac{1 \text{ mol } O_2}{32.00 \text{ g } O_2} \right) \left(\frac{4 \text{ mol } H_2O}{5 \text{ mol } O_2} \right) \left(\frac{18.02 \text{ g of } H_2O}{1 \text{ mol of } H_2O} \right) = 22.5 \text{ g } H_2O$$

Complete reaction of the given O_2 produces 22.5 g of H_2O, which is less than the 40.9 g produced from complete reaction of the C_3H_8. The O_2 limits the reaction, and a maximum of 22.5 g of H_2O can form.

Percent Yield

Often reactions do not go to completion for many possible reasons. Sometimes reactions are not run long enough. Some reactions simply do not go to completion for energetic reasons. The efficiency of a reaction is measured by the percent yield, defined as:

$$\% \text{ yield} = \frac{\text{actual yield}}{\text{theoretical yield}} \times 100\%$$

PROBLEM: 12.6 g of uranium (IV) oxide is reacted with excess hydrofluoric acid, yielding 13.1 g of uranium tetrafluoride. Calculate the percent yield. (Molar masses: $UO_2 = 270$ g/mol, $UF_4 = 314$ g/mol.)

SOLUTION:

$$UO_2(s) + 4HF(g) \rightarrow UF_4(g) + 2H_2O(l)$$
$$g \text{ of } UO_2 \rightarrow \text{mol of } UO_2 \rightarrow \text{mol of } UF_4 \rightarrow g \text{ of } UF_4$$

Calculate the theoretical yield:

$$12.6 \text{ g } UO_2 \left(\frac{1 \text{ mol } UO_2}{270 \text{ g } UO_2} \right) \left(\frac{1 \text{ mole } UF_4}{1 \text{ mol } UO_2} \right) \left(\frac{314 \text{ g } UF_4}{1 \text{ mol } UF_4} \right) = 14.7 \text{ g } UF_4$$

Calculate the percent yield:

$$\% \text{ yield} = \frac{\text{actual yield}}{\text{theoretical yield}} \times 100\%$$

$$\% \text{ yield} = \frac{13.1 \text{ grams}}{14.7 \text{ grams}} \times 100\% = 89.11\% \text{ yield.}$$

A helpful hint in solving these types of problems is to remember, "Number, unit, substance." Each calculation needs to have carefully tracked the value, unit, and substance involved.

CHAPTER 15

Solution Chemistry

Read This Chapter to Learn About

➤ Factors Affecting Solubility

➤ Concentration Units

➤ Colligative Properties

➤ Solubility of Ionic Compounds

➤ Solution Stoichiometry

Solution is another name for a homogeneous mixture, or a mixture with only one phase. The phase of a solution may be a gas such as air, which is a mixture of nitrogen, oxygen, and other gases; a liquid such as sugar water; or a solid such as 14-carat gold, which is a mixture of 14 parts gold and 10 parts other metals. In general, when one substance is dissolved in another, the substance that changes phase is the solute and the one that does not change phase is the solvent. Some may argue that the solvent is the substance in the greater amount, but beware, this can be proven wrong by the fact that 140 grams of KI(s) can dissolve in 100 grams of water at 15 degrees C.

Solutions form if the interactions between solute and solvent are stronger than the sum of the interactions between solute-solute or solvent-solvent. The forces between particles in solutions are similar to those in pure solids and pure liquids. One new type of interparticle force is possible in solutions. This force is an ion-dipole interaction, in which an ion interacts with polar molecules in an electrical attraction. The ion-dipole interaction between water and ions in an NaCl solution is shown in the following figure.

$$\text{Na}^+ \text{----} \overset{\text{H}}{\underset{\text{H}}{:\text{O}}} \qquad \text{Cl}^- \text{------ H} \text{---} \overset{}{\underset{\text{H}}{:\text{O}:}}$$

It has been found that substances with similar interparticle forces will be soluble in each other. For example, organic substances that can form hydrogen bonds such as ethyl alcohol, $CH_3\text{-}CH_2\text{-}OH$, or acetic acid, CH_3COOH, are readily soluble in water. Substances with only London dispersion forces are soluble in each other. For example, grease, a mixture of long-chain hydrocarbons, $CH_3\text{-}(CH_2)_x\text{-}CH_3$ (where x = from about 10 to 20), with only nonpolar C-C and C-H bonds, dissolves in octane, C_8H_{18}, one of the major components of gasoline. The generalizations of this paragraph are often summarized in the simple statement "like dissolves like." Hydrocarbon oils (only London forces) do not dissolve in water (hydrogen bonding forces).

FACTORS AFFECTING SOLUBILITY

The concentration of solutions can be described qualitatively as concentrated (more solute dissolved) or dilute (less solute dissolved). A solution with the maximum amount of a solute that can dissolve in a given amount of solvent under a given set of conditions is saturated. A supersaturated solution is an unstable state in which more solute is dissolved than in a saturated solution. If crystals start to form in a supersaturated solution, the solute precipitates until the solution becomes saturated.

Temperature affects solubility in the following ways:

➤ **Solid and liquid solutes:** solubility increases with increasing temperature, with some exceptions.
➤ **Gaseous solutes:** solubility generally decreases with increasing temperature.

Pressure affects solubility in the following ways:

➤ **Solid and liquid solutes:** changes in pressure have little effect.
➤ **Gaseous solutes:** solubility increases with increasing partial pressure of the gas according to Henry's law:

$$s_{gas} = k_H P_{gas}$$

CONCENTRATION UNITS

The concentration of a solution is measured quantitatively by several units. Each unit is generally an amount of solute per amount of solution or solvent. The definitions of the various concentration units are given here.

$$\text{Mass fraction} = \frac{\text{mass of solute}}{\text{mass of solution}}$$

$$\text{Mass percent (mass \%)} = \frac{\text{mass of solute}}{\text{mass of solution} \times 100\%}$$

The mass percent is often called the weight percent. For very small amounts of solute such as pollutants, parts per million or parts per billion are used.

$$\text{Parts per million (ppm)} = \frac{\text{mass of solute}}{\text{mass of solution} \times 10^6}$$

$$\text{Parts per billion (ppb)} = \frac{\text{mass of solute}}{\text{mass of solution} \times 10^9}$$

1 L of water has a mass of 1,000 g, and 1 mg = 0.001 g. For 1 mg solute, the ratio of solute to solvent is 0.001 g/1,000 g = 1/10^6, so 1 ppm is approximately 1 mg of solute per L of solution. Similarly 0.001 mg of solute per liter of solution is approximately 1 ppb.

$$\text{Molarity (M)} = \frac{\text{mol of solute}}{\text{L of solution}}$$

$$\text{Molality (m)} = \frac{\text{mol of solute}}{\text{kg of solvent}}$$

$$\text{Mole fraction } (\chi) = \frac{\text{mol of solute}}{\text{total moles in system}}$$

Conversion between units is often necessary.

PROBLEM: Calculate the mass percent, molarity, molality, and mole fraction of a solution prepared by mixing 210 g of water with 90.0 g of H_2SO_4. The density of the solution is 1.22 g/mL.

SOLUTION: First you must determine the values of the quantities needed for the calculations.

The solution has a total mass of 210 + 90.0 = 300 g.
The solution has a volume of 300 g × 1 mL/1.22 g = 246 mL.
The molar mass of water is 18.02 g/mol.
The molar mass of H_2SO_4 is 98.09 g/mol.
The solution contains $210.0 \text{ g } H_2O \times \dfrac{1 \text{ mole } H_2O}{18.02 \text{ g } H_2O} = 11.7 \text{ mol } H_2O$.

The solution contains $90.0 \text{ g } H_2SO_4 \times \dfrac{1 \text{ mole } H_2SO_4}{98.09 \text{ g } H_2SO_4} = 0.918 \text{ mol } H_2SO_4$.

$$\text{Mass percent (mass \%)} = \frac{90.0 \text{ g } H_2SO_4}{300 \text{ g soln}} \times 100\% = 30.0\% \ H_2SO_4.$$

$$\text{Molarity (M)} = \frac{0.918 \text{ mol } H_2SO_4}{0.246 \text{ L soln}} = 3.73 \text{ M } H_2SO_4.$$

$$\text{Molality (m)} = \frac{0.918 \text{ mol } H_2SO_4}{0.210 \text{ kg } H_2O} = 4.37 \text{ m } H_2SO_4.$$

$$\text{Mole fraction} = \frac{0.918 \text{ mol } H_2SO_4}{0.918 + 11.7 \text{ mol } H_2O} = 0.0728.$$

COLLIGATIVE PROPERTIES

Several physical properties of solutions differ from those of the pure solvent. Those properties that depend only upon the number of particles in solution and not the identity of the solute are called colligative properties. When compared to the pure solvent, solutions have:

➤ Lower vapor pressures
➤ Lower freezing points

➤ Higher boiling points
➤ Osmotic pressures

The lower vapor pressure of solutions is given by Raoult's law:

$$P_{soln} = \chi_{solvent} P_{solvent}$$

where P_{soln} is the vapor pressure of the solution, $\chi_{solvent}$ is the mole fraction of solvent (not solute), and $P_{solvent}$ is the vapor pressure of the pure solvent. If the solute is also volatile, the vapor pressure is the combination of the vapor pressure of both components. The equation becomes:

$$P_{soln} = \chi_1 P_1 + \chi_2 P_2$$

The freezing point depression of solutions is given by:

$$\Delta T_{fp} = K_{fp} m$$

where ΔT_{fp} is the freezing point depression, K_{fp} is the freezing point depression constant, and m is the molality of the solute. K_{fp} is dependent on the solvent (for water it is 1.86°C/m). The boiling point elevation of solutions is given by a similar expression:

$$\Delta T_{bp} = K_{bp} m$$

where ΔT_{bp} is the boiling point elevation, K_{bp} is the boiling point elevation constant, and m is the molality of the solute. K_{bp} is dependent on the solvent (for water it is 0.51°C/m).

A fourth colligative property is osmotic pressure. A semipermeable membrane is a barrier that allows flow of solvent but not solute. If there is a difference in concentration of a solute across a semipermeable membrane, the solvent flows in a direction to equalize the concentrations on the two sides of the membrane. In Figure 15.1, the solution within the membrane is placed into a more dilute solution or pure solvent.

Solvent flows into the membrane to equalize the concentrations. The flow continues until the pressure from the weight of the solution that has risen in the tube balances

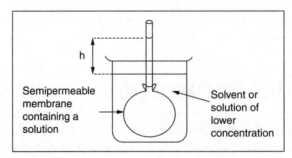

FIGURE 15.1 A semipermeable membrane.

with the osmotic pressure of the solution. Osmotic pressure is the pressure required to prevent the flow of the solvent into the membrane. It is given by:

$$\Pi = MRT$$

where Π is the osmotic pressure (atm), M is the molarity of the solute, R is the gas constant $0.08026 \, ^{L \, atm}/_{mol \, K}$, and T is the Kelvin temperature.

Because ionic compounds break down into ions in water, the colligative property equations must be multiplied by the van't Hoff factor, i, which is an experimental measure of the moles of particles in solution per mole of solute dissolved. Theoretically, sodium chloride has a van't Hoff factor of 2, but due to ion pairing the experimental value is less. A 0.10 m NaCl solution will have a lower vapor pressure, lower freezing point, higher boiling point, and greater osmotic pressure than a 0.10 m solution of sucrose, a molecular solid.

The ions in solutions of ionic compounds allow the solutions to conduct electricity. Ionic substances that completely dissociate into ions are called strong electrolytes. Most soluble ionic compounds are strong electrolytes. Substances that only partially dissociate into ions are called weak electrolytes.

In an ionic precipitation reaction, two solutions of ionic compounds are mixed and an insoluble compound called a precipitate forms that settles out of the solution. You may predict if a precipitate will form by using a simple set of solubility rules for ionic compounds in aqueous solutions.

SOLUBILITY OF IONIC COMPOUNDS

Following are the rules describing which compounds are usually soluble or insoluble:

1. All salts of Group 1 cations, Li^+, Na^+, and K^+, and the ammonium ion, NH_4^+, are soluble.
2. All nitrates, NO_3^-, and acetates, CH_3COO^-, are soluble.
3. All chlorides, Cl^-, bromides, Br^-, and iodides, I^-, are soluble except when combined with Ag^+, Pb^{2+}, or Hg_2^{2+}.
4. All sulfates, SO_4^{2-}, are soluble except when combined with Ca^{2+}, Sr^{2+}, Ba^{2+}, Pb^{2+}, Ag^+, or Hg_2^{2+}.
5. Compounds that are usually insoluble: all phosphates, PO_4^{3-}, carbonates, CO_3^-, hydroxides, OH^-, and sulfides, S^{2-}, are insoluble except when combined with Group 1 cations or ammonium. $Ca(OH)_2$, $Sr(OH)_2$, and $Ba(OH)_2$ are also soluble.

Most of the rules governing solubility concern anions. Only rule 1 focuses on the cations. To use these rules, first consider all ions that are in solution. Consider combinations of cations and anions and decide whether or not a precipitate will form.

PROBLEM: Predict whether a precipitate will form if barium nitrate is reacted with copper (II) sulfate.

$$Ba(NO_3)_2(aq) + CuSO_4(aq) \rightarrow ?$$

SOLUTION: The ions present in the reactant solutions that are formed by each soluble compound are $Ba^{2+}(aq)$, $NO_3^-(aq)$, $Cu^{2+}(aq)$, and $SO_4^{2-}(aq)$. Consider the possible combinations of cations and anions. Ignore reactant combinations. Ba^{2+} and SO_4^{2-} precipitate according to rule 4, and NO_3^- and Cu^{2+} are soluble according to rule 2.

The formulas for the products are as follows: Ba^{2+} and SO_4^{2-} will form $BaSO_4$, and NO_3^- and Cu^{2+} will form $Cu(NO_3)_2$. The balanced equation for this reaction, including the phases of the reactants and products, is as follows:

$$Ba(NO_3)_2(aq) + CuSO_4(aq) \rightarrow BaSO_4(s) + Cu(NO_3)_2(aq)$$

The actual state of the species in solution is shown in the total or overall ionic equation. Soluble compounds are broken down into ions. Precipitates are left intact.

$$Ba^{2+}(aq) + 2NO_3^-(aq) + Cu^{2+}(aq) + SO_4^{2-}(aq) \rightarrow BaSO_4(s) + Cu^{2+}(aq) + 2NO_3^-(aq)$$

The net ionic equation eliminates any species that are identical on the reactant and product side, which are called spectator ions. In this case, eliminate Cu^{2+} and NO_3^- to get a net ionic equation of:

$$Ba^{2+}(aq) + SO_4^{2-}(aq) \rightarrow BaSO_4(s)$$

SOLUTION STOICHIOMETRY

Remember that 1 liter equals 1,000 mL. This conversion factor will be used often with solutions. Solutions consist of some solute that is dissolved in a solvent. Rather than weighing out a specific quantity of a substance, you use the concentration of a solution (the amount of solute per unit volume) and measure out the desired amount by volume. The most useful solution concentration unit for chemical reactions is molarity (M), which is moles of solute per liter of solution. Note that this is per liter of solution, not per liter of solvent. Molarity is a conversion factor between the volume of solution and moles of solute.

PROBLEM: If 50.51 g of $Ca(NO_3)_2$ (molar mass = 164.1 g/mol) is dissolved in water and diluted to a final volume of 250.0 mL, what is the molarity of the solution?

SOLUTION:

$$g\ Ca(NO_3)_2 \rightarrow mol\ Ca(NO_3)_2 \rightarrow M\ of\ Ca(NO_3)_2\ solution$$

$$50.51\ g\ Ca(NO_3)_2 \times \frac{1\ mol\ Ca(NO_3)_2}{164.1\ g\ Ca(NO_3)_2} = 0.3078\ mol\ Ca(NO_3)_2$$

$$\frac{0.3078\ mol\ Ca(NO_3)_2}{0.2500\ L\ soln} = 1.231\ M\ Ca(NO_3)_2$$

Note that each mole of $Ca(NO_3)_2$ dissolves to form 1 mol Ca^{2+} and 2 mol of NO_3^-, so the solution is 1.231 M Ca^{2+} but is $2 \times 1.231 = 2.462$ M NO_3^-.

Once the molarity is known, a volume for a desired number of moles or the number of moles in a given volume may be calculated. For these calculations, molarity is most conveniently expressed by the unit mol/L, where mol is for the solute and L is for the solution.

PROBLEM: How many mL of 0.987 M NaOH solution will supply 0.345 mol of NaOH?

SOLUTION:

$$0.345\ mol\ NaOH \times \frac{1\ L\ soln}{0.987\ mol\ NaOH} = 0.350\ L\ or\ 350\ mL\ of\ 0.987\ M\ NaOH$$

PROBLEM: How many mol of NaOH are there in 150.0 mL of 0.345 M NaOH?

SOLUTION:

$$0.1500\ L\ soln \times \frac{0.345\ mol\ NaOH}{1\ L\ soln} = 0.0518\ mole\ of\ NaOH$$

Another important use of molarity is for calculating a solution's concentration upon dilution. When solvent is added to a solution, the number of moles of solute does not change, only the volume. Dilution spreads a given amount of solute into a larger volume. The molarity of the solution decreases upon dilution.

PROBLEM: If 50.00 mL of 0.673 M $FeCl_2$ is mixed with 75.00 mL of water, what is the final concentration of the solution? (Final volume of solution is 50.00 + 75.00 mL = 125.00 mL.)

SOLUTION:

$$V\ conc.\ solution \rightarrow mol\ solute \rightarrow M\ dilute\ solution$$

$$0.0500\ L\ soln \times \frac{0.673\ mol\ FeCl_2}{1\ L\ soln} = 0.0337\ mole\ of\ FeCl_2$$

$$Molarity = \frac{0.0337\ mol\ of\ FeCl_2}{0.12500\ L\ soln} = 0.270\ M\ FeCl_2$$

Because the number of moles can be obtained from the molarity, stoichiometry calculations may be done using volumes and molarity in a manner similar to that using grams and the molar mass.

PROBLEM: How many mL of 0.235 M K_3PO_4 are needed to completely precipitate the calcium in 40.0 mL of 0.125 M $CaCl_2$?

SOLUTION: Start with a balanced reaction:

$$3CaCl_2 + 2K_3PO_4 \rightarrow Ca_3(PO_4)_2 + 6KCl$$

$$0.0400 \text{ L soln} \left(\frac{0.125 \text{ mol } CaCl_2}{1 \text{ L soln}} \right) \left(\frac{2 \text{ mol } K_2CO_3}{3 \text{ mol } CaCl_2} \right) \left(\frac{1 \text{ L soln}}{0.235 \text{ mol } K_3PO_4} \right)$$

$$= 0.142 \text{ L of } 0.235 \text{ M } K_3PO_4, \text{ or } 142 \text{ mL}$$

In a titration, a solution of known concentration, the standard solution, is used to analyze other solutions of unknown concentrations. The equivalence point is reached when enough of the standard solution is added to completely react with the unknown.

PROBLEM: A 20.00 mL sample of HBr of unknown concentration required 29.63 mL of standard 0.9623 M NaOH to be neutralized. What is the molarity of the HBr solution?

SOLUTION:

$$HBr(aq) + NaOH(aq) \rightarrow H_2O(l) + NaBr(aq), \text{ so}$$
$$V \text{ of NaOH} \rightarrow \text{mol of NaOH} \rightarrow \text{mol of HBr} \rightarrow M \text{ of HBr}$$

$$0.02963 \text{ L NaOH} \left(\frac{0.9623 \text{ mol NaOH}}{1 \text{ L soln}} \right) \left(\frac{1 \text{ mol HBr}}{1 \text{ mol NaOH}} \right) \left(\frac{1}{0.02000 \text{ L soln}} \right) = 1.426 \text{ M HBr}$$

There is another method to solving this problem. Using the more familiar equation $M_aV_a = M_bV_b$, we can substitute and solve:

$$M_aV_a = M_bV_b \text{ becomes } (x \text{ M HBr})(20.00 \text{ ml}) = (0.9623)(29.63 \text{ ml})$$

Solving for x gives 1.426 M HBr.

The next question is to ask if this makes sense. Because less HBr was used, its concentration had to be greater. Because more NaOH was used in the titration, its concentration had to be lower.

CHAPTER 16

Chemical Kinetics and Equilibrium

> **Read This Chapter to Learn About**
> ➤ Kinetics
> ➤ Determining the Order of a Reaction
> ➤ Equilibrium
> ➤ Solubility Equilibria

KINETICS

Some chemical reactions are fast, such as the burning of iron powder in a sparkler. Some reactions are slow, such as the rusting of an iron gate. Both reactions are oxidation of iron to oxides or related compounds, but the form of the iron determines the speed at which it combines with oxygen. A rise in temperature speeds up a chemical reaction, such as the rate at which milk sours. The study of the rates of reactions is called kinetics.

In basic physics, the velocity or rate of an object is defined as the distance traveled per unit time, d = r × t. In the study of the rates of chemical reactions, the distance is replaced by concentration, and rates are given in units of concentration per unit time such as molar per second or molar per minute. The rate of a reaction depends upon what concentration is being measured. For the following sample reaction:

$$aA + bB \rightarrow cC + dD$$

the rate is defined with respect to the disappearance of a reactant, rate = $\dfrac{-\Delta[A]}{\Delta t}$, or the appearance of a product, rate = $\dfrac{+\Delta[D]}{\Delta t}$. The change for reactants is negative; for products, it is positive. The relationships of the reaction rates are related to the balanced equation. The mathematical relationships are:

$$\text{Rate} = -\left(\frac{(1)\Delta[A]}{(a)\Delta t}\right) = -\left(\frac{(1)\Delta[B]}{(b)\Delta t}\right) = +\left(\frac{(1)\Delta[C]}{(c)\Delta t}\right) = +\left(\frac{(1)\Delta[D]}{(d)\Delta t}\right)$$

Example: Write the relative rates for nitrogen and ammonia in the reaction $N_2(g) + 3H_2(g) \rightarrow 2NH_3(g)$.

$$\text{Rate} = -\left(\frac{(1)\Delta[N_2]}{(1)\Delta t}\right) = +\left(\frac{(1)\Delta[NH_3]}{(2)\Delta t}\right)$$

Ammonia is being formed at twice the rate that nitrogen is disappearing.

The kinetics of chemical reactions are generally studied early in the course of the reaction when the concentration of products is small. Under these conditions the reverse reaction is negligible, and the rate of reactions is given by a rate law:

$$\text{Rate} = k[A]^x[B]^y$$

where k is a rate constant that is fixed for a given reaction at a given temperature. The exponent x is the order of the reaction in A (y is the order of the reaction in B). Most chemical reactants have orders equal to 0, 1, or 2. During the reaction, the concentration of the reactants decreases and thus the rate decreases. Increasing the concentration of a substance in the rate law increases the rate of a reaction.

DETERMINING THE ORDER OF A REACTION

The order of the reaction may be determined by a technique called the method of initial rates. A reaction is run with variations in the concentrations of the reactants. In some reactions the concentration of one reactant is held constant:

$$2NO(g) + Cl_2(g) \rightarrow 2NOCl(g)$$

The initial rate is for the disappearance of Cl_2:

$$\text{Rate} = -\left(\frac{(1)\Delta[Cl_2]}{(1)\Delta t}\right)$$

Experiment	[NO]	[Cl$_2$]	Initial Rate (M/s)
1	0.020	0.010	8.27×10^{-5}
2	0.020	0.020	1.65×10^{-4}
3	0.020	0.040	3.31×10^{-4}
4	0.040	0.020	6.60×10^{-4}

For this reaction, the rate law is of the form:

$$\text{Rate} = k[NO]^x[Cl_2]^y$$

The concentrations were picked so that the concentration of one reactant doubles and one remains fixed. Examining the data in experiments 1 and 2, doubling the concentration of chlorine doubled the rate. This means that $y = 1$. Examining experiments 2 and 4, doubling the concentration of NO quadrupled the rate. This means that $x = 2$. The rate law is rate $= k[NO]^2[Cl_2]$. The order of the reaction is not related to the coefficients of the balanced equation and must be determined experimentally. Once you have the rate law, the value of k may be obtained from any of the experiments.

The Effect of Temperature on k

The rates of chemical reactions are explained by collision theory, which is an extension of the kinetic molecular theory first discussed in the description of gases in Chapter 13. Reactants will be successfully converted to products when the reactant molecules collide with sufficient energy and with the correct orientation. These two factors are incorporated into the Arrhenius equation, which gives the value of the rate constant as a function of the temperature:

$$k = Ae^{-(E_a/RT)}$$

where k is the rate constant, A is the frequency factor (a measure of the frequency of molecular collisions and the fraction with proper orientations), E_a is the activation energy (the minimum energy required for successful reaction to occur), R is the gas constant, and T is the Kelvin temperature.

Note: This equation indicates that as the temperature increases, the rate constant increases. The reverse is true for the activation energy. As the activation energy increases, the rate constant decreases and the reaction rate slows down.

Catalysts

Catalysts are substances that speed up the rate of a reaction but are not consumed during the reaction. Catalysts are used to make industrial preparations more efficient. Catalytic converters on automobiles convert exhaust gases to less toxic substances. Enzymes are natural catalysts that accelerate important biological reactions. For example, proteases in the stomach reduce the time required to break down proteins. Catalysts work by lowering the activation energy of reaction. The lower activation energy increases the value of the rate constant. Catalysts have no effect on the energies of the reactants or products, so the energy or enthalpy change of the reaction does not change. The concentrations at equilibrium (discussed in the next section) are also not affected by a catalyst.

EQUILIBRIUM

If a reaction goes on long enough, the concentration of products will increase and the reverse reaction will begin to occur. Eventually the rates of the forward and reverse reactions will become equal. The concentration of reactants and products will not change, even though both the forward and reverse reactions continue to occur. When forward and reverse rates of a reaction are equal, the reaction is at equilibrium. Equilibrium is dynamic. Because both reactions are occurring, equilibrium reactions are written with a double arrow. The equilibrium is characterized by the equilibrium constant, K. A capital K is used to distinguish this constant from the kinetic rate constant. For a gas phase reaction:

$$aA(g) + bB(g) \leftrightarrow cC(g) + dD(g)$$

The equilibrium constant K_c is given by:

$$K_c = \frac{[C]^c[D]^d}{[A]^a[B]^b}$$

All the concentrations are at equilibrium. The equilibrium expression may be written directly from the balanced equation. The units for K are usually ignored.

> **PROBLEM:** Consider an equilibrium obtained by introducing H_2, I_2, and HI into a 5.00 L flask at 825°K. At equilibrium, the flask contains 7.500 mol of HI, 1.875 mol of H_2, and 0.261 mol I_2. Calculate the equilibrium constant. The balanced equation is:
>
> $$H_2(g) + I_2(g) \leftrightarrow 2\,HI(g)$$

SOLUTION: Dividing the number of moles of each gas by 5.00 liters each gives us the molarity of each gas:

$$[HI] = 1.50\,M\,HI$$
$$[H_2] = 0.375\,M\,H_2$$
$$[I_2] = 0.0522\,M\,I_2$$

The equilibrium constant is:

$$K_c = \frac{[HI]^2}{[H_2][I_2]} = \frac{[1.50]^2}{[0.0522][0.375]} = 115$$

Pressures are usually easier to measure for gases, so a different equilibrium constant may be used, K_p. This constant has the same form as the regular equilibrium constant expression (which may be distinguished as K_c), except pressures are used.

$$K_p = \frac{[P\,HI]^2}{[P\,H_2][P\,I_2]}$$

Unless otherwise indicated, K means K_c. K_c and K_p will differ in number except when the number of gas molecules in the reactants equals the number of gas molecules in the products. Because the concentration of pure solids and liquids is fixed at a given temperature and pressure, these values are not incorporated into K. Pure solids and liquids are left out of the equilibrium constant expression.

The value of K indicates the relative amounts of products and reactants at equilibrium:

➤ K > 1: mostly products present at equilibrium
➤ K = 1: both reactants and products present at equilibrium
➤ K < 1: mostly reactants present at equilibrium

If an equation is altered, the form of the equilibrium constant expression is also changed.

PROBLEM: Consider the reaction for the formation of HI discussed earlier.

$$H_2(g) + I_2(g) \leftrightarrow 2HI(g)$$

SOLUTION: The reverse of the equation is:

$$2HI(g) \leftrightarrow H_2(g) + I_2(g)$$

The equilibrium constant expression for the reverse reaction is:

$$K_{rev} = \frac{[H_2][I_2]}{[HI]^2}$$

Clearly, $K_{rev} = \dfrac{1}{K_{for}}$. If a reaction is reversed, take the reciprocal of K to find its value.

Reaction Quotient

The reaction quotient (Q) has the same form as the equilibrium constant expression except that the concentrations used are the *initial concentrations*. For example:

$$aA + bB \leftrightarrow cC + dD$$

The reaction quotient is given by:

$$Q = \frac{[C]^c[D]^d}{[A]^a[B]^b}$$

The reaction quotient may be used to predict in which direction a reaction will proceed.

➤ Q = K: at equilibrium, no shift
➤ Q > K: too much of the products, shift to the reactants (left)
➤ Q < K: too little of the products, shift to the products (right)

PROBLEM: K = 115 at 825°K for the reaction:

$$H_2(g) + I_2(g) \leftrightarrow 2HI(g)$$

If [HI] = 2.00 M, [H$_2$] = 0.125 M, and [I$_2$] = 0.150 M, determine the direction the reaction will shift.

SOLUTION:

$$K = \frac{[HI]^2}{[H_2][I_2]} = \frac{[2.00]^2}{[0.125][0.150]} = 213 > K = 115$$

Q is greater than K, so the reaction shifts to the left to decrease the products and increase the reactants until Q = K.

Le Châtelier's Principle

The reaction quotient is also useful for predicting in which direction a reaction at equilibrium will shift if the conditions are altered. The general rule used to predict these changes is called Le Châtelier's principle. It states that a system at equilibrium that is changed so it is no longer at equilibrium will respond in a way that counteracts the change. A summary of important possible changes to equilibrium is given in the following table.

Change Direction	Counteraction	Shift
Reduce products	Increase products	Forward (right or to products)
Increase products	Reduce products	Reverse (left or to reactants)
Reduce reactants	Increase reactants	Reverse
Increase reactants	Decrease reactants	Forward
Increase temperature	Decrease heat	Forward for endothermic
		Reverse for exothermic
Decrease temperature	Increase heat	Reverse for endothermic
		Forward for exothermic
Increase pressure or decrease volume	Reduce pressure	To the side with fewer gas molecules
Decrease pressure or increase volume	Increase pressure	To the side with more gas molecules

Each of these entries can be justified by calculating Q after the given change to predict the direction the reaction will shift. For the temperature changes, consider that heat is a reactant in an endothermic reaction, and heat is a product in an exothermic reaction.

PROBLEM: Consider the formation of ammonia written as a thermochemical equation ($\Delta H = -92.2$ kJ):

$$N_2(g) + 3H_2(g) \leftrightarrow 2NH_3(g) + 92.2 \text{ kJ}$$

SOLUTION: If H_2 is added, the reaction will shift to the right to decrease the added H_2. If the temperature is increased, the reverse reaction will run to absorb the heat (shift left). If the volume is doubled, this lowers the pressure, and the system shifts to the left to increase the pressure by generating more gas molecules.

SOLUBILITY EQUILIBRIA

The equilibrium equation for sparingly soluble solids where M is a cation and A is the anion is:

$$M_xA_y = x[M^{y+}](aq) + y[A^{x-}](aq)$$

The resulting equilibrium expression is:

$$K_{sp} = [M^{y+}]^x[A^{x-}]^y$$

K_{sp} is called the solubility product constant. Some examples of K_{sp} equations, K_{sp} expressions, and numerical values are:

$$AgCl(s) \leftrightarrow Ag^+(aq) + Cl^-(aq) \qquad K_{sp} = [Ag^+][Cl^-] = 1.8 \times 10^{-10}$$
$$PbCl_2(s) \leftrightarrow Pb^{2+}(aq) + 2Cl^-(aq) \qquad K_{sp} = [Pb^{2+}][Cl^-]^2 = 1.7 \times 10^{-5}$$
$$Ag_2SO_4(s) \leftrightarrow 2Ag^+(aq) + SO_4^{2-}(aq) \qquad K_{sp} = [Ag^+]^2[SO_4^{2-}] = 1.2 \times 10^{-5}$$

Solubility is usually given in terms of g of solute per 100 g of water. This is taking into account the assumption that the density of the solution is very close to 1.00 g/mL, which is not unreasonable for slightly soluble salts. The K_{sp} may be determined through simple calculations.

PROBLEM: 0.123 g of $SrCrO_4$ (molar mass = 203.62 g/mol) dissolves in 100 g of water to produce a saturated solution. Find the K_{sp} for this substance. The appropriate equilibrium is:

$$SrCrO_4(s) \leftrightarrow Sr^{2+}(aq) + CrO_4^{2-}(aq) \text{ and } K_{sp} = [Sr^{2+}][CrO_4^{2-}]$$

SOLUTION:

$$0.123 \text{ g } SrCrO_4 \times \frac{1 \text{ mol } SrCrO_4}{203.62 \text{ g } SrCrO_4} = 0.000604 \text{ mol } SrCrO_4$$

A solution of 100 g would have a volume of 100 mL or 0.100 L. So,

$$\frac{0.000604 \text{ mol } SrCrO_4}{0.100 \text{ L}} = 0.00604 \text{ M } SrCrO_4$$

Because one mole of each ion is formed from each mol of $SrCrO_4$, $[Sr^{2+}] = [CrO_4^{2-}] = 0.00604$ M. (For other salts in which more than one ion forms per mole of solute, the molarity of that ion must be doubled, tripled, etc., depending on how many ions form per mol of solute.) You may now substitute ion concentrations into the K_{sp} expression:

$$K_{sp} = [Sr^{2+}][CrO_4^{2-}] = (0.00604)(0.00604) = 3.65 \times 10^{-5}$$

There are a number of factors affecting solubility equilibria. For example, CaF_2 is less soluble in solutions that contain either Ca^{2+} or F^- than in pure water, due to the common ion effect. If the anion of the solid is a Brønsted-Lowry base, it will be more soluble in an acid solution—in other words, the base will react with water to form the conjugate acid; this reduces the concentration of the anion, allowing more salt to dissolve.

PROBLEM: Consider CaF_2 dissolving in an acidic solution.

$$CaF_2(aq) \leftrightarrow Ca^{2+}(aq) + 2F^-(aq)$$

SOLUTION: If the solution is acidic, H_3O^+ will reduce the F^- concentration by the reaction:

$$F^-(aq) + H_3O^+ \leftrightarrow HF(aq) + H_2O(l)$$

Removing F^- allows more CaF_2 to dissolve to restore the equilibrium.

CHAPTER 17

Thermodynamics and Thermochemistry

Read This Chapter to Learn About

➤ Thermodynamics

➤ Calorimetry

➤ Bond Energies

➤ Thermochemical Equations

➤ Hess's Law

➤ Entropy and Free Energy

➤ The Second Law and Free Energy

THERMODYNAMICS

Chemical reactions and physical changes often involve a transfer of energy. The transfer of energy in chemical reactions usually takes the form of heat. Temperature is associated with heat, but these two concepts are not the same. As discussed in Chapter 16, temperature may be defined as being proportional to the average speed of gas molecules. Temperature is measured in units of Fahrenheit, Celsius, or Kelvin. Because heat is a measure of energy transfer, it has the same units as energy.

In the SI system, the unit of energy is the Joule: $1\,J = kg(m^2/s^2)$. Thermodynamics, as its name implies, is the study of the movement of heat. This section will discuss thermodynamics with respect to chemical reactions and physical changes such as melting or boiling.

Energy is defined as the ability to do work. Work is defined as a force acting on an object moving the object through some distance. Energy can take two basic forms:

➤ **Kinetic energy** is the energy of motion. It is determined by the formula $KE = \frac{1}{2}mv^2$, where KE is kinetic energy, m is the mass, and v is the velocity.

➤ **Potential energy** is energy due to position. Varieties of potential energy include solar, electrical, gravitational, and chemical. One form of potential energy is chemical energy, which is the energy stored in the bonds of molecules, such as the energy of a fuel like gasoline.

Two important concepts in thermodynamics are the system and the surroundings. The system is the part of the universe under study. The surroundings are everything else. For chemical reactions, the system is usually the compounds involved in a particular reaction.

The first law of thermodynamics states that the energy of the universe is fixed. This law is often called the law of conservation of energy. This law can be expressed mathematically as:

$$\Delta E_{univ} = \Delta E_{sys} + \Delta E_{surr} = 0, \text{ which implies } \Delta E_{sys} = -\Delta E_{surr}$$

where ΔE_{univ} is the energy change for the universe, ΔE_{sys} is the energy change for the system, and ΔE_{surr} is the energy change of the surroundings.

Energy lost by the system is gained by the surroundings and vice versa. The internal energy of the system can be described as the sum of the kinetic and potential energy contained in all the parts that make up the system. Changes in the energy of the system are the main concern of thermodynamics. The internal energy of the system may be changed in two ways: (1) by the flow of heat into or out of the system, or (2) by work done either to or by the system. This relationship is expressed in the following equation:

$$\Delta E = q + w$$

where q is the heat and w is the work.

➤ If heat is added to (absorbed by) the system, the energy increases. This is called an endothermic process.
➤ If heat is lost (released) from the system, the energy decreases. This is called an exothermic process.
➤ Work done on the system causes an increase in the energy of the system.
➤ Work done by the system causes a decrease in the energy of the system.

In chemical systems, the main type of work is so-called PV or pressure-volume work. The change in energy of the system may be rewritten as follows:

$$\Delta E = q - \Delta PV$$

The negative sign is present because a $\Delta V(+)$ means W $(-)$.

311

**CHAPTER 17:
THERMO-
DYNAMICS AND
THERMO-
CHEMISTRY**

Because most chemical reactions are carried out at constant pressure, the change in energy at constant pressure is:

$$\Delta E = q_p - P\Delta V$$

The subscript p refers to the heat transferred at constant pressure. One final rearrangement gives:

$$\Delta E + P\Delta V = q_p = \Delta H$$

Enthalpy, H, is the heat transferred at constant pressure. Enthalpy is one of the key properties in thermochemistry. To determine enthalpy, heat transferred at a constant pressure is measured. Volume changes do not have to be measured.

To measure a transfer of heat, we use the specific heat capacity, S (some books use C), which is the amount of heat needed to raise the temperature of 1 gram of a substance by 1 K (or °C). The equation used with the specific heat capacity is $q = mS\Delta T$ where q is heat, m is mass, and ΔT is the change in temperature.

> **PROBLEM:** 1,000 J of heat is added to 100.0 g of Fe(s) and Al(s), both at 25°C. What is the final temperature of each metal? The specific heat of Fe and Al are $\dfrac{0.444\,J}{g°C}$ and $\dfrac{0.900\,J}{g°C}$ respectively.

> **SOLUTION:**

For Fe	For Al
$1{,}000\,J = 100.0\,g\left(\dfrac{0.444\,J}{g°C}\right)\Delta T$	$1{,}000\,J = 100.0\,g\left(\dfrac{0.900\,J}{g°C}\right)\Delta T$
$22.5 = \Delta T$	$11.1 = \Delta T$
$T_f = T_i + \Delta T$	$T_f = T_i + \Delta T$
$T_f = 47.5°C$	$T_f = 36.1°C$

Notice that the same mass of both metals received the same amount of heat, but the one with the higher heat capacity increased less in temperature. Water has an unusually high heat capacity; this is important in regulating the temperature of living things, which are made up in large part of water.

CALORIMETRY

Calorimetry is the process of measuring heat. Even simple calorimeters such as the two coffee cups that are often used in chemistry labs can give good results. Inside the calorimeter, a chemical reaction or a physical change such as the melting of ice takes place. The calorimeter contains water, or in the case of soluble reactants, a solution. The Styrofoam cups and a cover prevent heat from escaping the calorimeter. The heat released (or absorbed) by the process under study will be transferred to the water (or solution) in the calorimeter. The heat gained or lost by the water or solution is equal and opposite in value to the heat released by the chemical or physical process. Heat transferred to the calorimeter is usually small and can be neglected.

The steps in calculating the q for a given process are:

$$q = 0 \text{ (total heat is zero because all the heat is held in the calorimeter)}$$
$$q = q_{rxn} + q_{soln}$$
$$q_{rxn} = -q_{soln}$$
$$q_{rxn} = -(mS\Delta T) \text{ (using the definition of heat capacity)}$$

q_{rxn} may be a physical process such as melting, dissolving, or simply a change in temperature of an object, or q_{rxn} may be a chemical reaction.

PROBLEM: A 80.0 g piece of metal at 90.0°C is added to a calorimeter with 100.0 mL of water at 25°C. The final temperature of the water after the metal is added is 26.6°C. What is the heat capacity of the metal?

SOLUTION:

$$q_{metal} = -q_{water}$$
$$m_m S_m \Delta T_m = -(m_w S_w \Delta T_w)$$
$$(80.0 \text{ g})(S_m)(26.6 - 90.0) = -\left[(100.0 \text{ g})\left(\frac{4.184 J}{g°C}\right)(26.6 - 25.0)\right]$$
$$S_m(-5,072 \text{ g°C}) = -669.4 \text{ J}$$
$$S_m = \frac{0.132 J}{g°C}$$

BOND ENERGIES

Average bond energies (BE) have been tabulated for a large number of bonds. These bond energies will not be exact for a specific compound but can be used for estimating enthalpy changes. Enthalpy of a reaction may be estimated by the formula:

$$\Delta H = \Sigma BE \text{ (bonds broken)} - \Sigma BE \text{ (bonds formed)}$$

Energy is required to break bonds. Energy is released when bonds form. The value obtained from this calculation is not as exact as would be obtained from calculations using ΔH values.

PROBLEM: Consider the combustion of methane with the associated bond energies:

$$CH_4(g) + 2O_2(g) \rightarrow 2H_2O(g) + CO_2(g)$$

SOLUTION: Bond energies (in kJ): C-H (416), O=O (498), C=O (803), O-H (467)

$$\Delta H_{rxn} \text{ (estimate)} = 4(C-H) + 2(O=O) - [4(O-H) + 2(C=O)]$$
$$= [4(416) + 2(498)] - [2(803) + 4(467)] \text{ kJ}$$
$$= 2,660 - 3,474 \text{ kJ}$$
$$= -814 \text{ kJ/mol}$$

Calculation of this value from ΔH_f gives −801 kJ, so the estimate has a 1.6 percent error.

313

**CHAPTER 17:
THERMO-
DYNAMICS AND
THERMO-
CHEMISTRY**

THERMOCHEMICAL EQUATIONS

Once the enthalpy is found, you can write a thermochemical equation. Following is the thermochemical equation for the burning of methane:

$$CH_4(g) + 2O_2(g) \rightarrow CO_2(g) + 2H_2O(l) \Delta H = -890 \text{ kJ/mol}$$

The enthalpy is for the number of moles in the balanced equation: 1 mol CH_4, 2 mol O_2, 1 mol CO_2, and 2 mol H_2O. The minus sign (−) means that the reaction is exothermic. Heat is released by the reaction, so heat is a product. Thus the equation can be rewritten:

$$CH_4(g) + 2O_2(g) \rightarrow CO_2(g) + 2H_2O(l) + 890 \text{ kJ/mol}.$$

If the reaction is reversed, the equation becomes:

$$890 \text{ kJ/mol} + CO_2(g) + 2H_2O(l) \rightarrow CH_4(g) + 2O_2(g).$$

For the reverse reaction, heat is a reactant and is absorbed during the course of the reaction, so $\Delta H = +890 \text{ kJ/mol}$. If you reverse the reaction, you must reverse the sign of ΔH. The equation may be multiplied by a number such as 3. This is equivalent to burning three times as much methane, so the heat is increased threefold.

$$3CH_4(g) + 6O_2(g) \rightarrow 3CO_2(g) + 6H_2O(l) + 2{,}670 \text{ kJ/mol}$$

When an equation is multiplied by some number, the ΔH of the equation must be multiplied by the same number. If ΔH is considered a reactant or product, it may be used in stoichiometry problems:

PROBLEM: How much heat is released through the burning of 135.0 g of C_4H_{10}?

SOLUTION:

$$2C_4H_{10}(g) + 13O_2(g) \rightarrow 8CO_2(g) + 10H_2O(l) \Delta H = -5{,}762 \text{ kJ/mol}$$

grams of C_4H_{10} are converted to moles of C_4H_{10}, then heat is calculated.

$$135.0 \text{ g } C_4H_{10} \left(\frac{1 \text{ mol } C_4H_{10}}{58.12 \text{ g } C_4H_{10}} \right) \left(\frac{5{,}762 \text{ kJ}}{2 \text{ mol } C_4H_{10}} \right) = 6{,}692 \text{ kJ heat released}$$

The heat was divided by 2 because the balanced equation contains 2 moles of C_4H_{10}.

HESS'S LAW

Hess's law states that if a series of reactions adds up to a total overall reaction, the enthalpy of the overall reaction is the sum of the enthalpies of the individual reactions. The first three of the following reactions sum up to the fourth. The sum of the ΔH for the reactions is calculated as shown.

PROBLEM: Given the following set of reactions:

$$3C(s) + 4H_2(g) \rightarrow C_3H_8(g)\ \Delta H_1 = -103.9 \text{ kJ}$$
$$C(s) + O_2(g) \rightarrow CO_2(g)\ \Delta H_2 = -393.5 \text{ kJ}$$
$$2H_2(g) + O_2(g) \rightarrow 2H_2O(l)\ \Delta H_3 = -571.6 \text{ kJ}$$

Calculate the enthalpy of the following reaction:

$$C_3H_8(g) + 5O_2(g) \rightarrow 3CO_2(g) + 4H_2O(l)\ \Delta H = ?$$

SOLUTION: The only place the reactant C_3H_8 appears is in reaction 1 on the products side, so the reaction and the enthalpy must be reversed. The reactant O_2 appears in two reactions, so it would be hard to balance. The products, CO_2 and H_2O, are in reaction 2 and 3, respectively, but each reaction must be multiplied by a number to obtain the desired number of molecules.

$-1 \times$ Rxn 1	$C_3H_8(g) \rightarrow 3C(s) + 4H_2(g)$	$-1 \times \Delta H_1 = -(-103.9 \text{ kJ}) = +103.9 \text{ kJ}$
$3 \times$ Rxn 2	$3C(s) + 3O_2(g) \rightarrow 3CO_2(g)$	$3 \times \Delta H_2 = 3(-393.5 \text{ kJ}) = -1,180.5 \text{ kJ}$
$2 \times$ Rxn 3	$4H_2(g) + 2O_2(g) \rightarrow 4H_2O(l)$	$2 \times \Delta H_3 = 2(-571.6 \text{ kJ}) = -1,143.2 \text{ kJ}$
	$C_3H_8(g) + 5O_2(g) \rightarrow 3CO_2(g) + 4H_2O(l)$	$\Delta H = -2,219.8 \text{ kJ}$

Hess's law is useful, but it can be used only when suitable equations are known that add up to the desired equation. Enthalpy values may also be calculated using the standard enthalpy of formation, $\Delta H°_f$, defined as the enthalpy for the formation of one mole of a substance from the elements in their standard states. Standard states for solids, liquids, and gases are the most stable form at 1 atm pressure and 25°C. Certain elements' standard state is molecular: H_2, N_2, O_2, F_2, Cl_2, P_4, Br_2, and I_2. Sulfur exists as S_8, but S is often used. The standard state of C is graphite. By definition, the standard enthalpy of formation of elements is zero. Some $\Delta H°_f$ reactions are shown here:

Elements	1 mole
$H_2(g) + \frac{1}{2}O_2(g)$	$\rightarrow H_2O(l)$
$C(s) + 2Cl_2(g)$	$\rightarrow CCl_4(l)$
$H_2(g) + \frac{1}{8}S_8(s) + 2O_2(g)$	$\rightarrow H_2SO_4(l)$
$6C(s) + 6H_2(g) + 3O_2(g)$	$\rightarrow C_6H_{12}O_6(s)$

The ΔH can be calculated for any reaction in which $\Delta H°_f$ values of all reactants and products are known. The formula for this calculation is:

$$\Delta H = \Sigma n_p \Delta H°_f \text{ (products)} - \Sigma n_r \Delta H°_f \text{ (reactants)}$$

(n_p and n_r are the number of moles of the products and reactants, respectively, in the balanced equation.)

315

**CHAPTER 17:
THERMO-
DYNAMICS AND
THERMO-
CHEMISTRY**

PROBLEM: Consider the following reaction:

$$2C_4H_{10}(g) + 13O_2(g) \rightarrow 8CO_2(g) + 10H_2O(g)$$
$$C_4H_{10}(g): \Delta H° = -126.2 \text{ kJ/mol}$$
$$CO_2(g): \Delta H°_f = -393.5 \text{ kJ/mol}$$
$$H_2O(g): \Delta H° = -241.8 \text{ kJ/mol}$$
$$\text{(Note: } O_2: \Delta H° = 0\text{)}$$

SOLUTION: $\Delta H_{rxn} = [8\Delta H°(CO_2) + 10\Delta H°(H_2O)] - [2\Delta H°(C_4H_{10})]$

$$= [8(-393.5) + 10(-241.8)] - [2(-126.2)] \text{ kJ}$$
$$= [-5,566] - [-252.4] \text{ kJ} = -5,313.6 \text{ kJ}$$

ENTROPY AND FREE ENERGY

Many chemical reactions start as soon as the reactants are brought together and continue until one or both reactants are used up. Other reactions require energy input for the reaction to occur:

➤ Reactions with large equilibrium constants are product-favored (or spontaneous) reactions.

➤ Reactions with small equilibrium constants are called reactant-favored (or non-spontaneous) reactions.

➤ It has been observed that reactions that lead to dispersal of energy tend to be product favored. Energy can also be dispersed if the volume of a system increases. This is especially true for gases. There are two main factors that control the dispersal of energy:

   ➤ An exothermic reaction transfers heat to the surroundings, thus dispersing energy over a wider number of particles. Most product-favored reactions are exothermic.

   ➤ Some endothermic processes are product favored. In these reactions, spreading out of matter increases disorder. This increase in disorder is measured by a quantity called entropy, S.

Certain qualitative generalizations can be made about entropy:

$$S(\text{solid}) < S(\text{liquid}) << S(\text{gas})$$

Gases often dominate entropy because the volumes of gases are about 1,000 times greater than those of solids and liquids. Reactions that increase the number of gas molecules have large entropy changes. The following have large positive entropy changes:

➤ $H_2O(l)$ becomes $H_2O(g)$
➤ $N_2O_4(g)$ becomes $2NO_2(g)$
➤ $2NH_3(g)$ becomes $3H_2(g) + N_2(g)$

For solid and liquid solutes, the entropy of the pure substance is less than the entropy of the mixture:

$$S(solute) + S(solvent) < S(solution)$$

For gaseous solutes dissolving in a liquid solvent, the opposite is true, because the volume is greatly decreased.

$$S(solute) + S(solvent) > S(solution)$$

In general, the entropy of mixtures is greater than the entropy of pure substances.

The more complicated a molecule is, the greater the entropy, because there are many more possible arrangements of the molecule.

Each substance has an entropy of formation, S_f, similar to an enthalpy of formation. Because the entropy of a perfect crystal of a substance at 0 K is defined as zero, even ΔH_f elements have entropies of formation values at temperatures greater than 0 K. Mathematically, the equation for the entropy of a reaction is analogous to that for ΔH_{rxn}:

$$\Delta S°_{rxn} = \Sigma n_p S°_f \text{ (products)} - \Sigma n_r S°_f \text{ (reactants)}$$

PROBLEM: Find $\Delta S°_{rxn}$ for the following reaction in the gas phase at 25°C:

$$2NH_3(g) \leftrightarrow 3H_2(g) + N_2(g)$$

SOLUTION:

$$S°_f NH_3: 192.5 \text{ J/mol K}$$
$$S°_f H_2: 130.7 \text{ J/mol K}$$
$$S°_f N_2: 191.6 \text{ J/mol K}$$
$$\Delta S°_{rxn} = [3 \times S°_f H_2 + S°_f N_2] - [2 \times S°_f NH_3]$$
$$[3(130.7) + (191.6)] - [2(192.5)] \text{ J/mol K}$$
$$= +198.7 \text{ J/mol K}$$

Note that the entropy change is positive (+) as would be expected with an increase in the number of gas molecules.

THE SECOND LAW AND FREE ENERGY

The second law of thermodynamics states that the total entropy of the universe is increasing. In other words, things are continuously becoming more disordered. The change in entropy for the universe is:

$$\Delta S_{universe} = \Delta S_{system} + \Delta S_{surroundings}$$
$$\Delta S_{surroundings} = -\Delta H_{rxn}/T, \text{ and the second law equation becomes:}$$
$$\Delta S_{universe} = \Delta S_{system} + (-\Delta H_{rxn}/T).$$

317

**CHAPTER 17:
THERMO-
DYNAMICS AND
THERMO-
CHEMISTRY**

This equation allows calculation of $\Delta S_{universe}$ from two quantities associated with the reaction of interest, ΔH_{rxn} and ΔS_{rxn}. A simpler quantity ΔG can be defined by multiplying this equation by $-T$ and rearranging, which gives:

$$-T\Delta S_{universe} = \Delta H_{rxn} - T\Delta S_{rxn} = \Delta G_{sys}.$$

The quantity ΔG is called the Gibbs free energy. Note that it will have units of J/mol or kJ/mol just like enthalpy. Because T is always positive, ΔG and $\Delta S_{universe}$ have opposite signs.

Sign of ΔH	Sign of ΔS	Sign of ΔG	Product Favored?
(−)	(+)	(−)	Yes
(−)	(−)	(−) at low T, (+) at high T	At low T
(+)	(+)	(+) at low T, (−) at high T	At high T
(+)	(−)	(+)	No

In the first entry, both ΔH and ΔS favor the reaction. The opposite is true for the last entry. In the second entry, ΔH is favorable and ΔS is not. At low temperature, ΔH dominates, and at higher temperature, ΔS dominates.

The standard free energy of formation is analogous to ΔH_f (ΔG_f of elements = 0).

PROBLEM: It is important to note that ΔH_{rxn} is usually given in kJ and ΔS_{rxn} is given in J/mol K. To convert both energy units to kJ, divide ΔS_{rxn} by 1,000.

SOLUTION: For the breakdown of NH_3 to H_2 and N_2 at 298 K ($\Delta H = 92.2$ kJ/mol):

$$\Delta G°_{rxn} = \Delta H°_{rxn} - T\Delta S°_{rxn}$$
$$= +92.2 \text{ kJ/mol} - (298 \text{ K})(+0.1987 \text{ kJ/mol K})$$
$$= +92.2 - 59.2 \text{ kJ/mol} = +33 \text{ kJ/mol}.$$

In this case, ΔH is unfavorable, but ΔS is favorable. At 298 K, the favorable effects of entropy are not large enough to overcome the unfavorable enthalpy. If the temperature is raised, the contribution of entropy becomes more important. At 500 K:

$$\Delta G°_{rxn} = \Delta H°_{rxn} - T\Delta S°_{rxn}$$
$$= +92.2 \text{ kJ/mol} - (500 \text{ K})(+0.1987 \text{ kJ/mol K})$$
$$= +92.2 - 99.4 \text{ kJ/mol} = -7.2 \text{ kJ/mol}.$$

If the $\Delta G°_f$ for all species in a reaction are known, the following equation may be used:

$$\Delta G_{rxn} = \Sigma n_p \Delta G_f \text{ (products)} - \Sigma n_r \Delta G_f \text{ (reactants)}$$

PROBLEM: Calculate the Gibbs free energy for $H_2(g) + CO_2(g) \leftrightarrow H_2O(l) + CO(g)$.

SOLUTION:

Substance	$\Delta G°_f$ in kJ/mol
H_2	0 by definition
CO_2	−394.4
H_2O	−237.1
CO	−137.2

$$\Delta G°_{rxn} = [G°_f\, H_2O + G°_f\, CO] - [G°_f\, CO_2]$$
$$[(-237.1) + (-137.2)] - [(-394.4)]\ kJ/mol = +20.1\ kJ/mol\ (\text{reactants favored})$$

Hess's law applies to $\Delta G°_{rxn}$ values. If a series of reactions add up to a total reaction, the $\Delta G°_{rxn}$ for the total reaction is the sum of the $\Delta G°_{rxn}$ of the individual reactions.

$$2S(s) + 2O_2(g) \leftrightarrow 2SO_2(g) \qquad \Delta G°_{rxn} = -600.4\ kJ/mol$$
$$\underline{2SO_2(g) + O_2 \leftrightarrow 2SO_3(g) \qquad \Delta G°_{rxn} = -141.6\ kJ/mol}$$
$$-742\ kJ/mol$$

To calculate the free energy, ΔG, for systems not at standard conditions, use the following equation:

$$\Delta G = \Delta G°_{rxn} + RT\ln Q$$

where R is the gas constant 8.314 J/mol K, T is temperature in K, and Q is the reaction quotient, which has the same form as K with initial concentrations.

$\Delta G°_{rxn}$ is related to the equilibrium constant. For a reaction with negative ΔG, spontaneous or product favored, the reaction tends to shift to the products ($K > Q$). For a reaction with positive ΔG, nonspontaneous or reactant favored, the reaction tends to shift to the reactants ($K < Q$). For a reaction with $\Delta G = 0$, there is no tendency to shift to either products or reactants ($K = Q$). This is a definition of equilibrium. So if $\Delta G = 0$, $Q = K$. Substitute into the equation for ΔG with concentration changes:

$$\Delta G = \Delta G°_{rxn} + RT\ln Q \text{ at equilibrium } \Delta G = 0 \text{ and } Q = K$$
$$\Delta G°_{rxn} = -RT\ln K, \text{ which may be rearranged to } K = e^{-(\Delta G°rxn/RT)}$$

While we addressed a number of factors and calculations in this chapter, always remember the basics and the changes in energy and entropy that drive a reaction.

CHAPTER 18

Acids and Bases

Read This Chapter to Learn About

➤ General Properties of Acids

➤ Acid-Base Equilibrium

➤ pH

➤ pH of Acid or Base Solutions

GENERAL PROPERTIES OF ACIDS

Acids are defined as substances that dissolve in water to produce H^+ ions. An H^+ ion (a proton) is so small it does not actually exist independently in water but is associated tightly with a water molecule. A better representation is $H^+(aq)$ or even better $H_3O^+(aq)$, which is the hydronium ion. Bases are defined as substances that dissolve in water to produce OH^- (hydroxide) ions.

➤ Acids that dissociate 100 percent are strong electrolytes and are termed strong acids. The six common strong acids are HCl, HBr, HI, $HClO_4$, HNO_3, and H_2SO_4.

➤ Acids that only partially disassociate are weak electrolytes and are called weak acids. A large class of weak acids are organic compounds that contain the group COOH. An example is the acid in vinegar, acetic acid, CH_3COOH. Other weak acids include HF, HCN, and H_3PO_4.

➤ Strong bases are strong electrolytes. Common strong bases are $NaOH$ and KOH.

➤ Weak bases are weak electrolytes. Weak bases include ammonia, NH_3.

Ammonia produces OH^- ions by removing a proton from water according to the following reaction:

$$NH_3(aq) + H_2O(l) \rightarrow NH_4^+(aq) + OH^-(aq)$$

Acids and bases react to produce an ionic solid (a salt) and water in a neutralization reaction.

$$HCl(aq) + NaOH(aq) \rightarrow NaCl(aq) + HOH(or\ H_2O)(l)$$

The water is initially written as HOH to emphasize the reaction as an exchange reaction. The ionic equation and net ionic equation can be written for a neutralization reaction.

PROBLEM: Consider the reaction between perchloric acid and potassium hydroxide:

$$HClO_4(aq) + KOH(aq) \rightarrow KClO_4(aq) + H_2O(l)$$

SOLUTION: Ionic equation:

$$H^+(aq) + ClO_4^-(aq) + K^+(aq) + OH^-(aq) \rightarrow K^+(aq) + ClO_4^-(aq) + H_2O(l)$$

Net ionic equation:

$$H^+(aq) + OH^-(aq) \rightarrow H_2O(l)$$

ACID-BASE EQUILIBRIUM

In the Arrhenius definition, acids form H^+ ions in water, and bases produce OH^- in water. A more general description is the Brønsted-Lowry theory of acids and bases, in which acids are defined as proton (H^+) donors and bases are defined as proton acceptors.

➤ A substance that is a Brønsted-Lowry acid must have a hydrogen atom in its formula. Not all hydrogen atoms are acidic; for example hydrogen atoms bound to carbon are generally not acidic.

➤ A substance that is a Brønsted-Lowry base must have a lone pair of electrons to accept the proton.

PROBLEM: A Brønsted-Lowry acid-base reaction is the ionization of HCl in water.

$$HCl(aq) + H_2O(l) \rightarrow Cl^-(aq) + H_3O^+(aq)$$

SOLUTION: The proton on HCl is donated to water, forming the hydronium ion, H_3O^+. This reaction goes nearly to completion, so the reaction is not written as an equilibrium. Acids that ionize nearly 100 percent such as HCl are strong acids. As a reminder, there are six common strong acids: HCl, HBr, HI, HNO_3, H_2SO_4, and $HClO_4$. Other acids that do not ionize 100 percent are called weak acids. An example is acetic acid:

$$CH_3COOH(aq) + H_2O(l) \leftrightarrow CH_3COO^-(aq) + H_3O^+(aq)$$

In a 1 M solution of acetic acid, only 4 out of every 1000 molecules ionize.

Ammonia functions as a weak base in water because it abstracts a proton from water leaving the hydroxide ion.

$$NH_3(aq) + H_2O(l) \leftrightarrow NH_4^+(aq) + OH^-(aq)$$

$$\text{Base} \qquad \text{Acid}$$

The reverse of the three preceding equations are also acid-base reactions. The reverse reactions involve a proton transfer back to the original acid. For example, this is illustrated in the acid-base reaction of HF, a weak acid.

$$HF(aq) + H_2O(l) \leftrightarrow F^-(aq) + H_3O^+(aq)$$

$$\text{Acid} \qquad \text{Base} \quad \text{Conj Base} \quad \text{Conj Acid}$$

Conjugate acid-base pairs are an acid and a related base that differs by one proton lost in the acid-base transfer. The conjugate base has a charge that is one less than the conjugate acid. The greater the tendency of an acid to donate a proton, the stronger the acid will be. An abbreviated table of relative acid strengths is shown.

Acid	Conjugate Base	Acid Strength
HCl	Cl^-	Strong
HNO_3	NO^{3-}	Strong
H_3PO_4	$H_2PO_4^-$	Weak
HF	F^-	Weak
HNO_2	NO_2^-	Weak
CH_3COOH	CH_3COO^-	Weak
NH_4^+	NH_3	Weak
HCN	CN^-	Weak
H_2O	OH^-	Water
OH^-	O_2^-	Very weak
H	H^-	Very weak

In the acid column, acid strength increases from the bottom to the top. In the base column, base strength increases from top to bottom. If an acid has a strong tendency to donate its proton, the conjugate base of this acid will have little affinity for protons. So the stronger the acid, the weaker the conjugate base will be. The relative strengths of the acids can be used to predict which side of an acid-base equilibrium will be favored.

$$H_3PO_4(aq) + CH_3COO^-(aq) \leftrightarrow H_2PO_4^-(aq) + CH_3COOH(aq)$$

H_3PO_4 is a stronger acid than CH_3COOH, so this equilibrium will favor the right side. This reaction may be thought of as a competition for the proton. The stronger base (in this case CH_3COO^-) is the conjugate of the weakest acid. In the competition for the proton, CH_3COO^- beats $H_2PO_4^-$ and the right side is favored. The acid-base equilibria will always favor the side with the weakest acid and weakest base pair.

A larger number of weak acids contain the carboxylic acid group (-COOH). Acetic acid and citric acid (shown here) are examples.

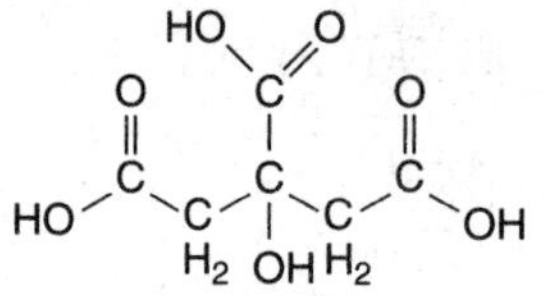

A large number of weak bases are derivatives of ammonia called amines in which the H atoms have been replaced by carbon-containing groups, such as methyl amine, CH_3NH_2, and trimethyl amine, $(CH_3)_3N$. The lone pair on the nitrogen atom of these molecules accepts a proton. In the table of relative acid and base strengths, water appears both as an acid and as a base. Such substances are called amphiprotic. The autoionization of water is an acid-base reaction between two water molecules.

$$H_2O(l) + H_2O \leftrightarrow OH^-(aq) + H_3O^+$$
$$K_w = [H_3O^+][OH^-] \text{ (at 25°C, } K_w = 10^{-14})$$

Note that the small value of K_w means that the concentration of water does not change significantly, so it is omitted from the equilibrium constant expression. An equal number of hydronium ions and hydroxide ions are formed by the ionization of water ($[H_3O^+]=[OH^-]$), which means $[H_3O^+]^2 = 1.0 \times 10^{-14}$. Taking the square root of both sides gives $[H_3O^+] = 1.0 \times 10^{-7} = [OH^-]$.

Aqueous solutions are either:

➤ neutral if $[H_3O^+] = [OH^-]$
➤ acidic if $[H_3O^+] > [OH^-]$
➤ basic if $[H_3O^+] < [OH^-]$

The product of $[H_3O^+][OH^-]$ must be 10^{-14}, so as $[H_3O^+]$ increases, $[OH^-]$ will decrease and vice versa.

$[H_3O^+]$	$[OH^-]$	Solution
10^{-1}	10^{-13}	Acidic
10^{-5}	10^{-9}	Acidic
10^{-7}	10^{-7}	Neutral
10^{-10}	10^{-4}	Basic
10^{-12}	10^{-2}	Basic

pH

The concentrations of H_3O^+ and OH^- tend to involve large negative exponents. Before pocket calculators, these numbers were cumbersome, so a more convenient quantity was defined by taking the negative logarithm of the H_3O^+ concentration. This is the pH scale. The term *pH* stands for "power of H," with H meaning H^+ or more correctly H_3O^+.

$$pH = -\log[H_3O^+], \text{ sometimes written } -\log[H^+]$$

It should always be understood that $H^+(aq)$ is a shorthand for $H_3O^+(aq)$. Aqueous solutions can be categorized as:

		Example	pH
< 7	$[H_3O^+] > [OH^-]$	Acidic $[H_3O^+] = 10^{-3} > [OH^-] = 10^{-11}$ M	3
= 7	$[H_3O^+] = [OH^-]$	Neutral $[H_3O^+] = 10^{-7} = [OH^-] = 10^{-7}$ M	7
> 7	$[H_3O^+] < [OH^-]$	Basic $[H_3O^+] = 10^{-9} < [OH^-] = 10^{-5}$ M	9

From the values and data above we can now construct a pH scale.

$$1 \longleftarrow 7 \longrightarrow 14$$

Acidic   Neutral   Basic

pH is often measured by pH paper, which has dyes that change color with changes in pH or by a meter. For pH values that are not even powers of 10, it is useful to bracket the pH value. For example, if $[H_3O^+] = 2.0 \times 10^{-4}$ the concentration is between 10^{-4} and 10^{-3}. The pH will be between 4.0 and 3.0, but closer to 4.0 (actual value, $pH = -\log(2.0 \times 10^{-4}) = 3.7$).

Acid Dissociation Constant, K_a

The equation for the ionization of an acid has a corresponding equilibrium constant called the acid dissociation constant, K_a. For a generic acid HA, the K_a equation is:

$$HA(aq) + H_2O(l) \leftrightarrow H_3O^+(aq) + A^-(aq)$$

The equilibrium constant expression that omits the solvent water is:

$$K_a = \frac{[H_3O^+][A^-]}{[HA]}$$

Likewise, the equation for the ionization of a base may be written with a corresponding equilibrium constant called the base dissociation constant, K_b. For a generic base B, the K_b equation is:

$$B(aq) + H_2(g) \leftrightarrow BH^+(aq) + OH^-(aq)$$

The equilibrium constant expression that omits the solvent water is:

$$K_a = \frac{[BH^+][OH^-]}{[B]}$$

K_a and K_b values vary over a wide range (from less than 10^{-20} to much greater than 1.0) depending on the relative strength of the acid or base. Some values illustrating the wide range are listed in the following table. The numerical values confirm the reciprocal nature of the strengths of conjugate acid-base pairs.

Acid	K_a	Conjugate Base	K_b
HCl	Very large	Cl^-	Very small
HF	7.2×10^{-4}	F^-	1.4×10^{-11}
CH_3COOH	1.8×10^{-5}	CH_3COO^-	5.6×10^{-10}
H_2O	1.0×10^{-14}	OH^-	1.0

Some acids have more than one acidic proton. For example, H_2SO_3 is a diprotic acid. Successive ionization constants decrease in value ($K_{a1} >$ etc.). HSO_3^- is about a 10^5 times weaker acid than H_2SO_3. Removal of the second proton is always more difficult because the second proton is taken from a species with one more overall negative charge.

pH OF ACID OR BASE SOLUTIONS

This section addresses how to determine the pH of acid or base solutions using strong or weak acids or bases, ionic compounds, or buffers.

Strong Acids

Because strong acids ionize 100 percent, $[H_3O^+] = [HA]_o$, and $pH = -\log[HA]_o$. A 0.015 M HNO_3 solution has $[H_3O^+] = 0.015$ M and $pH = -\log(0.015) = 1.82$.

Strong Bases

Strong bases such as sodium hydroxide ionize 100 percent, so $[OH^-] = [NaOH]$. A 0.00034 M NaOH solution has a hydroxide concentration $[OH^-] = 0.00034$ M.

$$[H_3O^+] = \frac{K_w}{[OH^-]} = \frac{1 \times 10^{-14}}{3.4 \times 10^{-4}} = 2.9 \times 10^{-11}$$
$$pH = -\log(2.9 \times 10^{-11}) = 10.54$$

The pOH is defined in a way analogous to pH; $pOH = -\log[OH^-]$. The quantities pH and pOH are related through K_w. Taking the $-\log$ of the K_w equilibrium expression gives:

$$-\log(K_w) = -\log([H_3O^+][OH^-]) \rightarrow 14.00 = pH + pOH$$

The pH of the NaOH solution could be calculated using pOH.

$$pOH = -\log(0.00034) = 3.46 \rightarrow pH = 14.00 - 3.46 = 10.54$$

Weak Acids

Weak acids do not ionize 100 percent. The concentration $[H_3O^+]$ and the pH depend upon the percent ionization. For example, consider a 2.00 M solution of an acid, HA, which ionizes 1 percent. Consider the process in two steps. The concentrations of interest can be recorded in a table.

	HA(aq) +	H$_2$O(l)	$\leftrightarrow$	A$^-$(aq) +	H$_3$O$^+$(aq)
Initial	2.00 M			0 M	0 M
Change	−0.02 M			+0.02 M	+0.02 M
Equilibrium	1.98 M			+0.02 M	+0.02 M

$$K_a = \frac{[H_3O^+][A^-]}{[HA]}$$

$$K_a = \frac{[0.02][0.02]}{[1.98]} = 2 \times 10^{-4}$$

The pH in this example is pH = −log(0.02) = 1.7.

Weak Bases

Weak base problems are similar to weak acid problems except for the K_b equation and equilibrium constant expression, K_b. The OH$^-$ concentration can be found using a table similar to that used in the previous example. pOH is calculated and converted to pH.

Salts

Salt is another name for ionic compound. A salt thus consists of a cation and an anion. Reaction of an acid with a base produces a salt and water. The acid-base properties of the salt formed will depend upon the nature of the acid or base that formed the salt. There are four possibilities.

Cation Source	Anion Source	Acidity	Equilibrium Salt
Strong base (NaOH)	Strong acid (HNO$_3$)	Neutral	NaNO$_3$
Strong base (NaOH)	Weak acid (HF)	Basic	NaF
Weak base (ammonia)	Strong acid (HCl)	Acidic	NH$_4$Cl
Weak base (ammonia)	Weak acid (HF)	Depends on K_a & K_b	NH$_4$F

Neither the cation nor the anion of a salt formed by a strong acid and a strong base has any acidity or basicity. These ions do not affect the pH. Anions from weak acids are conjugate bases, and these species will tend to make the solution basic by the following K_b reaction illustrated for F$^-$ from NaF:

$$F^-(aq) + H_2O(l) \leftrightarrow HF(aq) + OH^-(aq)$$

The $K_b = \dfrac{K_w}{K_a}$ (HF) = $\dfrac{1.0 \times 10^{-14}}{7.2 \times 10^{-4}}$ = 1.4×10^{-11}. F$^-$ is a very weak base.

Lewis Acids and Bases

Certain reactions behave in a similar fashion to the acid-base reactions described earlier but do not involve the transfer of a proton. Consider the following reaction.

$$NH_3(aq) + H_2O(l) \leftrightarrow NH_4^+(aq) + OH^-(aq)$$
$$NH_3 + BF_3 \leftrightarrow H_3N\text{-}BF_3$$

In both reactions, the lone electron pair of ammonia is reacting with an electron-poor species (H^+ in the first reaction and BF_3 in the second reaction) to form a new bond (N-H in the first and N-B in the second). The second reaction can be classified as an acid-base reaction if the definition of acids and bases is expanded to the Lewis theory:

➤ A Lewis base is defined as an electron pair donor.
➤ A Lewis acid is defined as an electron pair acceptor.

Lewis acids are electron-poor species such as H^+; highly charged transition metal ions such as Fe^{2+}, Ni^{2+}, and Co^{3+}; molecular oxides such as NO_2, SO_2, and CO_2; and certain electron-deficient compounds of elements such as Be, Al, or B. Lewis bases must, by definition, contain unshared pairs of electrons, such as NH_3, H_2O, and Cl^-.

Buffers

Solutions that are mixtures containing appreciable amounts of both a weak acid and its conjugate base are called buffers. A weak acid will dissociate into hydronium and its conjugate base to an extent determined by the value of K_a.

$$HA(aq) + H_2O(l) \leftrightarrow H_3O^+(aq) + A^-(aq)$$

Now consider the dissociation into a solution of low pH. This solution already contains hydronium ions. The equilibrium is still governed by K, but it will take less dissociation to reach the value of K_a because the $[H_3O^+]$ is initially nonzero. This suppression of the dissociation is called the common ion effect. The common ion in this case is H_3O^+, but it could just as well have been the conjugate base of the acid A^-. Buffer solutions resist changes in pH when strong acids or strong bases are added. This is especially important in biological systems because most biological molecules function best in a narrow pH range and do not tolerate large changes in pH well. The pH of a buffer can be calculated through the Henderson-Hasselbalch equation:

$$pH = pK_a + \log \frac{[A^-]}{[HA]}$$

where $pK_a = -\log K_a$. The pH is a function of the pK_a, which is fixed, and the ratio of the conjugate base to the weak acid. For example, consider a solution that has the following concentrations: $[HF] = 1.5$ M and $[F^-] = 0.50$ M. What is the pH of this solution?

The K_a of HF is 7.2×10^{-4} so $pK_a = -\log(7.2 \times 10^{-4}) = 3.14$. According to the Henderson-Hasselbalch equation, the pH of the buffer would be:

$$pH = 3.14 + \log \frac{[0.50]}{[1.5]} = 3.14 + \log 0.33 = 3.14 + (-0.48) = 2.66$$

Now consider a solution that has the composition $[HF] = [F^-] = 1.5$ M:

$$pH = 3.14 + \log \frac{[1.5]}{[1.5]} = 3.14 + \log 1 = 3.14 + (0) = 3.14$$

So:

➤ If $[A^-] = [HA]$, $pH = pK_a$
➤ If $[A^-] > [HA]$, $pH > pK_a$
➤ If $[A^-] < [HA]$, $pH < pK_a$

A buffer resists pH changes by reacting with the added strong acid or base to remove either species from the system. In the case of a HF/F⁻ buffer, the added strong base reacts with HF to form F⁻.

$$HF(aq) + OH^-(aq) \leftrightarrow F^-(aq) + H_2$$

This will increase F⁻ and decrease the HF in the buffer, so the solution is more basic, but the change will not be as large as if the added OH⁻ remained in solution.

Added strong acid will react with F⁻ to form HF.

$$F^-(aq) + H_3O^+(aq) \rightarrow HF(aq) + H_2O(l)$$

The solution becomes more acidic, but the change will be small. Buffers are most effective when the concentrations of weak acid and conjugate base are much greater than the concentration of the strong acid or base added to the buffer, and when the ratio of conjugate base to weak acid is between 0.1 and 10. The last condition means that a buffer has an effective range of $pK_a \pm 1.0$ pH units.

CHAPTER 19

Redox and Electrochemistry

Read This Chapter to Learn About

- ➤ Oxidation-Reduction Reactions
- ➤ Electrochemistry and Electrochemical Potentials
- ➤ The Relationships Between $E°_{cell}$, $\Delta G°$, and Q

OXIDATION-REDUCTION REACTIONS

In an oxidation-reduction reaction (redox for short), electrons are transferred. The species gaining electrons is reduced, and the species losing electrons is oxidized. An example is the formation of a metal oxide such as magnesium oxide:

$$2Mg(s) + O_2(g) \rightarrow 2\ MgO(s)$$

In this reaction Mg loses 2 electrons and forms a 2^+ ion, so Mg is oxidized. Simultaneously O gains two electrons and forms a 2^- ion, so O is reduced. The nature of the reaction is straightforward when ions are formed because the number of electrons lost or gained is clear. In other reactions, especially with molecular species, the transfer of electrons is not so apparent. The oxidation number is a bookkeeping method used to assign electrons to atoms to allow determination of the change in the number of electrons associated with an atom. An increase in oxidation number is oxidation. A decrease in oxidation number is reduction. In order to assign an oxidation number to an atom, follow these rules:

- ➤ The oxidation number of an atom of an element in its elemental form is zero.
- ➤ The oxidation number of a monoatomic ion is equal to the charge on the ion.

➤ Fluorine in compounds is assigned the oxidation number –1.

➤ Oxygen in compounds is assigned the oxidation number –2 unless combined with fluorine. In the peroxide ion O_2^-, oxygen has an oxidation number of –1.

➤ Hydrogen in compounds has an oxidation number of +1 except when combined with a metal, where it has an oxidation number of –1.

➤ The oxidation number of other elements is determined by the fact that the sum of the oxidation numbers of all the atoms in a species is equal to the ionic charge. For neutral molecules or atoms the sum is zero.

Ionic examples:

NaCl $Na^+ = +1$ $Cl^- = -1$
Ca_3N_2 $Ca^{2+} = +2$ $N^{3-} = -3$

Elemental symbols in parentheses represent an oxidation number

NO_2 $[(O) = -2]$ $(N) + 2(O) = 0$ $(N) = +4$
HCOOH $[(O) = -2, (H) = +1]$ $2(H) + 2(O) + (C) = 0$ $(C) = +2$
PO_4^{3-} $[(O) = -2]$ $(P) + 4(O) = -3$ $(P) = +5$
$C_2O_4^{2-}$ $[(O) = -2]$ $2(C) + 4(O) = -2$ $(C) = +3$

By looking at the change in oxidation number during the course of a reaction, you can determine which atom is oxidized or reduced.

$$2C_2H_6(g) + 7O_2(g) \rightarrow 4CO_2(g) + 6H_2O(l)$$

Assigning oxidation numbers:

C_2H_6 $[(H) = +1]$ $2(C) + 6(H) = 0$ $(C) = -3$
O_2 $[(O) = 0]$
CO_2 $[(O) = -2]$ $(C) + 2(O) = 0$ $(C) = +4$
H_2O $[(O) = -2, (H) = +1]$

Element	Reactant	Product	Change	Process
C	–3	+4	+7	Oxidation
H	+1	+1	0	None
O	0	–2	–2	Reduction

In terms of oxidation numbers, 4 carbon atoms lost 7 electrons each for a total of 28 electrons transferred, and 14 oxygen atoms gained 2 electrons each for a total of 28 electrons accepted. Oxidation and reduction must occur together. The substance that brings about oxidation is called the oxidizing agent (in this example O_2), and the substance that causes reduction is called the reducing agent (in this case C_2H_6). The oxidation agent is reduced, and the reducing agent is oxidized.

ELECTROCHEMISTRY AND ELECTROCHEMICAL POTENTIALS

In an oxidation-reduction reaction that is product favored, electrons are transferred as soon as the reactants are mixed. If the half reactions are separated, the electrons will flow through a wire and the ions will flow through the salt bridge. This current may be used to do electrical work. Such a setup is called an electrochemical or galvanic cell. An example is shown in the following figure. Many other arrangements are possible.

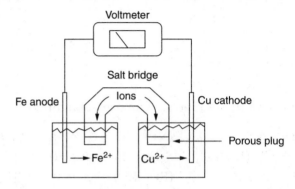

Metal or other material is often used to connect the external circuit to the two half cells. These connectors are called electrodes. The electrode for the oxidation cell is the anode, and the one for the reduction cell is the cathode. Sometimes an unreactive metal like platinum may be used as an electrode. In this cell the anode (oxidation reaction) is:

$$Fe(s) \rightarrow Fe^{2+}(aq) + 2e^-$$

And the cathode (reduction reaction) is:

$$Cu^{2+}(aq) + 2e^- \rightarrow Cu(s)$$

Electrons flow from the iron anode, where Fe^{2+} ions go into solution, through the wire to the copper cathode, where Cu^{2+} ions are reduced and deposited as Cu on the cathode. At the same time, ions move through the salt bridge to keep the charges balanced. The electrochemical cell is often represented by the notation:

anode | solution species || solution species | cathode

The double line represents the salt bridge. For this cell this representation is:

$$Fe(s) \mid Fe^{2+}(aq) \mid\mid Cu^{2+}(aq) \mid Cu(s)$$

A voltage arises when there is a difference in electrical potential. Electrons move from regions of high electrical potential to regions of low electrical potential. A positive voltage for an electrochemical cell means there is a tendency for the reaction to proceed in the direction as written. A negative voltage means the reaction has a strong tendency to proceed in the reverse direction. Charge is measured in Coulombs (C). An electron has a charge of 1.602×10^{-19} C. A volt (V) is defined as one Joule of work done when one Coulomb of charge moves through a potential of one volt.

$$1\,V = \frac{1\,J}{1\,C}$$

The standard reduction potential ($E°$) is defined as the voltage of an electrochemical cell written as a reduction reaction. For example, for iron and copper the standard reduction potentials are:

$$Fe^{2+}(aq) + 2e^- \rightarrow Fe(s) \qquad E° = -0.440 \text{ V}$$
$$Cu^{2+}(aq) + 2e^- \rightarrow Cu(s) \qquad E° = +0.337 \text{ V}$$

If you reverse a half cell, the potential is multiplied by −1. The values are referenced to the standard hydrogen electrode, which has a voltage defined to be zero.

$$E°_{cell} = E°_{cathode} - E°_{anode}$$

For this cell, Fe functions as the anode (oxidation). Its potential must be made the negative of its standard reduction potential. The Cu functions as the cathode (reduction), so its standard potential is used as is.

$$E°_{cell} = E°_{cathode} - E°_{anode} = (+0.337 \text{ V}) - (-0.440 \text{ V}) = +0.777 \text{ V}$$

Finally, when calculating $E°_{cell}$ values, never multiply the $E°_{cell}$ values by the number that the half reaction was multiplied by to balance the equation.

THE RELATIONSHIPS BETWEEN $E°_{CELL}$, $\Delta G°$, AND Q

The standard cell potential is a measure of the direction of an oxidation-reduction reaction. It has been found that the relationship between $\Delta G°$ and $E°_{cell}$ is:

$$\Delta G° = -nFE°_{cell}$$

where n is the number of moles of electrons transferred in the oxidation-reduction reaction and F is Faraday's constant. $F = \dfrac{96500 \text{ C}}{\text{mol } e^-}$. The minus sign (−) is necessary because $\Delta G°$ is negative and $E°_{cell}$ is positive for a product-favored reaction. Consider the following oxidation-reduction reaction. Recall that five electrons ($5e^-$) are transferred in this reaction.

$$MnO_4^-(aq) + 8H_3O^+(aq) + 5Fe^{2+}(aq) \rightarrow Mn^{2+}(aq) + 12 H_2O(l) + Fe^{3+}(aq)$$
$$E°_{cell} = +0.739 \text{ V}$$

You can calculate $\Delta G°$ using the relationship $\Delta G° = -nFE°_{cell}$

$$= \left(\frac{-5 \text{ mol } e^-}{\text{mol}}\right)\left(\frac{96,500 \text{ C}}{1 \text{ mol } e}\right)\left(\frac{0.739 \text{ J}}{1 \text{ C}}\right)\left(\frac{1 \text{kJ}}{1000 \text{ J}}\right) = -357 \text{ kJ/mol}$$

The mol in the denominator of the first term means per mole of the reactants and products (1 mol MnO_4^-(aq), 8 mol H_3O^+(aq), etc.). The standard free energy, $\Delta G°$, has been related to the equilibrium constant, Q, and the standard electrochemical cell potential, $E°_{cell}$. These two relationships may be combined to relate Q and $E°_{cell}$:

$$\Delta G° = -nFE°_{cell} \text{ and } \Delta G° = -RT \ln Q$$

Equating these two equations and solving for $E°_{cell}$ gives: $E°_{cell} = \dfrac{RT}{nF}(\ln Q)$ where R, T, and F are constants. If their values are substituted into the equation, the equation simplifies to:

$$E°_{cell} = \frac{0.0257 \text{ V}}{n}(\ln Q)$$

or in base 10 logarithms,

$$E°_{cell} = \frac{0.0592 \text{ V}}{n}(\ln Q)$$

Cell potential under nonstandard conditions may be calculated according to the Nernst equation:

$$E_{cell} = E°_{cell} - \frac{0.0592 \text{ V}}{n}(\log Q)(T = 298 \text{ K})$$

A summary of the relationships between values of $E°_{cell}$, $\Delta G°$, and Q and the favored side of the equation is shown in the following table.

Q	$\Delta G°$	$E°_{cell}$	Side Favored
$Q \gg 1$	$\Delta G° < 0$	$E°_{cell} > 0$	Product favored
$Q \approx 1$	$\Delta G° = 0$	$E°_{cell} = 0$	Neither
$Q \ll 1$	$\Delta G° > 0$	$E°_{cell} < 0$	Reactant favored

So the next time you use a battery to power a device, keep in mind the chemistry taking place inside it.

CHAPTER 20

Nuclear Chemistry

Read This Chapter to Learn About

- ➤ Radioactive Isotopes
- ➤ Nuclear Fission and Fusion

RADIOACTIVE ISOTOPES

As an overview, radioactive materials have the ability to undergo a change in the composition of their nucleus and become a new element. This type of a change is called a transmutation. Besides the formation of a new element or a nucleus with a new composition, there is also attention drawn to what is ejected from the nucleus, either energy or a particle.

The Belt of Stability

Not all isotopes of the elements are radioactive and undergo a decay of the nucleus. However, all elements with an atomic number of 84 or greater are guaranteed to be radioactive. What serves as an indicator as to which elements will be radioactive? The belt of stability is a good indicator as to whether a particular isotope will be stable or radioactive. Isotopes that have the ratio of neutrons to protons that falls on this belt will be stable. On the other hand, the vast majority of all radioactive isotopes do not fall on the belt of stability (which explains their unstable nucleus). Also, the belt of stability and the N/Z ratio can be used to predict what the decay mode will be for a particular isotope. In general:

- ➤ A higher ratio of neutrons to protons will dictate beta decay.
- ➤ A lower ratio of neutrons to protons will dictate positron decay or electron capture.
- ➤ An atomic number of 84 or greater will dictate alpha decay.

For example,

Isotope	Number of Neutrons	Number of Protons	Ratio of N/Z	Decay Mode	Type of Decay
U-238	146	92	1.59	Alpha	Atomic #92
C-12	6	6	1.00	Stable	N/Z = 1
C-14	8	6	1.33	Beta	Higher N/Z
Rn-222	136	86	1.58	Alpha	Atomic #86
H-3	2	1	2.00	Beta	Higher N/Z

Transmutation and Decay Modes

Before going any further, let us first reexamine the decay modes mentioned previously. Each type has its own unique properties, which are summarized here:

Decay Mode	Symbol	Mass	Charge
Alpha particle	α or $_2^4He$	4 amu	+2
Beta particle	β^- or $_{-1}^0e$ or $_{-1}^0\beta$	1/1836 amu	−1
Gamma radiation	γ or $_0^0\gamma$	0 amu	0
Positron	β^+ or $_{+1}^0e$ or $_{+1}^0\beta$	1/1836 amu	+1

Additional particles will be analyzed as we come across them in the transmutations that follow.

Besides the use of the belt of stability to determine the decay mode, we can also use the law of conservation of mass to determine the decay mode of an isotope. Consider the following transmutation:

$$_{91}^{234}Pa \rightarrow\ _{90}^{243}\text{Th} + \text{X}$$

What is the particle labeled X? Inspection of the mass numbers of the isotopes involved shows that the mass number of the reactant is 234 as is the mass number of one of the products. Because mass is conserved (along with charge and energy), the mass of X is 0. The equation also shows that a nuclear charge of 91 entered the reaction and a nuclear charge of 90 is present for the Th. In order to obey conservation of charge, X has to have a nuclear charge of +1. X is $_{+1}^0\beta$, a positron.

PROBLEM: Find X in $_6^{14}C + _1^1H \rightarrow\ _7^{14}N + \text{X}$.

SOLUTION: X must have a mass number of 1 and nuclear charge of 0. Do we know a particle with a mass of 1 amu and no charge? A neutron is $_0^1n$.

PROBLEM: Find X in $^{35}_{17}Cl + ^1_0n \rightarrow ^{35}_{16}S + X$.

SOLUTION: X must have a mass number of 1 and a nuclear charge of 1. A particle that weighs 1 amu and has a +1 charge is a proton, ^1_1H, p^+, or ^1_1p.

Another concept that can be learned from the two problems above is the concept of the artificial transmutation. Consider the nuclear transmutation $^{234}_{19}Pa \rightarrow ^{234}_{90}Th + ^0_{+1}\beta$. In this problem the protactinium decayed without having to be bombarded by another particle. In the previous two examples we see that the carbon-14 and chlorine-35 needed to be bombarded to cause a transmutation. In this case we call the transmutation an artificial transmutation.

NUCLEAR FISSION AND FUSION

Stemming from the concepts of bombardment and artificial transmutation is the bombardment of U-235 by a neutron to give the following reaction: $^{235}U + ^1_0n \rightarrow ^{141}Ba + ^{92}Kr + 3 ^1_0n + $ energy. Take note of how the addition of one neutron causes the release of three neutrons. These three neutrons can split an additional three U-235 atoms and cause nine neutrons to be released. The process continues where more neutrons are released exponentially, setting off what is called a chain reaction. This concept explains why nuclear weapons and nuclear reactors can give off the amount of energy that they do.

On the other hand, there is nuclear fusion. An excellent example of this process is the nuclear reaction that occurs in stars: $4 ^1_1H \rightarrow ^4_2He + 2 ^0_{+1}e$. Again, we have witnessed the heat and energy that the sun can give off from 93,000,000 miles away—further confirming the powerful energy associated with a nuclear reaction. What is the source of this energy? In these cases we are not looking at the endo- and exothermic reactions that occur from the breaking and formation of chemical bonds. Enter Einstein for an answer.

Examine the nuclear reaction below and take note of the masses of the reactants and products:

	$^1_1H +$	$^7_3Li \rightarrow$	$2 ^4_2He + $ energy
Atomic masses	1.00728	7.01601	8.00520
Total mass	8.02329	$\rightarrow$	8.00520

What happened to the missing 0.01809 amu? Has the concept of conservation of mass been violated? According to Einstein and the equation $E = mc^2$, it has! The missing 0.01809 amu is called the mass defect and is the mass that has been converted to energy. Remember that c^2 is $(3 \times 10^8 \text{ m/s})^2$, which is $9 \times 10^{16} \text{ m}^2/\text{s}^2$. This helps to explain why 1.6×10^{12} J of energy is released in this reaction.

Half-Life

Keeping life simple, let us take a look at the following situation: A 100-gram sample of Ag-112 is allowed to decay naturally over time. After 3.10 hours, 50 grams of the sample remains. After 6.10 hours just 25 grams, or one-fourth of the original amount, remains. With each half-life of 3.10 hours, we see that one-half of the mass of the substance remains. This leads us to the definition of half-life: the time it takes for half of the mass of a sample to decay. The half-life is a unique time for each isotope that undergoes decay, and it cannot be changed.

Stepping it up a notch, we can now use rates to calculate the half-life of a substance. But first we must revisit rate laws. The integrated rate law gives the concentration as a function of time. Derivation of the integrated rate law requires calculus, so the results will simply be stated. Two cases will be considered for a single reactant-producing product: the first order and second order.

$$A \rightarrow products$$

For a first-order reaction, the rate law is rate $= k[A]$. Integrating this equation gives:

$$\ln[A]_t = -kt + \ln[A]_o$$

where $[A]t$ is the concentration at time t, $[A]_o$ is the concentration at time 0, k is the rate constant, and t is the time. An equivalent representation is $[A]_t = [A]_o e^{-kt}$. Either form may be used. The first form is convenient for plotting an equation because it is in the form $y = mx + b$, so a plot of $\ln[A]_t$ as y and t as x will have slope of $-k$ and a y intercept of $\ln[A]_o$. The second form is probably easier for calculations.

A convenient quantity to use for a first-order reaction is the half-life $(t_{\frac{1}{2}})$, which is defined as the time required for the initial concentration of a reaction to be reduced by one-half. Half-life for a first-order reaction is easily obtained. The concentration at $t_{\frac{1}{2}}$ is one-half the initial concentration:

$$[A]_{t1} = \frac{1}{2}[A]_0$$

Substituting in the integrated rate law equation:

$$\ln\left(\frac{[A]_0}{2}\right) = -kt_{\frac{1}{2}} + \ln[A]_0$$

Rearranging the equation gives:

$$\ln\left(\frac{[A]_0}{2}\right) - \ln[A]_0 = -kt_{\frac{1}{2}}$$

Using one of the laws of logarithms, the equation can be solved for the half-life:

$$= \frac{\ln 2}{k} \quad t_{\frac{1}{2}} \ln(2) = 0.693, \text{ so } \frac{0.693}{k} = t_{\frac{1}{2}}$$

The half-life of the decomposition of SO_2Cl_2 with a k of 2.83×10^{-3} 1/min is:

$$\frac{0.693}{2.83 \times 10^{-3} \text{ 1/min}} = t_{\frac{1}{2}} = 245 \text{ mins}$$

The half-life is independent of the concentration (this is true only for a first-order reaction). The half-life remains constant during the course of the reaction. The percentage remaining as a function of number of half-lives is given in the following table:

Number of Half-Lives Elapsed	Percentage Remaining
0	100
1	50
2	25
3	12.5
4	6.25
5	3.13

This table allows you to estimate the fraction left by the number of half-lives that have elapsed. For example, what percentage of SO_2Cl_2 remains after 600 minutes of reaction? Two half-lives is $2 \times 245 = 490$ minutes, and three half-lives is $3 \times 245 = 785$ minutes. Because 600 minutes of the reaction is between 490 and 735 minutes, the percentage remaining is between 12.5 percent and 25 percent.

A second-order rate law has the form rate $= k[A]^2$. Integrating the rate law for this reaction gives:

$$\frac{1}{[A]_t} = kt + \frac{1}{[A]_0}$$

For a second-order reaction, a plot of $\frac{1}{[A]_t}$ as y and t as x will have slope of $+k$ and a y intercept of $\frac{1}{[A]_0}$. The half-life of a second-order reaction can also be derived by substituting $\frac{[A]_0}{2}$ for $[A]_t$:

$$\frac{1}{\frac{[A]_0}{2}} = kt_{\frac{1}{2}} + \frac{1}{[A]_0}$$

Solving for $t_{\frac{1}{2}}$ gives $\frac{1}{[A]_0 k} = t_{\frac{1}{2}}$.

The half-life depends on the initial concentration. Because the concentration decreases over the course of a reaction, the half-life of a second-order reaction increases with time.

Dangers and Benefits of Radioisotopes

It doesn't take much to cause alarm with the use of the word *nuclear*. While one could understand the concern from the public, nuclear materials can be used to benefit society as well. To be fair, let us examine both points of view:

Positive Aspects

Radiometric dating	C-14 is used in dating artifacts of living organisms.
	U-235 is used to date even the oldest rocks on earth.
Food preservation	Radiation can be used to kill bacteria on food and extend shelf life.
Radiotracers	I-131 can be used to diagnose thyroid disorders.
	Tracers can be used to follow certain elements in a chemical reaction.
Biological uses	Radiation can be used to overcome cancer.
	Xe-133 can be used to image the lungs.
Power	Radiation can be used as an alternative to fossil fuels.

Negative Aspects

Nuclear accidents or leaks	Three Mile Island (1979)
	Chernobyl (1986)
	Fukushima (2011)
Terrorism	Threat from nuclear weapons, dirty bombs
Biological damage	Can cause cancer
Reactor waste	Can pollute, make areas uninhabitable

The debate will continue over the use of nuclear materials. In the end it comes back to the same point—if used properly and kept properly contained, nuclear materials can be a benefit. As seen in the list, that has not always been the case, and so the debate continues.

General and Organic Chemistry Laboratory Skills

Read This Chapter to Learn About

➤ Laboratory Safety
➤ Percent Error
➤ Extraction
➤ Chromatography
➤ Distillation and Sublimation
➤ Recrystallization
➤ Combustion
➤ Chemical Tests

LABORATORY SAFETY

Let us use this chapter to bridge general and organic chemistry because both organic and general chemistry laboratory experiments add excitement (and at times disappointment) to their course. Before we examine the joy of the laboratory, let us first examine safety:

➤ Wear goggles and protective clothing at all times.
➤ Never consume food or drink in the laboratory.
➤ Pour all aqueous chemicals over a sink. Know where the inorganic/organic waste jars are located.
➤ Perform your experiments under a fume hood.
➤ Always point a test tube away from yourself or others while heating. Never stopper the test tube while heating.

➤ Know where to locate a fire extinguisher, eyewash station, and fire blankets in case of emergency.

➤ Read all labels carefully to avoid confusion.

➤ Bottle tops or stoppers placed on the table top will contaminate the contents of the bottle.

➤ Always add acid to water—never the other way around.

➤ Handle hot materials with an appropriate holder.

➤ Flush all chemicals with water when they come in contact with your skin.

➤ Note the odors of substances cautiously by gently fanning the odor toward your nose.

PERCENT ERROR

The percent error is a calculation that allows us to see how close we have come to the actual value (usually a value that our laboratory teacher has been hiding from us). The percent error can be calculated with the following equation:

$$\frac{\text{Experimental value} - \text{Accepted value}}{\text{Accepted value}} \times 100\%$$

Example: A student finds the melting point of benzoic acid to be 120°C. The actual or accepted value is 122.4°C. What is the percent error?

Using the preceding equation, we get: $\frac{120°\text{C} - 122.4°\text{C}}{122.4°\text{C}} \times 100\% = -1.96\%$, showing that the student was off by about 2°C.

Accuracy Versus Precision

Chemists are constantly repeating experiments to collect a number of results. In fact, take a course in quantitative analysis and you'll see that one must repeat an experiment at least four times. At times it has been seen where students repeated a titration nine times! Why so much data? A larger sample of data allows one to determine if the findings are precise—that is, if the data is clustered together with a minimal range. Let us examine the following data for the melting point of citric acid:

Trial 1: 153°C   Trial 2: 154°C   Trial 3: 150°C   Trial 4: 151°C

Not only is this data precise, but it is also accurate in that the data all come very close to the accepted melting point of 153°C. Again, an A in organic lab!

EXTRACTION

The basis of extraction techniques is the "like dissolves like" rule. Water typically dissolves inorganic salts (such as lithium chloride) and other ionized species, while organic solvents (ethyl acetate, methylene chloride, diethyl ether, etc.) dissolve neutral

341

**CHAPTER 21:
GENERAL AND
ORGANIC
CHEMISTRY
LABORATORY
SKILLS**

organic molecules. However, some compounds (e.g., alcohols) exhibit solubility in both media. Therefore, it is important to remember that this method of separation relies on partitioning—that is, the preferential dissolution of a species into one solvent over another. For example, 2-pentanol is somewhat soluble in water (about 17 grams per 100 mL H_2O), but infinitely soluble in diethyl ether. Thus, 2-pentanol can be preferentially partitioned into ether.

One of the most common uses of extraction is during aqueous workup as a way to remove inorganic materials from the desired organic product. On a practical note, workup is usually carried out using two immiscible solvents—that is, in a biphasic system. If a reaction has been carried out in THF, dioxane, or methanol, then it is generally desirable to remove those solvents by evaporation before workup because they have high solubilities in both aqueous and organic phases and can set up single-phase systems (that is, nothing to separate) or emulsions. Typical extraction solvents include ethyl acetate, hexane, chloroform, methylene chloride, and diethyl ether. All of these form crisp delineations between phases.

While extractions are usually carried out with a neutral aqueous phase, sometimes pH modulation can be used to advantage. For example, a mixture of naphthalenesulfonic acid and naphthalene can be separated by washing with bicarbonate, in which case the sulfonic acid is deprotonated and partitioned into the aqueous phase. Similarly, a mixture of naphthalene and quinoline can be separated by an acid wash (Figure 21.1), taking advantage of the basic nature of the heterocyclic nitrogen (pKa 9.5). If it is necessary to isolate the quinoline, it is neutralized with bicarbonate and extracted back into an organic solvent.

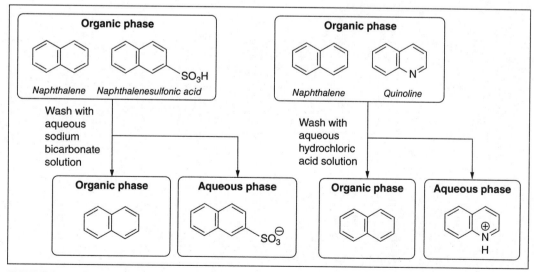

FIGURE 21.1 Two pH-controlled extractions.

CHROMATOGRAPHY

Chromatography represents the most versatile separation technique readily available to the organic chemist. Conceptually, the technique is very simple—there are two components: a stationary phase (usually silica or cellulose) and a mobile phase (usually a solvent system). Any two compounds usually have different partitioning characteristics between the stationary and mobile phases. Since the mobile phase is moving (thus the name), then the more time a compound spends in that phase, the farther it will travel.

Chromatographic techniques fall into one of two categories: analytical and preparative. Analytical techniques are used to follow the course of reactions and determine purity of products. These methods include gas chromatography (GC), high-performance liquid chromatography (HPLC), and thin-layer chromatography (TLC). Sample sizes for these procedures are usually quite small, from microgram to milligram quantities. In some cases, the chromatographic method is coupled to another analytical instrument, such as a mass spectrometer or NMR spectrometer, so that the components that elute can be easily identified. Preparative methods are used to purify larger quantities of a compound for further use.

By far the most common chromatographic technique used in the laboratory is TLC. Figure 21.2 depicts a typical TLC plate developed in a 1:1 mixture of ethyl acetate and hexane, which exhibits two well-separated components. The spots can be characterized by their R_f value, which is defined as the distance traveled from the origin divided by the distance traveled by the mobile phase. Generally speaking, the slower-moving component (R_{f1} 0.29) is either larger, more polar, or both. If we wanted a larger R_f value, we could boost the solvent polarity by increasing the proportion of ethyl acetate in the mobile phase. Conversely, more hexane would result in lower-running spots.

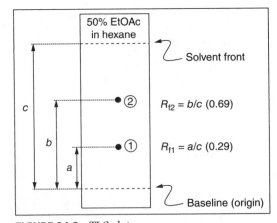

FIGURE 21.2 TLC plate.

343

**CHAPTER 21:
GENERAL AND
ORGANIC
CHEMISTRY
LABORATORY
SKILLS**

DISTILLATION AND SUBLIMATION

If chromatography is the most versatile separation method in the laboratory, it might be argued that distillation is the most common. This technique is used very frequently for purifying solvents and reagents before use. When volatile components are being removed from nonvolatile impurities, the method of *simple distillation* is employed (Figure 21.3). In this familiar protocol, a liquid is heated to a boil, forcing the vapor into a water-cooled condenser, where it is converted back to a liquid and conveyed by gravity to a receiving flask.

When separating two liquids with similar boiling points—or substances that tend to form azeotropes—*fractional distillation* is used. In this method, a connector with large surface area (such as a Vigreux column) is inserted between the still pot and the distillation head. The purpose of this intervening portion is to provide greater surface area upon which the vapor can condense and revolatilize, leading to greater efficiency of separation. In more sophisticated apparatus, the Vigreux column and condenser are separated by an automated valve that opens intermittently, thus precisely controlling the rate of distillation. For compounds with limited volatility, the technique of *bulb-to-bulb distillation* (Figure 21.4) is sometimes successful. In this distillation, the liquid never truly boils—that is to say, the vapor pressure of the compound does not reach the local pressure of the environment. Instead, the sample is placed in a flask (or bulb) and subjected to high vacuum and heat, which sets up a vapor pressure adequate to equilibrate through a passage to another bulb that is cooled with air, water, or dry ice.

Another way to distill sparingly volatile compounds is by *steam distillation*. The underlying principle of steam distillation is that an azeotrope forms with water that has a lower boiling point than the pure compound itself. For example, naphthalene has a boiling point of 218°C, but in the presence of steam an azeotrope is formed that contains 16%

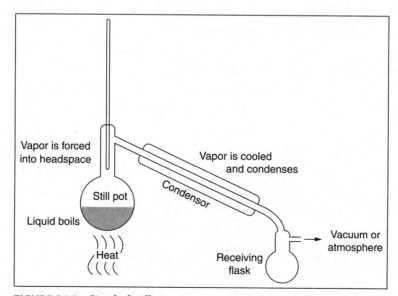

FIGURE 21.3 Simple distillation.

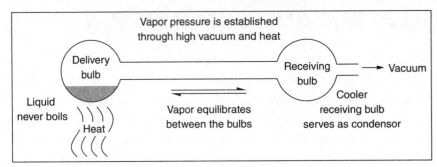

FIGURE 21.4 Bulb-to-bulb distillation.

naphthalene and boils at 99°C. In addition, the continual physical displacement of the headspace by water vapor aids in the collection of slightly volatile components.

The method of *sublimation* is identical in principle to distillation, the only difference being that the material to be purified is a solid. For example, potassium *tert*-butoxide (KO*t*-Bu) is a solid at room temperature (melting point 257°C), but at 1 torr it can be sublimed at 220°C. Because most sublimations are carried out under vacuum at high temperature, the necessary safety requirements limit the availability of a large apparatus. Further, since the cooling surface is quickly covered with solid—unlike a distillation, in which the liquid is removed from the condenser by gravity—the amount of material recoverable from a single sublimation tends to be small.

RECRYSTALLIZATION

Chromatography is the most versatile method of purification, and distillation the most common, but recrystallization is the most elegant. Unfortunately, it is also the hardest to master and the most poorly comprehended by the beginning experimentalist. In essence, the principle is quite simple: coax one compound out of solution while leaving any impurities or by-products dissolved, then separate the newly formed crystals from the solution. Consider a 10 g sample of a substance (Compound A) that is contaminated with a 5% impurity (Compound B). Another way to express this is to say that we have a mixture of 9.5 g Compound A and 0.5 g Compound B. For the sake of discussion, let us say that both compounds happen to have the same solubility characteristics in methanol: 20 g/L at room temperature and 400 g/L at the boiling point of methanol. Therefore, 25 mL of boiling methanol should be sufficient to completely dissolve the sample, since it would have the capacity to dissolve 10 g of each substance (400 g/L × 0.025 L = 10 g). After the solution has cooled to room temperature, however, the methanol can only hold 0.5 g in solution (20 g/L × 0.025 L = 0.5 g). Inasmuch as 0.5 g of each compound remains dissolved, 9.0 g of Compound A and *none* of Compound B should be present as a precipitate. Thus, by simple filtration of this mixture, Compound A can be obtained in pure form and 95% recovery $\left(\dfrac{9.0 \text{ g recovered}}{9.5 \text{ g originally}} = 0.95 \right)$.

With this example in mind, it is easy to see that recrystallization works best if the sample is already relatively pure. Since Compound B is present in comparatively small amounts, its concentration is significantly lower than that of Compound A. In fact, paradoxically, we can sometimes remove a *less soluble component* by this method if it is present in small enough quantity. However, if we were presented with a 1:1 mixture of the compounds described, the situation would not have been so straightforward.

COMBUSTION

Combustion analysis data is presented as weight percent of each given element, as shown in the boxed area of Figure 21.5. To be useful, though, this data must be converted to mole ratios of elements. The first thing to recognize here is that the weight percent values for carbon, hydrogen, and nitrogen do not add up to 100%. Given the practical considerations, we shall assume the balance is made up by oxygen (in this case, 12.58%), unless we have evidence from alternative analyses that other elements are present. Next, since we must leverage the mass quantities into molar ratios, a third column is introduced containing the atomic weights of all elements involved. Dividing the weight percent by the atomic weight gives a modified value designated χ, or molar contribution (fourth column), which has no particular meaning on its own; however, if we divide each χ value by the sum of all the χ values, we can express the elemental abundance as a mole percent value (fifth column). The final step is to find the molar ratio—the best way to approach this is to divide all mole percent values by the smallest value. For example, carbon is present in 31.80 mol% and nitrogen is present in 4.54 mol%; dividing 31.80 by 4.54, we can say that the molar ratio of carbon to nitrogen is 7.00:1.00 (sixth column).

The empirical formula already can tell us much about the structure of the molecule, aside from the obvious benefit of knowing the identity and ratio of elements on board. One useful feature we can extract from the elemental data is the degree of unsaturation (DoU), also known as the index of hydrogen deficiency (IHD). Each double bond or ring in a compound confers one degree of unsaturation (Figure 21.6). For example, benzene has four degrees of unsaturation—one for the ring, and one for each double bond in the ring.

Element	Weight %	Atomic weight	χ	Mol%	Mol ratio
C	66.10	12.011	5.503	31.80	7.00
H	10.31	1.0079	10.229	59.11	13.02
N	11.01	14.007	0.786	4.54	1.00
O	12.58	15.999	0.786	4.54	1.00
Total	100.00		17.305	100.00	

FIGURE 21.5 Treatment of combustion analysis data.

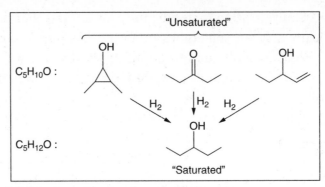

FIGURE 21.6 Degrees of unsaturation.

When presented with a molecular formula, the following method is useful in determining the degree of unsaturation:

1. Calculate the hydrogen count for the corresponding saturated molecule:
    ➤ Number of hydrogens = 2(number of carbons) + 2
    ➤ Oxygen (or any divalent species) has no effect on this count.
    ➤ For every nitrogen (or any trivalent species) add 1.
    ➤ For every halogen (or any monovalent species) subtract 1.
    These calculations can be summarized with the equation $C_aH_bN_cO_dX_e$ and
    $$= \frac{1}{2}(2 + 2a - b + c - e).$$

2. Compare the actual hydrogen count to the saturated hydrogen count:
    ➤ Divide the difference by 2 to get the DoU.
    ➤ If the difference is an odd number, recheck the math in step 1.

Applying these guidelines to an example, let us consider the empirical formula $C_5H_7N_2OCl$. Since the formula has 5 carbons, we would predict 12 (2n + 2) hydrogen atoms for a simple hydrocarbon. The presence of oxygen has no effect on this value, but we adjust the hydrogen count up by two on account of the two nitrogen atoms, and then down by one because of the monovalent chlorine. The adjusted saturation count for hydrogen is thus 13. The empirical formula has only 7, for a difference of 6—dividing this value by 2 gives 3 degrees of unsaturation. With this in hand, we can limit our consideration to those molecules that exhibit the proper degree of unsaturation—one such example is shown in Figure 21.7.

DoU Calculation for $C_5H_7N_2OCl$		
"Normal" saturation count	12	
Modification for oxygen	0	
Modification for nitrogen	+2	
Modification for chlorine	−1	
Adjusted saturation count	13	
Actual hydrogen count	7	
Δ between actual and saturated	6	
Degrees of unsatuaration (Δπ 2)	3	

One of many structures consistent with the empirical formula

FIGURE 21.7 Sample calculation for degrees of unsaturation.

347

**CHAPTER 21:
GENERAL AND
ORGANIC
CHEMISTRY
LABORATORY
SKILLS**

CHEMICAL TESTS

Chemical tests are a magnificent way of confirming the presence of a functional group. Coupled with IR and other various spectra and the classification via solubility, confirmation of a functional group is almost 100 percent guaranteed—the first step in deciding on an appropriate derivative to confirm the compound in question. Table 21.1 briefly summarizes a few chemical tests and the results of their positive tests.

Table 21.1 Chemical Tests for Organic Functional Groups		
Functional Group	**Name of Chemical Test**	**Positive Test Result**
Alkenes/alkynes	Bromine water	Brown-orange color of the bromine water will become clear.
Aldehydes	Tollen's	Formation of a silver "mirror" on the bottom of the test tube.
Aldehydes/ketones	2,4-dinitrophenylhydrazine (DNPH)	A precipitate forms. Yellow indicates the aldehyde or ketone is most likely aliphatic/non-conjugated. Orange-red color indicates conjugation/aromaticity bonded to C=O.
Ketones (R-C(=O)-CH$_3$)/ alcohols (R-CHOH-CH$_3$)	Iodoform	Formation of a yellow solid that has a melting point of 119°C.
Secondary or tertiary alcohols	Lucas	Tertiary alcohols will result in a cloudy solution almost immediately. Secondary alcohols will cloud the solution in about five minutes.
Phenols	Iron (iii) chloride	Produces a blue, violet, or purple solution.
Carboxylic acids	Sodium bicarbonate	Production of carbon dioxide gas.

CHAPTER 22

The Basics: Nomenclature, Stereochemistry, Properties

Read This Chapter to Learn About

➤ Nomenclature
➤ Stereochemistry
➤ Bonding
➤ Molecular Geometries
➤ Trends in Physical Properties
➤ Trends in Acid-Base Properties

NOMENCLATURE

Straight-chain hydrocarbons are named according to the number of carbons in the chain (Table 22.1). If used as a substituent, the names are modified by changing the suffix *-ane* to *-yl*; thus, a two-carbon alkane is *ethane*, but a two-carbon substituent is *ethyl*. In the event of branched hydrocarbons, rules established by IUPAC (International Union of Pure and Applied Chemists) dictate that the longest possible chain be used as the main chain, then all remaining carbons constitute substituents. If two different chains of equal length can be identified, then the one giving the greatest number of substituents should be chosen.

Table 22.1 Naming Straight-Chain Alkanes		
Name	**Number of Carbons**	**Formula**
Methane	1	CH_4
Ethane	2	CH_3CH_3
Propane	3	$CH_3CH_2CH_3$
Butane	4	$CH_3(CH_2)_2CH_3$
Pentane	5	$CH_3(CH_2)_3CH_3$
Hexane	6	$CH_3(CH_2)_4CH_3$
Heptane	7	$CH_3(CH_2)_5CH_3$
Octane	8	$CH_3(CH_2)_6CH_3$
Nonane	9	$CH_3(CH_2)_7CH_3$
Decane	10	$CH_3(CH_2)_8CH_3$

When molecules contain functional groups, then the parent chain is defined as the longest possible carbon chain that contains the highest-priority functional group (Table 22.2). Once that parent chain is identified, then all other functionalities become substituents (modifiers). For example, consider the two compounds in Figure 22.1. Both contain the hydroxy (-OH) functional group, but in the left it defines the parent chain. Therefore, the *-ol* form is used, and the compound is named *propan-2-ol*. However, the right compound has both the hydroxy and the carbonyl functional groups. Since the carbonyl has the higher IUPAC priority, it defines the parent chain; the hydroxy group thus serves only as a modifier, and the *-ol* suffix is not used.

Table 22.2 The Suffixes Used for Certain Functional Groups			
Functional Group	**Formula**	**As Parent**	**As Modifier**
Carboxylate ester	$R\text{-}CO_2R'$	alkyl-oate	—
Carboxylic acid	$R\text{-}CO_2H$	-oica cid	carboxy
Acyl halide	R-COX (Cl, Br, I)	-oyl halide	—
Amide	$R\text{-}CONH_2$	-amide	—
Nitrile	R-CN	-nitrile	cyano-
Aldehyde	R-COH	-al	oxo-
Ketone	R-C(O)-R'	-one	oxo-
Alcohol	–OH	-ol	hydroxy-
Amine	$–NH_2$	-amine	-amino
Ether	R–OR'	(Only used as modifiers)	alkoxy-
Nitro	$R–NO_2$		nitro-
Halide	R-X(F, Cl, Br, I)		halo- (e.g., chloro-)

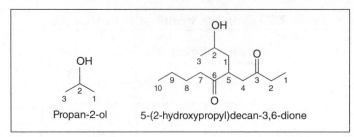

FIGURE 22.1   Functional groups in the main chain and as substituent.

STEREOCHEMISTRY

There are also IUPAC rules governing the nomenclature of stereoisomers, or absolute stereochemistry. Since any chiral carbon is surrounded by four different groups, the first order of business is to prioritize the substituents according to the IUPAC convention known as the Cahn-Ingold-Prelog (CIP) rules. The algorithm for CIP prioritization is as follows:

➤ Examine each atom connected directly to the chiral center (we shall call these the *field atoms*); rank according to atomic number (high atomic number has priority).

➤ In the event of a field atom tie, examine the substituents connected to the field atoms. (1) Field atoms with higher atomic number substituents have priority. (2) If substituent atomic number is tied, then field atoms with more substituents have priority.

For the purposes of prioritization, double and triple bonds are expanded—that is, a double bond to oxygen is assumed to be two oxygen substituents. If two or more field atoms remain in a tie, then the contest continues on the next atom out for each center, following the path of highest priority.

The next step is to orient the molecule so that the lowest-priority field atom is going directly away from us, as is shown on the right side of Figure 22.2 (atom d). Viewing this projection, we observe whether the progression of a → b → c occurs in a clockwise or counterclockwise sense. If clockwise, the enantiomer is labeled *R* (from the Latin *rectus*, proper); if counterclockwise, *S* (sinister, Latin *sinistrorsus*, to the left).

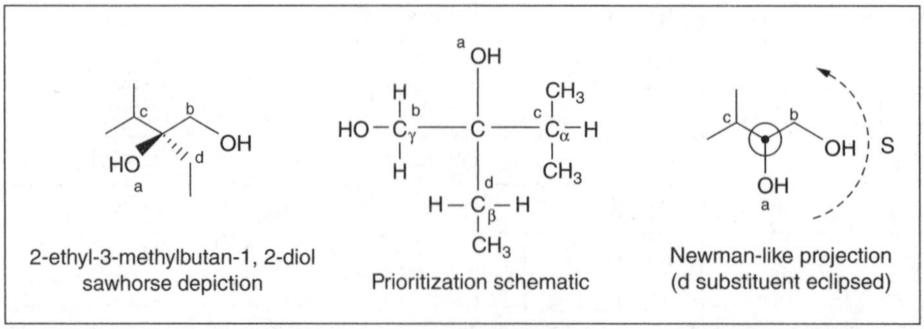

**2-ethyl-3-methylbutan-1, 2-diol
sawhorse depiction**

Prioritization schematic

**Newman-like projection
(d substituent eclipsed)**

FIGURE 22.2   R/S designation.

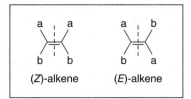

FIGURE 22.3 Stereochemistry of alkenes.

The stereochemistry of double bonds is also specified using CIP priorities. In this protocol, each double bond examined and the substituents on each side are prioritized according to the CIP rules illustrated in Figure 22.3. If the two high-priority substituents (a) are pointing in the same direction, the double bond is specified as Z (from the German, *zusammen*, or together); if they point in opposite directions, the double bond is designated E (German *entgegen*, or across from). Adding this stereochemical information to the chemical name proceeds exactly as described for *R/S* designation.

BONDING

Chemical bonds conventionally fall into one of two categories: ionic and covalent. When the electronegativity difference between the atoms is quite small, the electron density is equally distributed along the internuclear axis, and it reaches a maximum at the midpoint of the bond. Such a bond is said to be purely covalent. On the other hand, when the two nuclei have widely divergent electronegativities, the electron density is not "shared" at all: two ionic species are formed and the electron density approaches zero along the internuclear axis at the edge of the ionic radius. Polar covalent bonds result from an uneven sharing of electron density, a situation that sets up a permanent dipole along the bond axis. The O-H and C-F bonds are examples of polar covalent bonds. Such bonds are stronger than one would expect because the covalent attraction is augmented by the coulombic forces set up by the dipole.

With respect to global connectivity, the Lewis dot diagram represents a simple but powerful device. These diagrams are built up by considering the valence electrons brought to the table by each atom and forming bonds by intuitively combining unpaired electrons. For example, formaldehyde (H_2CO) is constructed in Figure 22.4.

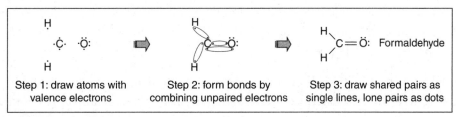

FIGURE 22.4 Lewis structure of formaldehyde.

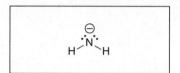

FIGURE 22.5 Lewis structure
of the amide ion.

There are two types of electron pairs in the molecule in Figure 22.4: (1) shared pairs (or bonds), which are represented by lines (each line representing two shared electrons), and (2) lone pairs, which are depicted using two dots. When calculating formal charges, assign to a given atom all of its lone pair electrons and half of each shared pair; then compare the sum to the number of valence electrons normally carried. For example, consider the amide anion (Figure 22.5). The nitrogen atom is surrounded by two lone pairs (nitrogen "owns" all four) and two shared pairs (nitrogen "owns" only one in each pair), giving a total of six electrons assigned to nitrogen. Compared to the five valence electrons normally carried by nitrogen, this represents an excess of one electron; therefore, a formal charge of −1 is given to the nitrogen atom.

Often, molecules can be represented by multiple Lewis structures. These are known as resonance forms, and while all reasonable candidates tell us something about the nature of the molecule in question, some resonance structures are more significant contributors than others. In making such an assessment, the following guidelines are helpful:

Rules of Charge Separation

➤ All things being equal, structures should have minimal charge separation.
➤ Any charge separation should be guided by electronegativity trends.

Octet Rules

➤ **Little octet rule:** all things being equal, each atom should have an octet.
➤ **Big octet rule:** no row 2 element can accommodate more than eight electrons.

Of all these, only the big octet rule is inviolable. Structures that break the first three rules are less desirable—those that break the last one are unreasonable and unsupportable. However, even when one structure satisfies all the rules, other resonance forms may need to be considered to predict the properties of a molecule.

Double bonds are formed by the interaction of two adjacent p orbitals. Similarly, extended π systems develop when three or more adjacent p orbitals are present, as is the case with butadiene (Table 22.3). Such double bonds are said to be *conjugated*, a term that stems from their tendency to undergo reactions as an interconnected system rather than as isolated double bonds.

Molecules with multiple double bonds are more stable if those bonds are arranged in alternating arrays so that extended π systems can be formed. For example, 1,3-pentadiene is more stable than 1,4-pentadiene. A similar (but weaker) effect can arise from the interaction of p orbitals with adjacent σ bonds. For example, the methyl cation is not a

Table 22.3 Pi Molecular Orbitals for Butadiene				
LCAO	**Schematic**	**Nodes**	**Population**	**Frontier**
$+\varphi_1-\varphi_2+\varphi_3-\varphi_4$		3	——	
$+\varphi_1-\varphi_2-\varphi_3+\varphi_4$		2	——	LUMO
$+\varphi_1+\varphi_2-\varphi_3-\varphi_4$		1	⇅	HOMO
$+\varphi_1+\varphi_2+\varphi_3+\varphi_4$		0	⇅	

very stable species, owing to the empty p orbital on the carbon and the resulting violation of the octet rule. However, the ethyl cation is a bit more stable because the C-H sigma bond on the methyl group can spill a bit of electron density into the empty p orbital, thereby stabilizing the cationic center (Figure 22.6). This is an effect known as *hyperconjugation*, and while the sharing of electron density is not nearly as effective here as in true conjugation, it is still responsible for the following stability trend in carbocations and radicals: methyl < primary < secondary < tertiary.

Aromaticity is a special form of conjugation that confers particular stability to compounds, and it arises only from systems possessing a cyclic, contiguous, and coplanar array of p orbitals (Figure 22.7). But this arrangement can also result in antiaromaticity, whereby molecules are less stable than expected. The difference between aromaticity and antiaromaticity lies in the number of π electrons housed in the cyclic array. This can be predicted using Hückel's rule, which states that systems having $4n$ π electrons

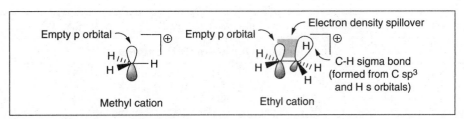

FIGURE 22.6 Hyperconjugation in the ethyl cation.

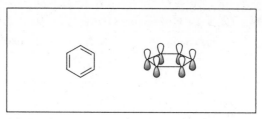

FIGURE 22.7 Contiguous P orbitals in benzene.

(4, 8, 12 electrons, etc.) tend to be antiaromatic, and those having $(4n + 2)\,\pi$ electrons (2, 6, 10 electrons, etc.) tend to be aromatic.

Electronic systems can be strongly impacted by substituents, which are generally designated either electron withdrawing (EW) or electron donating (ED). There are two components of electron-withdrawing and electron-donating behavior: resonance and induction. As the term suggests, the resonance effect can be represented by electron-pushing arrows to give different resonance forms. This effect may be weak or strong, but it can exert influence over very large distances through extended π systems. The inductive effect stems primarily from electronegativity; it can be quite strong, but its influence is local—the magnitude drops off sharply as distance from the functional group increases. Table 22.4 summarizes these effects for some common functional groups. In most cases the inductive and resonance effects work in concert, while in some instances they are at odds.

Table 22.4 Some Common ED and EW Groups			
Functional Group	**Formula**	**Resonance Effect**	**Inductive Effect**
Net Electron-Withdrawing (EW) Groups			
Acetyl	$-COCH_3$	EW	EW
Carbomethoxy	$-CO_2CH_3$	EW	EW
Chloro	$-Cl$	ED	EW
Cyano	$-CN$	EW	EW
Nitro	$-NO_2$	EW	EW
Phenylsulfonyl	$-SO_2Ph$	EW	EW
Net Electron-Donating (ED) Groups			
Amino	$-NH_2$	ED	EW
Methoxy	$-OCH_3$	ED	EW
Methyl	$-CH_3$	ED	EW

MOLECULAR GEOMETRIES

There are three frequently encountered central-atom geometries in organic chemistry: digonal (or linear), trigonal planar, and tetrahedral (Figure 22.8). Each atom within a molecule is almost always characterized by one of these geometries, the chief hallmark of which is the associated bond angle: 180° for linear arrays, 120° for trigonal planar centers, and 109.5° for tetrahedral arrangements. One classical approach to rationalize these geometries is through hybridization of atomic orbitals, as shown in Figure 22.9.

In cases where a tetrahedral center is surrounded by four uniquely different groups, the center is said to be asymmetric, or chiral. Molecules containing asymmetric centers (chiral centers, or stereocenters) are themselves usually chiral, and therefore exist in two enantiomeric forms that are nonsuperimposible mirror images (Figure 22.10). Enantiomers are identical in almost all physical properties with one notable exception. A chiral compound rotates plane-polarized light that passes through it, a phenomenon

Geometry	Arrangement	Bond angle	Hybridization of x
Digonal	a — x — b	180°	sp
Trigonal	$\overset{a}{\underset{c}{\diagdown}}$ x — b	120°	sp^2
Tetrahedral	$\overset{a}{\underset{c}{d \text{—} x}} \text{— b}$	109.5°	sp^3

FIGURE 22.8 Common molecular geometries in organic chemistry.

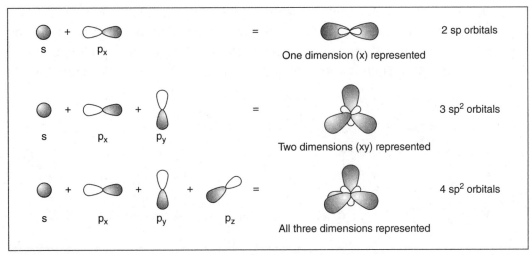

FIGURE 22.9 Central atom geometry as described by orbital hybridization.

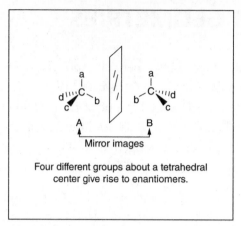

FIGURE 22.10 Tetrahedral centers and enantiomerism.

known as optical rotation. Its enantiomer rotates plane-polarized light to the same degree, but in the opposite direction. Racemic mixtures, which contain exactly equal amounts of enantiomers, do not exhibit optical activity.

Compounds with more than one chiral center can form diastereomers, as is the case with the naturally occurring sugar D-ribose (Figure 22.11). Since there are three chiral centers, the total number of unique permutations is $2^3 = 8$. D-ribose represents one such permutation, and the enantiomer of D-ribose is l-ribose. Notice that *each and every chiral center is inverted*—this is true for any set of enantiomers. Thus, l-ribose accounts for one stereoisomer of D-ribose, but there are six others—all of them diastereomers of D-ribose. Thus, a diastereomer is a stereoisomer in which one or more, *but not all*, chiral centers have been inverted.

Once connectivity has been established, molecular conformation must be considered, and this can be examined in several ways. For example, the sawhorse projection (Figure 22.12) views the molecule from the side, whereas a Newman projection looks at the molecule along a carbon-carbon bond (indicated by the observer's eye). Newman projections are useful for examining the difference between staggered and eclipsed conformations.

In staggered conformations, any two substituents are characterized by one of two relationships. Substituents are gauche with respect to each other if they are side by side. In the illustration, there are six gauche relationships: a-e, e-c, c-f, f-b, b-d, and d-a. The other relationship is antiperiplanar, in which case the two substituents are

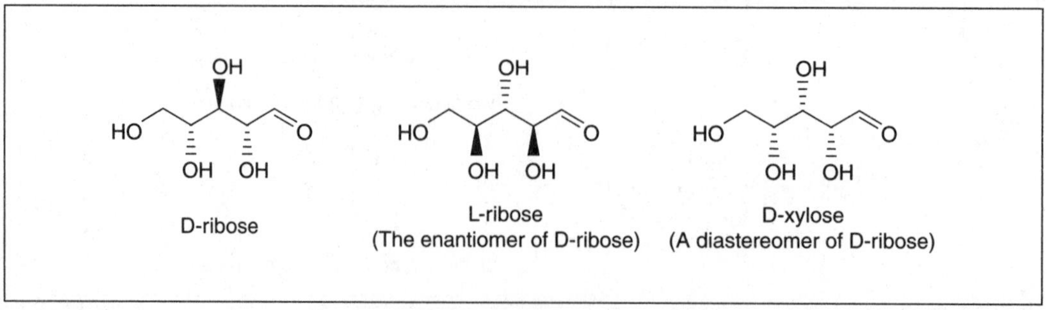

OH
HO O
OH OH
D-ribose

OH
HO O
OH OH
L-ribose
(The enantiomer of D-ribose)

OH
HO O
OH OH
D-xylose
(A diastereomer of D-ribose)

FIGURE 22.11 Enantiomers vs. diastereomers.

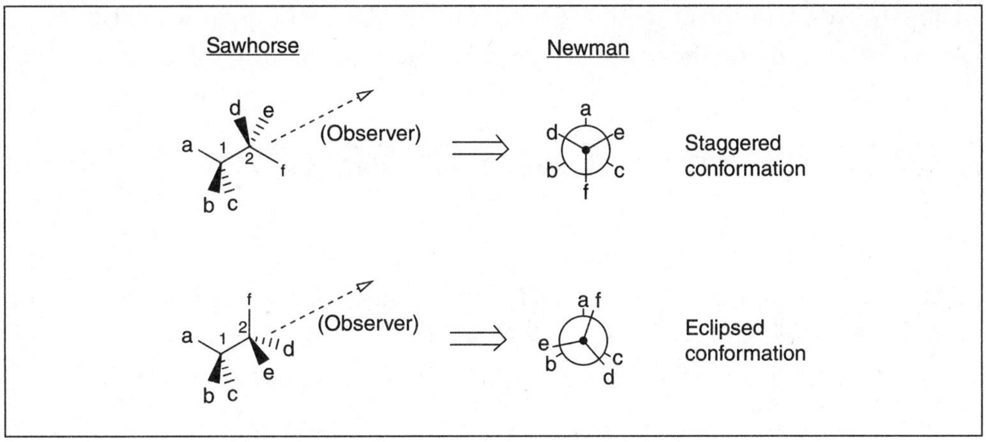

FIGURE 22.12 Sawhorse and Newman projections.

as far away as possible from each other. In eclipsed conformations, the only type of relationship between substituents is that in which they are eclipsed to one another. It should come as no surprise that eclipsed conformations are of higher energy than staggered conformations. By the same token, staggered conformations that place large groups in a gauche arrangement are of higher energy than those that have those groups antiperiplanar with respect to each other.

Cyclic molecules are less flexible than their open-chain analogs, and they can adopt far fewer conformations. For example, the most stable arrangement in cyclohexane is the so-called chair conformation (Figure 22.13), in which substituents can adopt one of two attitudes: axial (shown as triangles in the left chair) or equatorial (shown as squares in the left chair)—every chair conformation has six of each type. Note that a chair flip interchanges axial and equatorial substituents, so that all of the triangles become equatorial on the right side. As a general rule, the bulkiest substituent prefers the equatorial position.

Cyclic molecules can experience bond angle strain and torsional strain. The former is caused by a deviation from the ideal sp^3 bond angle (109.5°). This is worst for the three-membered ring and almost nil for five- and six-membered rings. Torsional strain, on the other hand, derives from the torque on individual bonds from eclipsed substituents trying to get out of each other's way. Again, this is most pronounced in cyclopropane, and all the other cycloalkanes twist in ways to minimize or eliminate this strain. In general, ring strain decreases according to the trend: 3 > 4 > > 5 > 6.

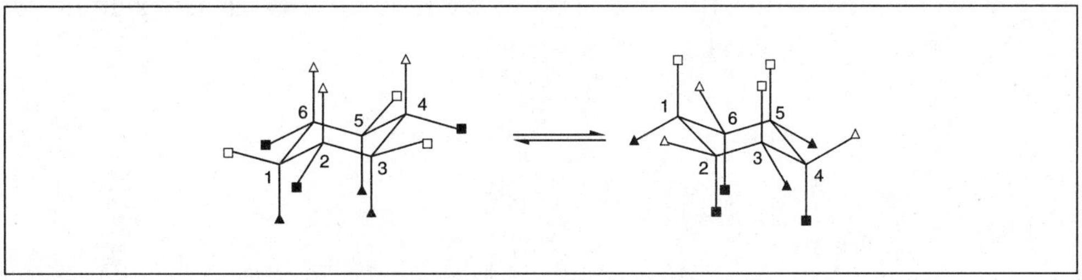

FIGURE 22.13 The chair flip of cyclohexane.

Knowing the trends of the functional groups and structures of organic molecules is just as important as studying the periodic trends in a general chemistry course.

TRENDS IN PHYSICAL PROPERTIES

When examining the melting and boiling points of hydrocarbons, one must keep in mind that we are dealing with nonpolar hydrocarbons and that dispersion forces come into play. With that we know the obvious: as the molecular mass of the compound increases, the boiling and melting points will increase, as evidenced here:

Compound	Melting Point °C	Boiling Point °C
Methane	−183	−162
n-Hexane	−95	69
n-Decane	−30	174

We can also compare straight-chain hydrocarbons to their corresponding branched hydrocarbon and see that the branched isomer has a lower boiling point than the straight chain:

Compound	Boiling Point °C
n-Butane	0
Isobutane	−12
n-Pentane	36
Isopentane	28
Neopentane	9.5

Because the branched isomers cannot pack together as effectively as the straight-chain isomer, they do not experience as many dispersion forces as the corresponding straight-chain alkane.

TRENDS IN ACID-BASE PROPERTIES

Keeping in mind that a larger K_a value for an acid means that an acid is stronger, a larger pK_a value means that the acid is weaker. Knowing this, let us examine some trends that occur regarding acid-base properties.

Hydrocarbon	pK_a Value
Ethane	50
Ethene	44
Ethyne	25

The terminal alkyne is more acidic than the alkane and alkene. This allows a terminal alkyne to react with $NaNH_2$ in NH_3 to yield $H-C\equiv C:^-$, making it available for further syntheses. This leads us to the general rule that the more s character on an anion, the more stable the anion will be.

We can also study the inductive effects that highly electronegative atoms have on the acidity of a molecule. For example, compare the pK_a values of acetic acid and ethanol:

Acetic Acid	**Ethanol**
$pK_a = 4.7$	$pK_a = 16$

While both groups have an -OH group on them, the presence of a carbonyl, C=O, withdraws electron density, allowing the H^+ to separate more easily. It should also be noted that when comparing the anions that form when these molecules lose an electron, the acetate ion will be more stable because of possible resonance stabilized structures. To take it one step further, compare the pK_a values of acetic acid to chloroacetic acid.

Acetic Acid	**Chloroacetic Acid**
$pK_a = 4.7$	$pK_a = 2.9$

Again, we see that the highly electronegative chlorine atom is creating a highly electron-attracting inductive effect causing the proton to separate from the molecule. This brings us to trichloroacetic acid and its use. A dermatologist uses this compound to remove warts. Thanks to the three chlorine atoms withdrawing electrons, the pK_a of this compound is approximately 0.70—warts beware!

We can also look at inductive effects with regard to the distance from the carboxylic acid. In general, inductive effects lose their effect with distance. For example, consider butanoic acid, $CH_3CH_2CH_2COOH$. If the chlorine atom were placed on the carbon atom (carbon #2) next to the -COOH, its effect on making the molecule a stronger acid would be greater than if it were placed on the third carbon atom (carbon #4). In fact, when the chlorine atom is four carbon atoms away from the -COOH group, its electron-attracting forces are rarely of importance.

PROBLEM: Which of the following compounds would you expect to have a lower pK_a value?

$$F-CH_2-COOH \text{ or } Br-CH_2-COOH$$

SOLUTION: There is no contest: fluorine is more electronegative and will be able to withdraw electrons better than the bromine, causing the carboxyl group to lose the proton. The fluorinated compound will be more acidic and have a lower pK_a.

Our last look at acidity of compounds will look at ethanol and phenol. There is a huge difference in the pK_a values of these two compounds:

Phenol, C_6H_5-OH $pK_a = 9.8$
Ethanol, CH_3CH_2OH $pK_a = 16$

These numbers show that phenol is 10^6 times more acidic than ethanol. Why? Aren't they both alcohols? Phenol is 10^6 times more likely to lose its proton because the benzene ring will have resonance stabilized structures. This stabilization does not occur with ethanol. Taking a look at benzyl alcohol:

$$C_6H_5\text{-}CH_2\text{-}OH$$

we see that the OH group is not directly bonded to the benzene ring and will *not* be stabilized via resonance structures. The pK_a value of this alcohol is about 16, the same as that of ethanol.

Please keep in mind that this chapter is a foundation for the remaining organic chemistry chapters to come. Refer to it as needed.

CHAPTER 23

Reactions and Mementos Mechanisms

RADICAL REACTIONS

Generally speaking, mechanistic steps fall into three broad categories:

➤ **Radical reactions**, which involve species with unpaired electrons and the motion of single electrons
➤ **Polar reactions**, which engage the activity of electron pairs and usually involve coulombic charges in the mechanistic pathway
➤ **Pericyclic reactions**, in which electrons move in concert without the generation of charge

Within the radical paradigm, there are three important generic reactions as shown in Figure 23.1: atom abstraction, addition to a pi bond, and fragmentation. Note that in each case the number of radical centers is constant in going from left to right. That is, the radical count neither increases nor decreases.

But what is the origin of the first radical center? One of the most common radical-producing processes is the homolytic cleavage of σ bonds, in which the two electrons of the shared pair go in separate directions to produce two new radicals (Figure 23.2).

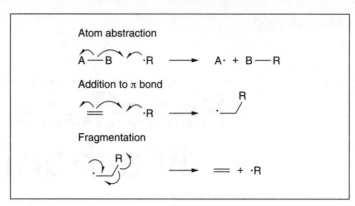

FIGURE 23.1 Three basic radical processes.

As part of a mechanism, this would fall under the heading of an initiation step. By the same token, the combination of any two radicals to form a new molecule would constitute a termination sequence (Figure 23.2).

Between initiation and termination there is propagation, and any of the processes shown in Figure 23.1 can serve as propagation steps. Since homolytic cleavage requires quite a bit of energy, if we relied on the stoichiometric generation of radicals through this process, the rate would be so slow as to be synthetically useless. Instead, once a single radical is formed, it can engage in a series of self-sustaining propagation steps to generate new compounds. This is nicely illustrated with the radical bromination of methane (Figure 23.3). The initiation step involves the homolytic cleavage of molecular bromine into two bromine radicals. In principle, this step (at a costly 46 kcal/mol) must only occur once. Afterward, the bromine radical attacks methane, engaging in hydrogen atom abstraction to form hydrobromic acid and methyl radical (Step 1). The methyl radical, in turn, attacks molecular bromine (present in stoichiometric quantity), which suffers bromine atom abstraction and produces methyl bromide and regenerates bromine radical (Step 2). Notice that each of the propagation steps consumes stoichiometric reactant and generates stoichiometric product.

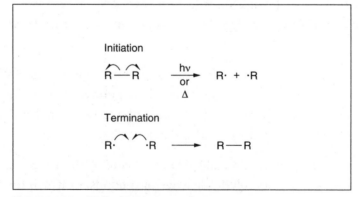

FIGURE 23.2 Radical initiation and termination.

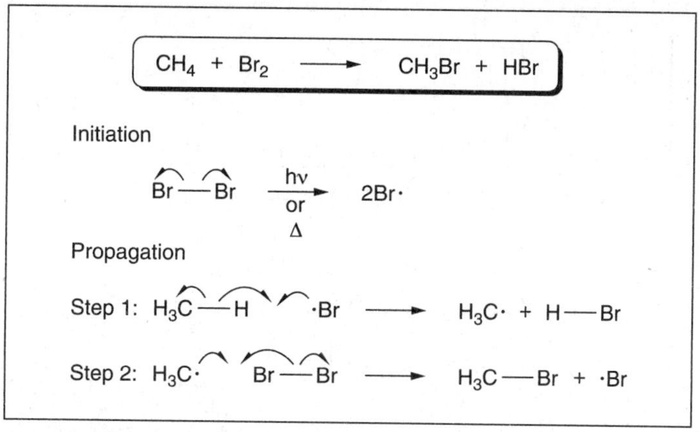

FIGURE 23.3 Radical bromination of methane.

POLAR REACTIONS

Turning our attention to polar chemistry, the most common representative of this class is the proton transfer, otherwise known as acid-base reactions. There are three general paradigms of acid-base chemistry, as shown in Table 23.1. We will use the Lewis acid-base concept as a workhorse for understanding much of the mechanistic underpinnings of polar chemistry. However, proton transfer is best treated using the Brønsted notion of acids and bases. For example, we can represent the experimentally derived equilibrium constant for the ionization of acetic acid (AcOH) as shown in Figure 23.4, where the equilibrium constant bears the special designation of acidity constant (K_a).

We can also express the acidity constant in terms of the chemical species involved, which has the generic form:

$$K_a = \frac{[H^+][A^-]}{[HA]} = \frac{[H^+][AcO^-]}{[HOAc]}$$

Table 23.1 Three Acid-Base Paradigms				
Paradigm	**Acid**		**Base**	
	Definition	**Example of Species Embraced**	**Definition**	**Example of Species Embraced**
Arrhenius	Proton donor	HCl	Hydroxide donor	NaOH
Brønsted	Proton donor	HCl	Pronor donor	NaOH, **NH$_3$**
Lewis	Electron density acceptor	HCl, **Fe^{3+}**, **BF$_3$**	Electron density donor	NaOH, NH$_3$

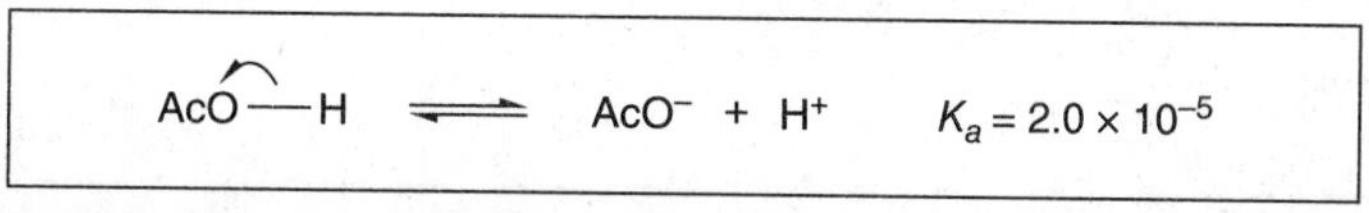

FIGURE 23.4 The ionization of acetic acid.

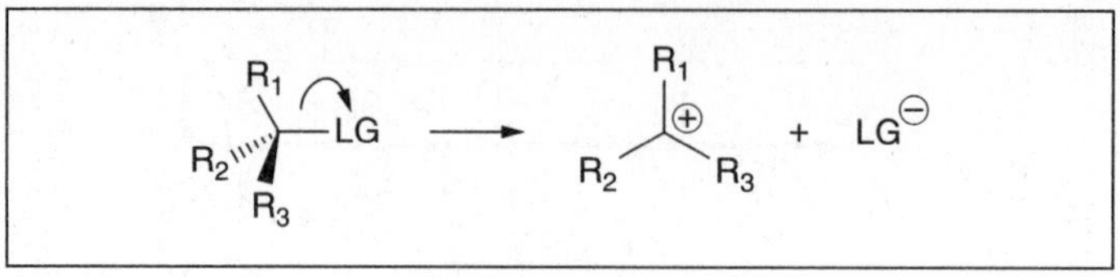

FIGURE 23.5   Unimolecular ionization.

In addition, an analogous scale of pK_a can be used to express the numerical values of the acidity constant according to the relationship:

$$pK_a = -\log_{10}(K_a)$$

Therefore, using $K_a = 2.0 \times 10^{-5}$, acetic acid is associated with a pK_a value of 4.7.

Another form of ionization is also frequently encountered in organic chemistry (Figure 23.5). Here a sigma bond is cleaved heterolytically to form an anion and a carbocation (carbon-centered cation). For this reaction to be kinetically relevant, the leaving group (LG) must provide a very stable anion, and the carbocation must be secondary, tertiary, or otherwise stabilized (for example, allylic or benzylic). Good leaving groups (such as chloride or water) are generally species with strong conjugate acids (HCl and hydronium, respectively). Once a carbocation has been formed, it can suffer subsequent capture by a nucleophile to form a new bond. In principle, any species that would be classified as a Lewis base is a potential nucleophile, since a nucleophile is also a source of electron density.

When ionization is followed by nucleophilic capture, an overall process known as unimolecular substitution (S_N1) occurs. An illustrative example is the solvolysis reaction, in which solvent molecules act as the nucleophilic species. Thus, when 2-bromobutane is dissolved in methanol, ionization ensues to form a secondary carbocation, which is captured by solvent to give (after proton loss) 2-methoxybutane (Figure 23.6). Note that even though optically pure (S)-2-bromobutane is used, the product is obtained as a racemic mixture.

Another characteristic of this mechanism—as the name implies—is the unimolecular nature of its kinetics. In other words, the rate of the reaction is dependent only upon the concentration of the substrate, according to the rate law:

$$rate = k[\text{2-bromobutane}]$$

Since ionization involves breaking a bond, it is the most demanding step energetically. It is therefore the slowest, or rate-determining step. Furthermore, since this step involves only the substrate, it is the only component of the overall rate law.

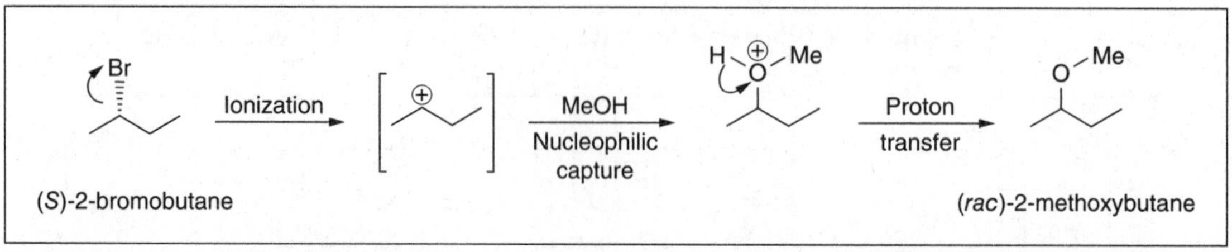

FIGURE 23.6   The S_N1 mechanism.

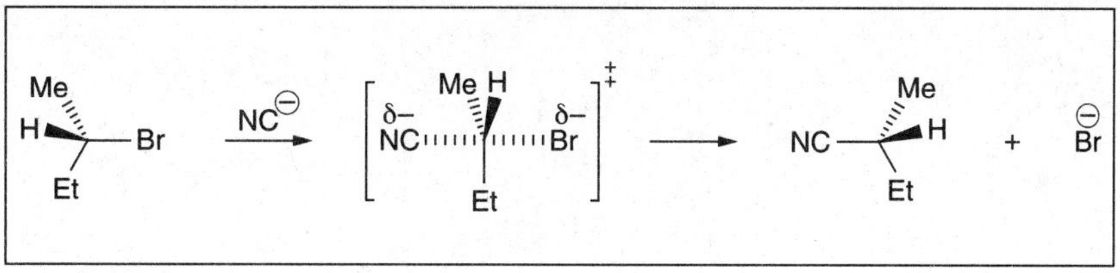

FIGURE 23.7 Inversion of stereochemistry in S_N2.

When the nucleophile is strong enough, substitution can take place directly, without the need for prior ionization. For example, treatment of 2-bromobutane with sodium cyanide leads to direct displacement in one step via an S_N2 mechanism (Figure 23.7).

The S_N2 reaction proceeds by a concerted mechanism, unlike the stepwise S_N1 sequence. Thus, there is a single activation energy that governs the kinetics of the process. Since the transition state involves both the substrate and the nucleophile, the rate law must also include terms for both species, as follows:

$$\text{rate} = k[\text{2-bromobutane}][\text{NaCN}]$$

For this reason, S_N2 reactions are particularly sensitive to concentration effects—a twofold dilution of each reagent results in a fourfold decrease in rate. Aside from concentration, the rate of the S_N2 reaction also depends upon the nature of the two species involved. Since the backside attack is sterically demanding, S_N2 reactivity drops off as substitution about the electrophilic center increases. Therefore, primary centers react faster than secondary, and tertiary centers are generally unreactive toward S_N2 displacement.

Elimination is another common process, and it is often in competition with substitution (Figure 23.8). This is exemplified by the methanolysis of t-butyl bromide, a process that is often accompanied by the generation of 2-methylpropene. Both products arise from a common intermediate—the initially formed t-butyl carbocation can be captured by methanol to give the corresponding ether (S_N1 product), or it can suffer direct proton loss to form a double bond. The combination of ionization followed by proton loss constitutes the E1 mechanism. Like the S_N1 mechanism, it is stepwise and is encountered only when a relatively stable carbocation can be formed.

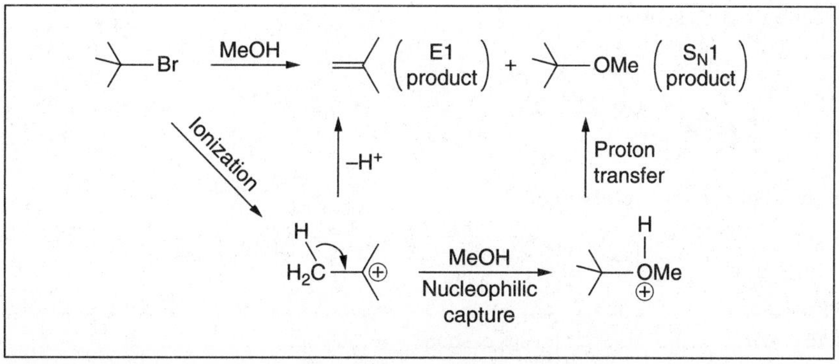

FIGURE 23.8 Competition between E1 and S_N1 mechanisms.

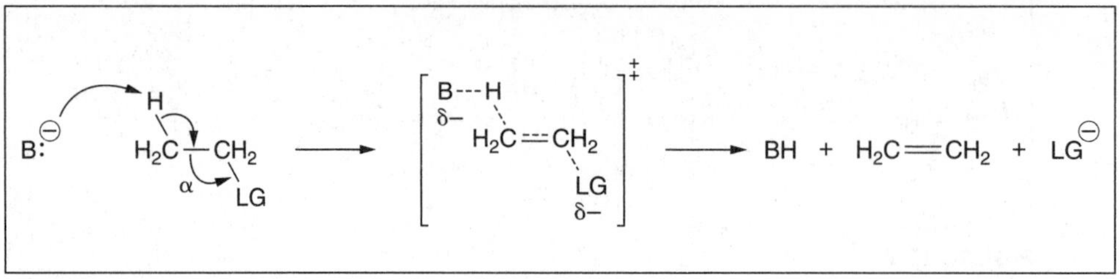

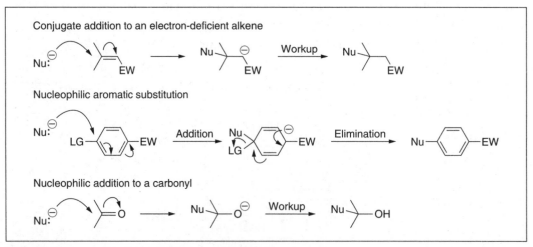

FIGURE 23.9 The E2 mechanism.

With stronger bases another eliminative pathway becomes feasible, namely bimolecular elimination (E2). This is a concerted process in which the base removes a β-proton as the leaving group leaves. Like the S_N2 reaction, the E2 has a single transition state involving both the base and the substrate; therefore, the observed kinetics are second order and the rate is dependent upon the concentration of both species (Figure 23.9). Note that as the reaction progresses, two molecules give rise to three molecules, a very entropically favorable result. Therefore, like the E1 mechanism, bimolecular elimination is made much more spontaneous with increasing temperature. Moreover, E2 eliminations tend to be practically irreversible.

So far we have discussed nucleophilic attack at an sp^3-hybridized electrophilic center bearing a leaving group. However, we can imagine another way to push electrons to form a stabilized anionic charge. Figure 23.10 shows two such possibilities. In the first, a nucleophile adds to an electron-deficient double bond in such a way as to place the anionic center adjacent to the stabilizing electron-withdrawing group. This type of reaction is often called conjugate addition, since the stabilizing group is usually a π system in conjugation with the double bond. It is also the basis for nucleophilic aromatic substitution. The other common mode of addition onto an sp^2 center is by nucleophilic attack onto a carbonyl carbon (Figure 23.10). This provides, after aqueous workup, an alcohol—and various modes of carbonyl addition are frequently used for the synthesis of complex alcohols.

FIGURE 23.10 Nucleophilic attack at an sp^2 carbon.

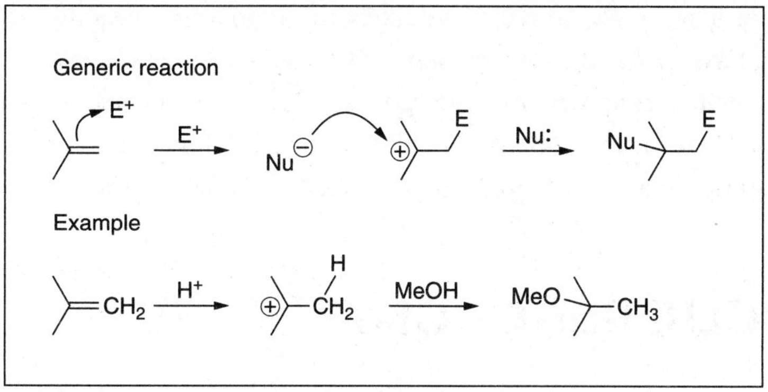

FIGURE 23.11 Electrophilic attack of an alkene.

In the absence of electron-withdrawing groups, alkenes are actually somewhat nucleophilic. The π electron density is somewhat far removed from the coulombic tether of the nuclei. It seems intuitively supportable, then, to posit that the π bond might be polarized toward electropositive species, and in some cases undergo electrophilic capture, as illustrated in Figure 23.11. The carbocation generated by the electrophilic attack is usually trapped by some weak nucleophile (solvent, for example), much like the second step of an S_N1 reaction. If the alkene is unsymmetrical (differently substituted on either side of the double bond), then the electrophilic attack will occur in such a way as to give the more substituted (hence, more stable) carbocation. Thus, the pendant nucleophile is generally found at the more substituted position. This regiochemical outcome is said to follow the Markovnikov rule, and the more substituted product is dubbed the Markovnikov product.

This mode of reactivity is also enormously important in aromatic chemistry. As shown in Figure 23.12, an aromatic ring can capture an electrophile to form a doubly allylic carbo-cationic intermediate, which quenches the positive charge by loss of a proton to form a new aromatic species. The first step is energetically challenging, since it destroys aromaticity; consequently, only very strong electrophiles engage in aromatic substitution. By the same token, proton loss to regain aromaticity is usually far more preferred than the nucleophilic capture observed in nonaromatic π systems (Figure 23.11).

Before moving on, it is worth summarizing E1, E2, S_N1, and S_N2 reactions:

➤ A leaving group on a methyl group will most likely undergo an S_N2 reaction.
➤ A primary leaving group will undergo an S_N2 reaction because of the nucleophile's ability to reach the carbon atom that holds the leaving group. A strong base that is sterically hindered will give an E2 reaction.

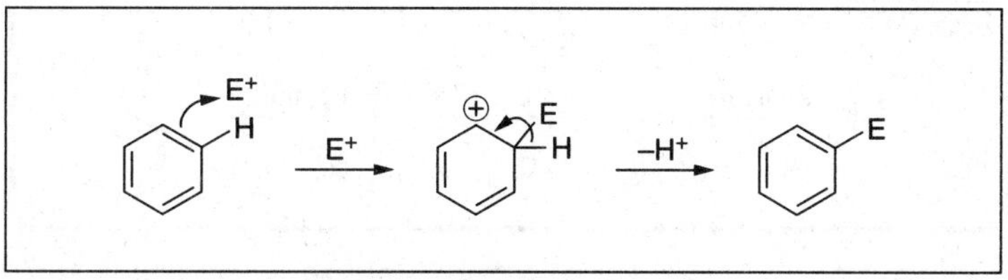

FIGURE 23.12 Electrophilic aromatic substitution.

➤ A secondary leaving group will more likely undergo an E2 reaction in the presence of a strong base, but S_N2 in the presence of a weak base.

➤ A tertiary leaving group will not undergo an S_N2 reaction because of steric hindrance. In the presence of a strong base, E2 will be the favored mechanism. In solvolysis, E1 and S_N1 can take place with S_N1 favored at a lower temperature.

PERICYCLIC REACTIONS

Finally, we consider the pericyclic reactions, to which the sigmatropic rearrangements belong. Figure 23.13 illustrates one example, known as the Cope rearrangement. At face value, a σ bond has moved from the right side to the left—however, there are actually six electrons in play. Formally, these processes are known as [3,3] rearrangements because there is a three-atom array walking across a three-atom array. Atoms other than carbon are also fair game. For example, oxygen can replace one of the sp³ carbons in what is known as the Claisen rearrangement (Figure 23.14). Unlike the Cope, which converts a diene to another diene, the Claisen actually provides different functionality. Thus, we start with an allyl vinyl ether, and the rearrangement results in a γ, δ-unsaturated carbonyl compound. In the case of the allyl phenyl ethers, the initially formed rearrangement product tautomerizes to restore aromaticity.

Two types of pericyclic reactions are particularly important for their ring-forming capabilities. One is the Diels-Alder reaction, also known as the [4 + 2] cycloaddition. Here the formal nomenclature is not based on the number of atoms involved, but the

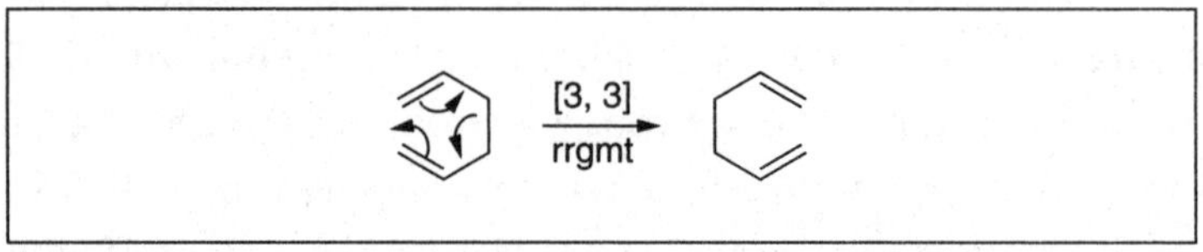

FIGURE 23.13   Cope rearrangement.

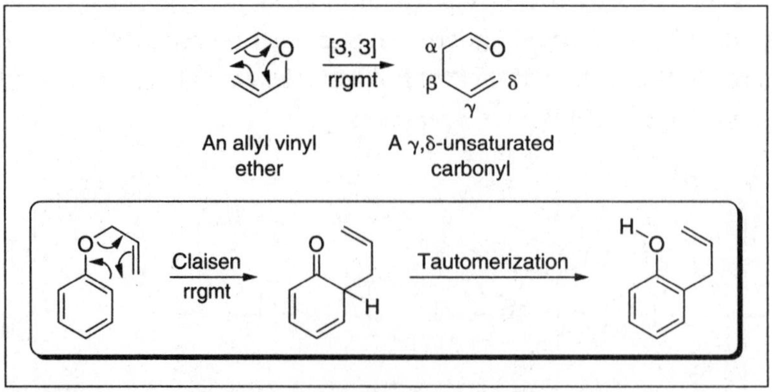

FIGURE 23.14   Claisen rearrangement.

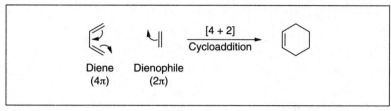

FIGURE 23.15 The prototypical Diels-Alder reaction.

number of electrons. Thus, a 4π component (called the diene) and a 2π component (called the dienophile) come together to form a cyclohexene, as shown in Figure 23.15. Again, we can see that the reaction involves the concerted motion of six electrons—this is important, because the transition state has considerable aromatic character, an outcome that provides for a particularly low activation barrier.

Another way to produce cyclic molecules from acyclic precursors is through electrocyclization. This is a process involving an extended π system and could encompass a rather large array of p orbitals. We consider here two types: 4π and 6π. The overall process is the conversion of a conjugated diene to a cyclobutene (4π) or a conjugated triene to a cyclohexatriene (6π), as shown in Figure 23.16. Both are best considered equilibrium reactions, and the reverse process is known as a cycloreversion.

The stereochemistry of this reaction is remarkably fixed and predictable. In fact, the observation that the stereochemical outcome always fell into certain patterns opened up many of the applications of molecular orbital (MO) theory that we use today (and also earned a Nobel Prize for Fukui and Hoffmann in 1981). For example, if *trans,trans*-2,4-hexadiene (Figure 23.17) is subjected to photochemical conditions, only *cis*-3,4dimethylbutadiene is formed.

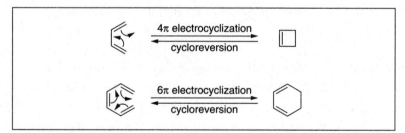

FIGURE 23.16 Two types of reversible electrocyclization.

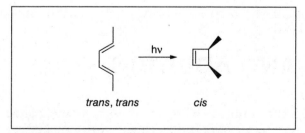

FIGURE 23.17 The stereochemical outcome of photochemical 4π electrocyclization.

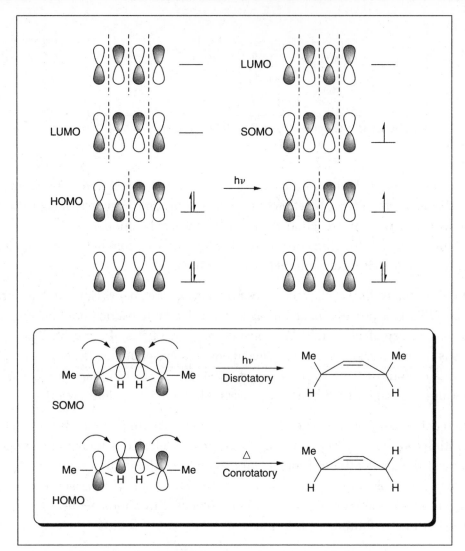

FIGURE 23.18   The molecular orbital underpinnings of electrocyclization.

An examination of molecular orbital theory provides some insight (Figure 23.18). Light promotes an electron into the lowest unoccupied molecular orbital (LUMO) thus converting it to a singly occupied molecular orbital (SOMO), which now controls the course of the reaction. If we superimpose the SOMO onto a depiction of the diene (inset), we see that the two end lobes must turn in toward each other to enjoy constructive orbital overlap. This is known as a disrotatory ring closure, since the right orbital is turning counterclockwise and the left orbital is turning clockwise, thus in opposite senses.

SYN AND ANTI ADDITION

When reacting with the double bond of an alkene, the mechanisms of the reaction can orient the reactants to react to the same face of the alkene or to react with opposite faces of the alkene. These are called syn and anti addition reactions, respectively.

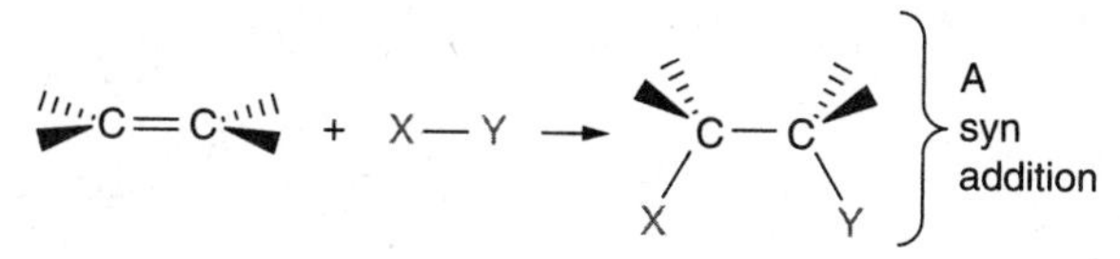

FIGURE 23.19 Syn addition.

The case of hydrogen gas reacting with ethene in the presence of a catalyst demonstrates syn addition (Figure 23.19).

The story changes dramatically when diatomic chlorine or bromine are added to the alkene. In this case they will add in an anti-addition fashion that includes a halonium ion as an intermediate (either bromonium or chloronium). Figure 23.20 demonstrates the reactants, intermediate, and product.

Should anti addition take place with, for example, cis-2-butene, then the products would be a racemic mixture of enantiomers. Should the anti addition take place with trans-2-butene, then the product (singular) would be a meso compound. These can be seen in Figure 23.21.

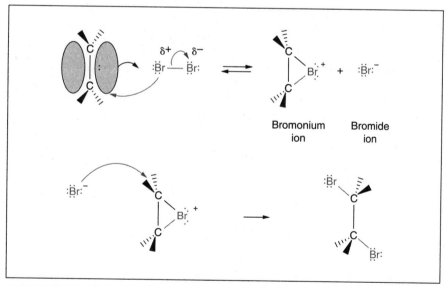

FIGURE 23.20 Mechanism for anti addition.

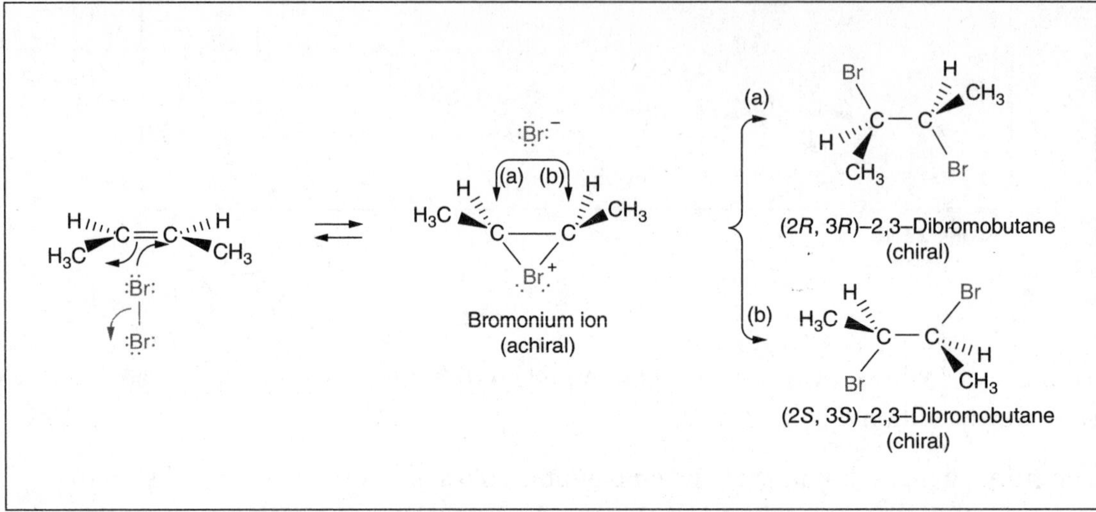

FIGURE 23.21   Anti addition to cis-2-butene.

As you continue to encounter stereochemistry, the use of a model kit will help with the visualization involved.

Reactions of Major Functional Groups

Read This Chapter to Learn About

➤ Alcohols and Ethers

➤ Ketones and Aldehydes

➤ Alkenes and Alkynes

➤ Carboxylic Acids and Derivatives

➤ Expoxides

➤ Amines

ALCOHOLS AND ETHERS

Part of the joy of organic chemistry is learning how to manipulate compounds and make them work for you. The ability to do so is what has changed the quality of life for humans over the past century. We've even gotten to the point where just about any biological organic compound can be manipulated like any other chemical in the laboratory. Keep this in mind when reviewing syntheses and reactions.

An organic chemist should be familiar with the following reactions involving alcohols and ethers. Keep in mind that Markovnikov reactions dictate that the carbon atom with more hydrogen atoms to start will receive the hydrogen.

➤ Simple Markovnikov hydration of alkenes (acid-catalyzed hydration):

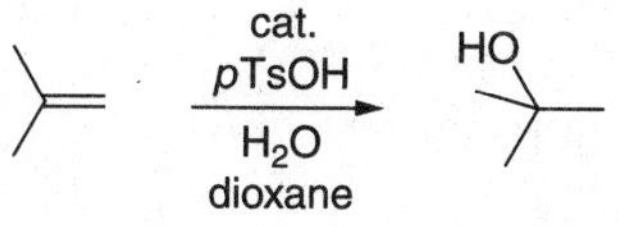

$$\text{alkene} \xrightarrow[\substack{H_2O \\ \text{dioxane}}]{\substack{\text{cat.} \\ p\text{TsOH}}} \text{alcohol}$$

➤ Oxymercuration-demercuration (also results in Markovnikov hydration):

$$\ce{>=} \quad \underset{\underset{\text{dioxane}}{\text{H}_2\text{O}}}{\overset{\text{Hg (OAc)}_2}{\longrightarrow}} \quad \overset{\text{NaBH}_4}{\longrightarrow} \quad \ce{HO-}$$

➤ Anti-Markovnikov hydration of alkenes (hydroboration):

$$\ce{>=} \quad \underset{\text{THF}}{\overset{\text{BH}_3}{\longrightarrow}} \quad \underset{\text{H}_2\text{O}_2}{\overset{\text{NaOH}}{\longrightarrow}} \quad \ce{-OH}$$

Functional groups containing a carbonyl group will also, many times, involve an alcohol.

➤ Treatment of ketones and aldehydes with hydride reagents (reduction):

$$\ce{O} \quad \underset{\underset{\text{LAH}}{\text{or}}}{\overset{\text{NaBH}_4}{\longrightarrow}} \quad \ce{OH}$$

➤ Treatment of ketones and aldehydes with organometallic reagents (for example, the Grignard reaction):

$$\ce{O} \quad \underset{\text{THF}}{\overset{\text{RMgBr}}{\longrightarrow}} \quad \ce{OH / R}$$

➤ Reduction of esters to primary alcohols:

$$\ce{O-OR'} \quad \underset{\text{THF}}{\overset{\text{LAH}}{\longrightarrow}} \quad \ce{OH}$$

➤ S_N2 reaction of hydroxide with alkyl halides, tosylates, or mesylates (works best with primary substrates):

$$\text{R-CH}_2\text{-X NaOH/Dioxane} \longrightarrow \text{R-CH}_2\text{-OH}$$

Reactions involving reagents that are oxygen-rich will give an oxidation reaction where oxygen atoms are added and/or hydrogen atoms are removed.

➤ Jones oxidation of secondary alcohols to ketones:

$$\ce{OH} \quad \underset{\underset{\text{H}_2\text{O}}{\text{H}_2\text{SO}_4}}{\overset{\text{K}_2\text{Cr}_2\text{O}_7}{\longrightarrow}} \quad \ce{O}$$

➤ Jones oxidation of primary alcohols to carboxylic acids:

$$\ce{R-OH} \quad \underset{\underset{\text{H}_2\text{O}}{\text{H}_2\text{SO}_4}}{\overset{\text{K}_2\text{Cr}_2\text{O}_7}{\longrightarrow}} \quad \ce{R-C(=O)-OH}$$

375

**CHAPTER 24:
REACTIONS OF
MAJOR
FUNCTIONAL
GROUPS**

➤ PCC oxidation of primary alcohols to aldehydes:

➤ Conversion to the corresponding halides or tosylates (good leaving groups):

$$R\text{-}CH_2\text{-}OH + PBr_3 \longrightarrow R\text{-}CH_2\text{-}Br$$

$$R\text{-}CH_2\text{-}OH + SOCl_2 \longrightarrow R\text{-}CH_2\text{-}Cl$$

$$R\text{-}CH_2\text{-}OH + TsCl \longrightarrow R\text{-}CH_2\text{-}OTs$$

$$R\text{-}CH_2\text{-}OH + MsCl \longrightarrow R\text{-}CH_2\text{-}OMs$$

➤ Acid-catalyzed dehydration:

➤ Reaction with acyl chlorides to form esters:

There are a number of ways to form ethers.

➤ The alkylation of alkoxide anions (Williamson ether synthesis):

➤ The acid-catalyzed addition of alcohols across alkenes:

➤ Ethers tend to be relatively inert. However, the acid-catalyzed elimination of tertiary ethers to form alkenes is sometimes synthetically useful:

KETONES AND ALDEHYDES

The following reactions involve ketones and aldehydes. Again, take note of the use of oxidizing agents.

➤ Jones oxidation of secondary alcohols to form ketones:

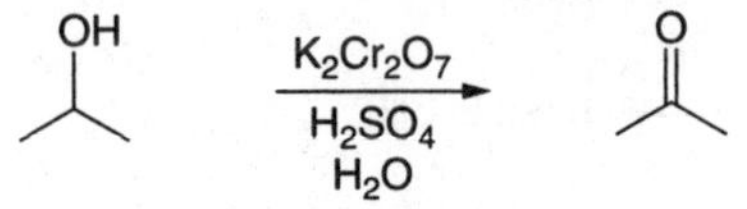

➤ PCC oxidation of primary alcohols to aldehydes:

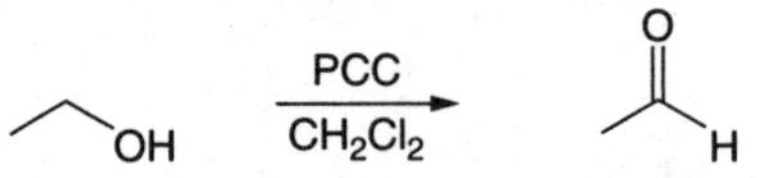

➤ Selective oxidation of benzylic alcohols with manganese dioxide (most other alcohols are unaffected):

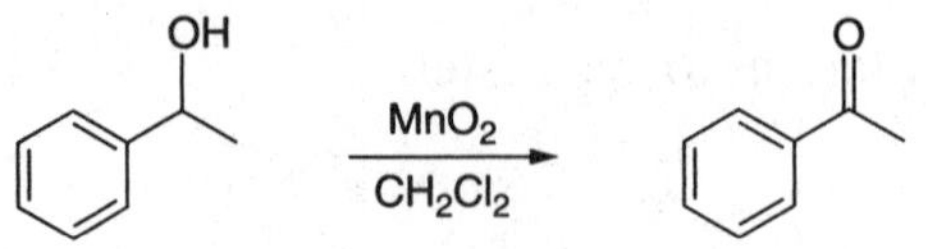

➤ Ozonolysis of alkenes to form carbonyls:

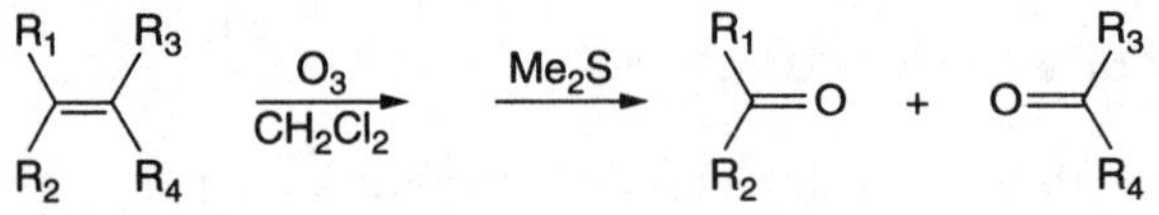

➤ Oxidative cleavage of vic-diols with periodic acid:

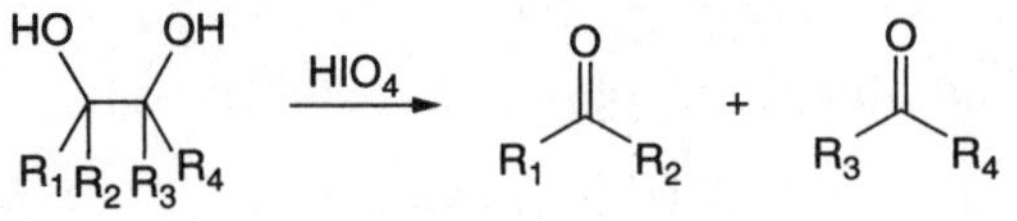

The reduction of compounds includes the addition of hydrogen and/or the removal of oxygen. Reducing reagents usually involve a B or Al and a number of hydrogen atoms.

➤ Reduction of acyl chlorides to aldehydes using lithium tri(t-butoxy)aluminum hydride:

R-C(=O)-Cl + LiAl(O-t-Bu)$_3$H in THF yields R-CHO.

➤ DIBAL reduction of esters to aldehydes:

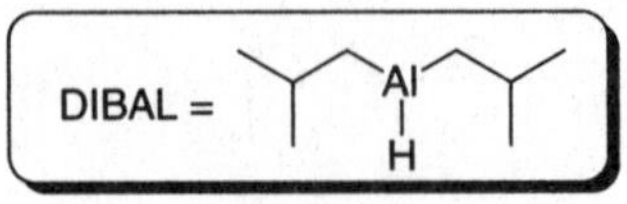

R-C(=O)-OR' + DIBAL in THF yields R-CHO.

377

**CHAPTER 24:
REACTIONS OF
MAJOR
FUNCTIONAL
GROUPS**

➤ Anti-Markovnikov hydration of terminal alkynes to aldehydes:

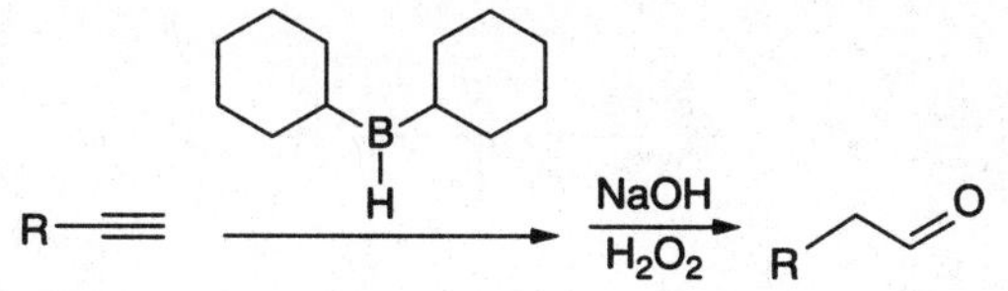

➤ Hydride reduction to alcohols:

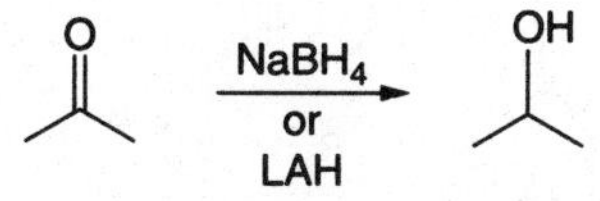

➤ Nucleophilic addition of organometallics (Grignard reaction):

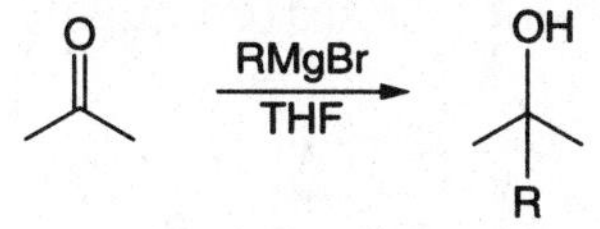

➤ Conversion to alkenes with phosphonium ylides (Wittig reaction):

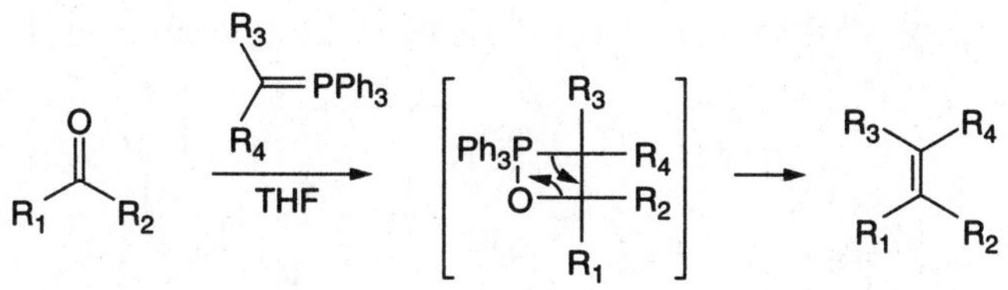

➤ Acid-catalyzed formation of acetals:

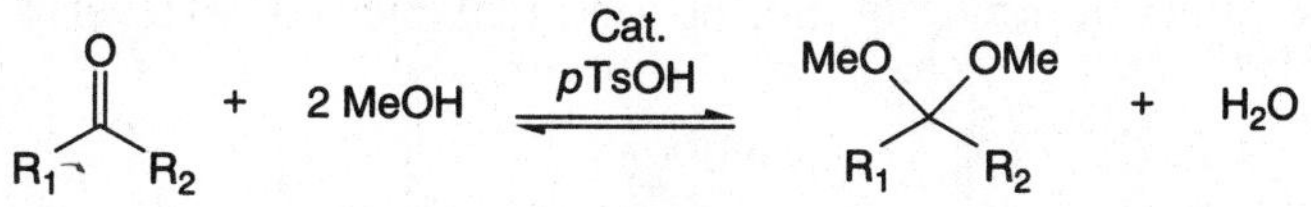

There are a number of reactions that are pertinent to nitrogen and a carbonyl group.

➤ Condensation with primary amines to form imines:

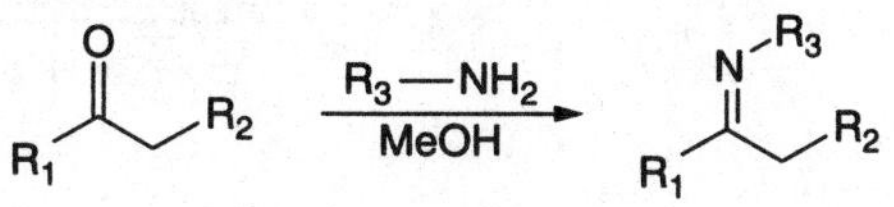

➤ Condensation with secondary amines to form enamines:

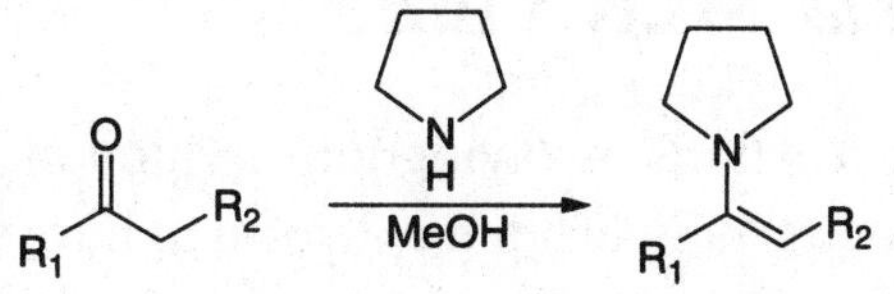

➤ Reaction with amines in the presence of sodium cyanoborohydride to form amines (reductive amination):

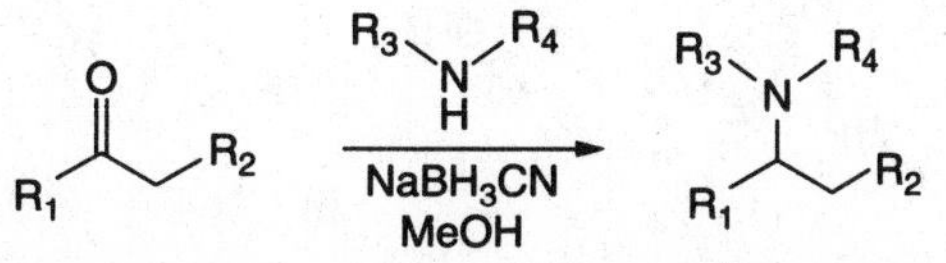

➤ Alkylation of enolate carbanions:

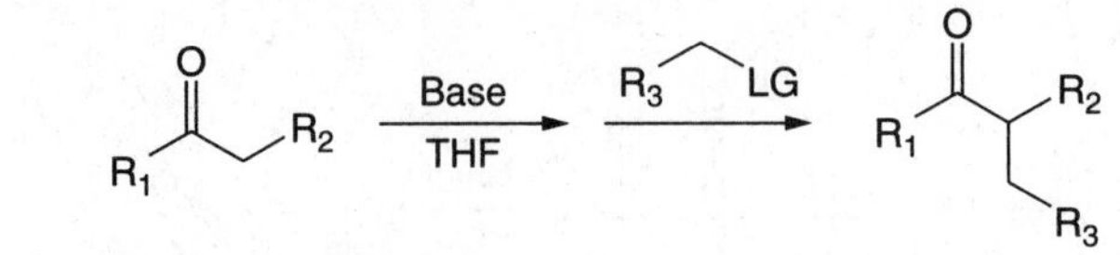

➤ Condensation with other carbonyl compounds (aldol condensation):

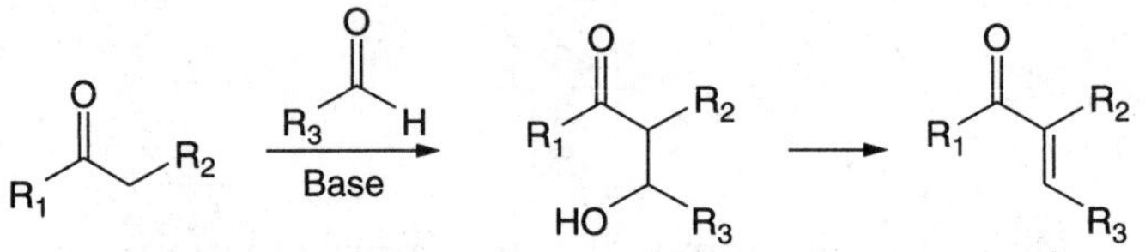

➤ Addition onto electron-deficient alkenes (conjugate addition):

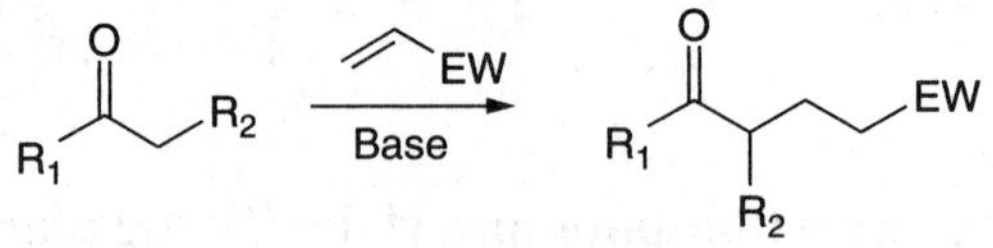

➤ Tandem conjugate addition/aldol condensation (Robinson annulation):

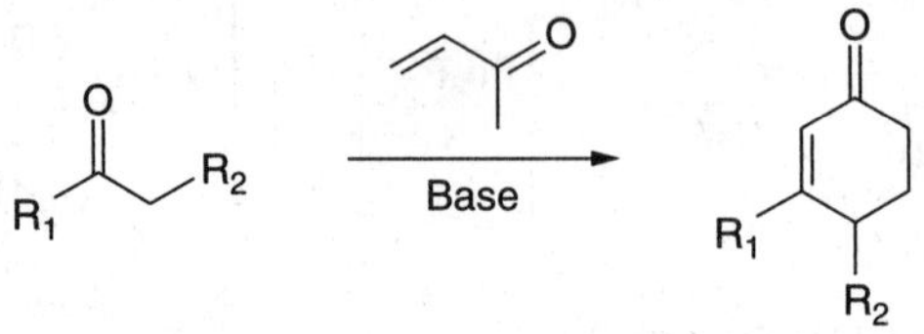

➤ Conversion to esters by action of *m*-chloroperbenzoic acid (Baeyer-Villiger oxidation):

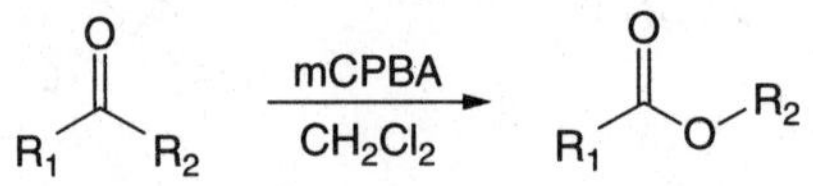

➤ Markovnikov hydration of terminal alkynes to methyl ketones:

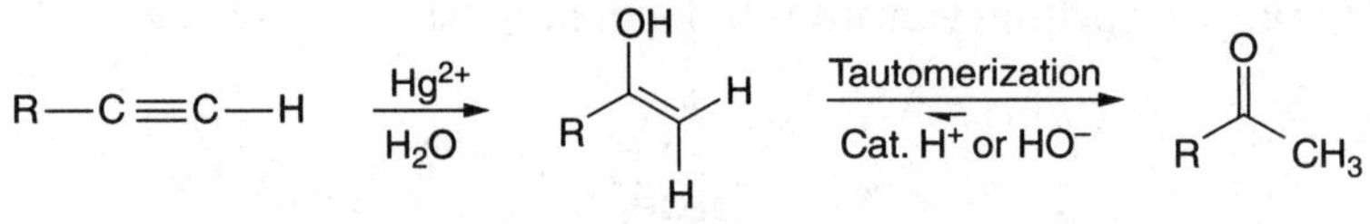

ALKENES AND ALKYNES

Following are important reactions involving alkenes and alkynes. Keep in mind that Zaitseff's rule dictates that the double bond will form to have the most R groups on the double-bonded carbon atoms.

➤ Acid-catalyzed dehydration of alcohols (E1 elimination):

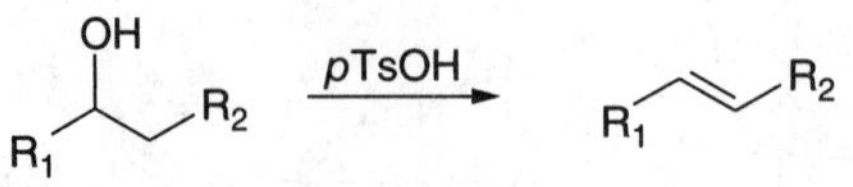

379

**CHAPTER 24:
REACTIONS OF
MAJOR
FUNCTIONAL
GROUPS**

➤ Base-catalyzed elimination (E2 elimination):

➤ Reaction of carbonyl compounds with phosphonium ylides (Wittig reaction):

➤ Conversion of alkynes to cis-alkenes using catalytic hydrogenation / reduction of internal alkynes to cis-alkenes by hydrogenation using Lindlar's catalyst:

➤ Conversion of alkynes to trans-alkenes using dissolving metal reduction / reduction of internal alkynes to trans-alkenes by dissolving metal reduction:

➤ Acid-catalyzed Markovnikov hydration to form alcohols:

➤ Mercury-catalyzed Markovnikov hydration (oxymercuration/demercuration):

➤ Anti-Markovnikov hydration (hydroboration):

➤ Markovnikov hydrobromination:

➤ Anti-Markovnikov hydrobromination in the presence of radical initiators:

➤ Dibromination with bromine in an inert solvent:

$$\text{Br}_2 / \text{CCl}_4$$

➤ Formation of bromohydrins by reaction with bromine in the presence of water:

$$\text{Br}_2 / \text{H}_2\text{O}$$

➤ Catalytic hydrogenation to form alkanes:

$$\text{H}_2 / \text{Cat}$$

➤ Ozonolysis with reductive workup to form carbonyl compounds:

$$\frac{\text{O}_3}{\text{CH}_2\text{Cl}_2} \quad \text{Me}_2\text{S}$$

➤ Osmium tetroxide-mediated syn-dihydroxylation:

$$\frac{\text{OsO}_4}{\text{H}_2\text{O}_2}$$

➤ Epoxidation with oxygen transfer reagents, such as dimethyldioxirane (DMD) or m-chloroperbenzoic acid (mCPBA):

$$\text{DMD/acetone} \quad \text{or} \quad \text{mCPBA} \quad \text{CH}_2\text{Cl}_2$$

➤ Cyclopropanation using carbene precursors, such as diazomethane or diiodomethane and zinc/copper couple (Simmons-Smith reaction):

$$\text{CH}_2\text{I}_2 \quad \text{Zn-Cu} \quad \text{or} \quad \text{CH}_2\text{N}_2 \quad \text{Cu}^0$$

➤ Conversion of alkenes to alkynes by dibromination followed by double elimination:

$$\frac{\text{Br}_2}{\text{CCl}_4} \quad \left[\right] \quad \frac{\text{xs LDA}}{\text{THF}} \quad R\!-\!\!\equiv$$

➤ Alkylation of alkynyl anions:

$$R\!-\!\!\equiv\!-\!H \quad \frac{\text{LDA}}{\text{THF}} \quad R'\!\frown\!\text{LG}$$

381

**CHAPTER 24:
REACTIONS OF
MAJOR
FUNCTIONAL
GROUPS**

➤ Markovnikov hydration of terminal alkynes to form methyl ketones:

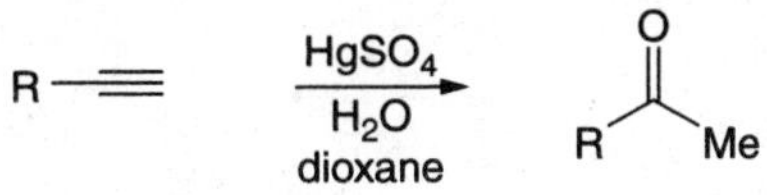

➤ Anti-Markovnikov hydration of terminal alkynes to form aldehydes:

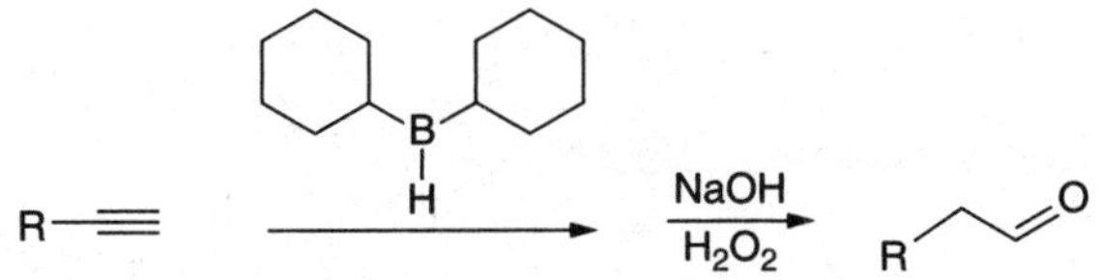

CARBOXYLIC ACIDS AND DERIVATIVES

This section lists some important reactions involving carboxylic acids and derivatives.

➤ Jones oxidation of primary alcohols or aldehydes:

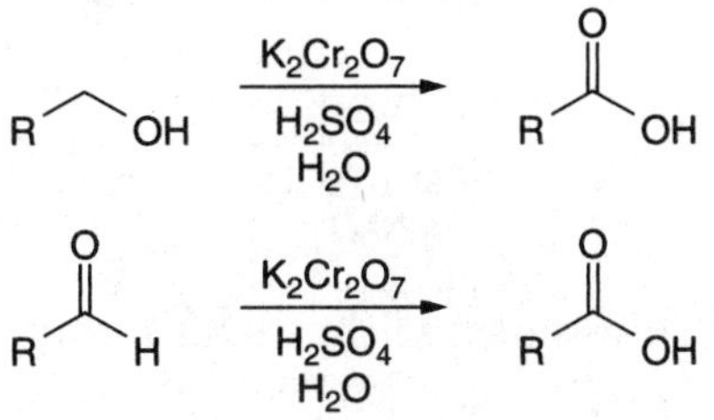

➤ Base-catalyzed hydrolysis of esters (saponification):

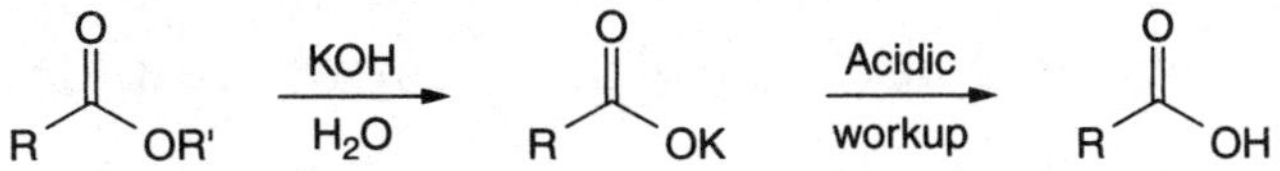

➤ Acid-catalyzed hydrolysis of nitriles:

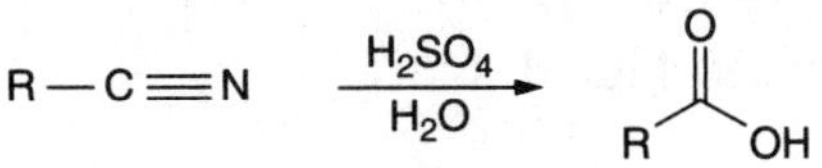

➤ Action of Grignard reagents on carbon dioxide:

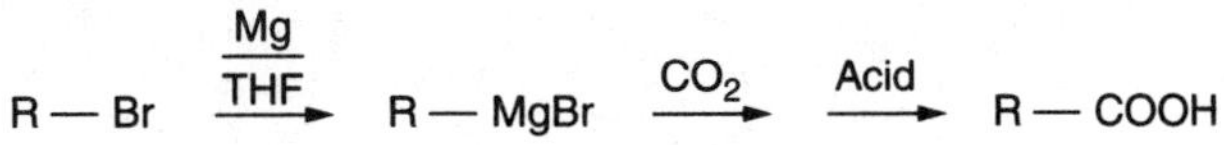

➤ Conversion to acyl chlorides using thionyl chloride or oxalyl chloride:

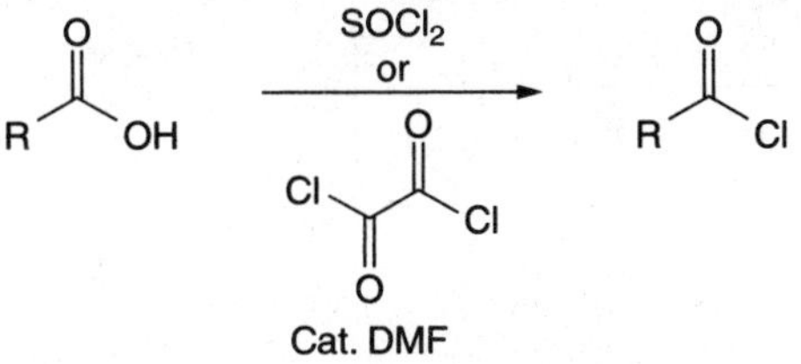

➤ Reduction to alcohols using lithium aluminum hydride:

➤ Acid-catalyzed esterification in an alcohol solvent:

R-COOH + R'-OH (cat. H$^+$) yields RCOOR'.

➤ Reaction of alcohols with acyl halides:

➤ Reaction of carboxylic acids with diazomethane to form methyl esters:

➤ Transesterification under acidic or basic conditions:

➤ Reduction to primary alcohols using lithium aluminum hydride:

➤ Reduction to aldehydes using diisobutylaluminum hydride (DIBAL):

➤ Reaction of amines with acyl halides:

➤ Conversion of ketones to hydroxylamines, followed by Beckmann rearrangement:

383

**CHAPTER 24:
REACTIONS OF
MAJOR
FUNCTIONAL
GROUPS**

➤ Conversion to amines by amide reduction:

➤ Conversion of amides to carboxylic acids:

➤ Reduction with diisobutylaluminum hydride (DIBAL) to form aldehydes:

➤ Conversion to amines with one less carbon through the Hofmann rearrangement:

EXPOXIDES

Following are important reactions involving expoxides.

➤ Oxidation of alkenes with oxygen transfer reagents:

➤ Base-catalyzed ring closure of halohydrins:

X = Br, Cl

➤ Base-catalyzed nucleophilic ring-opening at the less hindered carbon:

➤ Acid-catalyzed nucleophilic ring-opening at the more substituted site:

AMINES

This section lists important reactions involving amines.

➤ Using phthalimide (the Gabriel synthesis):

➤ Direct alkylation of amide anions:

➤ Reaction of azide anion with electrophiles, followed by reduction (the Staudinger reaction):

➤ Reduction of carboxamides using lithium aluminum hydride:

➤ Reaction of ketones with amines in the presence of sodium cyanoborohydride (reductive amination):

➤ From carboxamides via the Hofmann rearrangement:

➤ From carboxylic acids via the Curtius rearrangement:

➤ Conjugate addition onto electron-deficient double bonds:

385

**CHAPTER 24:
REACTIONS OF
MAJOR
FUNCTIONAL
GROUPS**

➤ Reaction with acyl chlorides to form amides:

➤ Conversion to alkenes via Hofmann elimination (forms least substituted alkene):

When considering reactions of major functional groups, keep in mind the following:

➤ Reducing agents are rich in H atoms and will add hydrogen and/or remove oxygen.
➤ Oxidizing agents are rich in O atoms and will add oxygen and/or remove hydrogen.
➤ Many of the reactions listed involve the removal of water or HCl. Usually an OH or Cl comes from one reactant while H atoms come from the other reactant.
➤ Be aware of Markovnikov's rule, Zaitseff's rule, and the conditions for anti-Markovnikov to take place.

CHAPTER 25

Aromaticity and Reactions of Benzene

Read This Chapter to Learn About

➤ Aromaticity
➤ Reactions and Directing Groups

AROMATICITY

Michael Faraday was the first to arrive at the formula for benzene, C_6H_6, but it was Friedrich August Kekule von Stradonitz who discovered benzene's structure. Initial examination by a beginning chemist would lead one to believe that benzene has three double bonds:

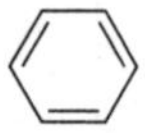

But there was something different about this molecule. An unsaturated hydrocarbon, such as an alkene or alkyne, should decolorize bromine in CH_2Cl_2. However, benzene does not, suggesting that there aren't any double bonds at all. Also interesting is that the bond lengths of the carbon-to-carbon bonds in benzene (1.4 angstroms) are exactly between the lengths of the carbon-to-carbon bonds of alkanes (1.5 angstroms) and alkenes (1.3 angstroms). Furthermore, if one were to examine the fingerprint region of

C-H stretching in an IR spectrum, one would find a trend where benzene falls in between that of an alkane and alkene:

Alkane	-C-H stretch	$3,000-2,850$ cm^{-1}
Aromatic	*C-H stretch*	*$3,050$ cm^1*
Alkene	=C-H stretch	$3,100-3,050$ cm^{-1}
Alkyne	$\equiv$C-H	$3,300$ cm^{-1}

More of these trends in the IR will be discussed later on.

So what is it that makes benzene different? Delocalized pi electrons that form resonance structures give benzene and other aromatic compounds a highly stabilized structure. But this does not mean that every conjugated system is aromatic. Instead, it was the work of Erich Hückel that determined cyclic, planar, fully conjugated molecules with $4n + 2$ π electrons (where n is any integer) are classified as being aromatic. As one can see, when n equals 1, we get a value of 6. Sure enough, there are 6 pi electrons in benzene. Naphthalene, $C_{10}H_8$ (which also follows the general formula of C_nH_{2n-6}), is also aromatic and has 10 pi electrons. Naphthalene follows Hückel's rule in that n = 2. Finally, much like benzene has two resonance structures, naphthalene has three resonance structures. Can you draw them?

REACTIONS AND DIRECTING GROUPS

Let us begin with the basics of the reactions that occur on a benzene molecule to make the benzene functional.

Nitration	$C_6H_6 + HNO_3/H_2SO_4$	Yields $C_6H_5NO_2$
Sulfonation	$C_6H_6 + SO_3/H_2SO_4$	Yields $C_6H_5SO_3H$
Halogenation	$C_6H_6 + Cl_2/AlCl_3$	Yields C_6H_5Cl
Friedel-Crafts alkylation	$C_6H_6 + R\text{-}Cl/AlCl_3$	Yields $C_6H_5\text{-}R$
Friedel-Crafts acylation	$C_6H_6 + Cl\text{-}C(=O)\text{-}R/AlCl_3$	Yields $C_6H_5\text{-}C(=O)\text{-}R$

Once these or other functional groups are on the benzene, they too can be reacted to form other compounds:

$C_6H_5SO_3H$	+ molten NaOH	Yields $C_6H_5\text{-}OH$
$C_6H_5NO_2$	+ H_2/cat. or Fe/HCl	Yields $C_6H_5NH_2$
$C_6H_5\text{-}C(=O)\text{-}R$	+ H_2/cat. or Zn(Hg)/HCl	Yields $C_6H_5CH_2R$
$C_6H_5CH_2R$	+ PCC or CrO_3/HOAc	Yields $C_6H_5\text{-}C(=O)\text{-}R$
$C_6H_5\text{-}R$	+ 1. Alkaline hot $KMnO_4$ / 2. H_2SO_4	Yields $C_6H_5\text{-}COOH$

When the benzene ring already bears a substituent, as a general rule, electron-donating (ED) substituents (methoxy, amino, etc.) have an activating influence on the aromatic ring, and they also direct electrophiles to the ortho and para sites. Conversely, electron-withdrawing (EW) groups (nitro, carbonyl, etc.) have a deactivating influence on the ring, and they direct electrophiles to the meta positions. The halogens exhibit unique behavior: they are deactivating, but ortho/para directing (Table 25.1).

Table 25.1 Substituent Effects on Electrophilic Aromatic Substitution	
Electron-Donating Groups	**Electron-Withdrawing Groups**
Activating o,p-directing	Deactivating m-directing
-NH$_2$ / -NR$_2$ (amino, amido) -OR / -OH (alkoxy, hydroxy) -R (alkyl)	-NO$_2$ (nitro) -COOR (esters, acids) -C(=O)-R (ketones, aldehydes) -SO$_3$H (sulfo) -CN (cyano)
Halogens	
Deactivating o,p-directing -F, -Cl, -Br, -I	

PROBLEM: What is/are the major product/s of the nitration of anisole ($C_6H_5OCH_3$)?

SOLUTION: The -OR group on the benzene means that any group that is placed on the anisole will be placed ortho or para to the -OR group. Because of steric effects, this reaction is more likely to go to the para product. It turns out that the products will be approximately 30% ortho, 2% meta, and 68% para.

PROBLEM: Starting with benzene, outline a synthesis for m-chlorobenzoic acid.

SOLUTION: Plan ahead! The chlorine will need to be placed on the benzene last because we need to establish the meta directing -COOH group first.

First perform a Friedel-Crafts acylation:

$$C_6H_6 + CH_3COCl/AlCl_3 \text{ yields } C_6H_5\text{-CO-CH}_3$$

Second, oxidize the acetyl group to a -COOH group:

$$C_6H_5\text{-CO-CH}_3 + 1. \text{ Alkaline hot } KMnO_4 / 2. H_2SO_4 \text{ yields } C_6H_5\text{-COOH}$$

Now that we have a meta director on the benzene, you can perform the chlorination:

$$C_6H_5\text{-COOH} + Cl_2/AlCl_3 \text{ yields m-ClC}_6H_4\text{COOH}$$

When dealing with benzene reactions it is important to remember the basic reactions, the directing influence of each functional group, and the ability a group has to be activating or deactivating.

CHAPTER 26

Spectrometric Methods

Read This Chapter to Learn About

➤ UV-Vis

➤ Mass Spectrometry

➤ Infrared Spectroscopy

➤ Proton NMR Spectroscopy

➤ Carbon NMR Spectroscopy

UV-VIS

This method allows the characterization of extended π systems. Through the examination of many experimentally derived values, sets of rules have been developed for predicting the wavelength of maximum absorbance (λ_{max}) for various substrates as a function of structure. This work was carried out primarily by Woodward, Fieser, and Nielsen. A brief summary of these rules is presented in Figure 26.1. While not immediately intuitive, they are straightforward to apply once the framework is understood, and they are very powerful predictive tools.

Two specialized terminologies also deserve mention. First, a *homoannular diene* refers to any two double bonds that are incorporated into the same ring. Therefore, 1,3cyclohexadiene would be considered a homoannular diene, but cyclohex-2-enone would not, since only one double bond is incorporated into the ring itself. For every instance of a homoannular component, we add 39 nm to the base absorbance. Second, even though the etymology of an exocyclic double bond means "outside the ring," it is best thought of as a double bond that terminates in a ring. Each time this occurs, we add 5 nm to the base absorbance.

To get some practice in applying these rules, consider the tricyclic enone shown in Figure 26.2. We choose the base absorption of 215 (six-membered-ring enone) and tack on three double bonds to extend the conjugation (30 nm each for 90 nm total).

	Dienes	Enones and enals			Benzophenones, benzaldehydes, and benzoic acids	
Base chromophore	(diene)	(cyclopentenone) α β	(cyclohexenone) α β	(open enone) α β' R	(benzophenone) O R, o m p	(benzoate) O OR, o m p
Base absorbance λ_{max} (nm)	214	202	215	245 / 208 (R=H)	246 / 250 (R=H)	230

Modifications to the base absorbance

	Position	All	α	β	γ	δ	o	m	p
Substituents	-R	5	10	12	18	18	3	3	10
	-OR	6	35	30	17	31	7	7	25
	-Br	5	25	30	25	25	2	2	15
	-Cl	5	15	12	12	12	0	0	10
	-NR₂	60	95				20	20	85
π system architecture	Double bond extending conjugation	+ 30 nm				Not typically relevant		
	Exocyclic character of a double bond	+ 5 nm						
	Homoannular diene component	+ 39 nm						

FIGURE 26.1 Abbreviated rules for predicting λ_{max} for UV-Vis absorptions.

We have thus established the domain of the chromophore. It is often helpful to high-light the chromophore for accounting purposes, even by darkening in with a pencil. Examination of the chromophore thus reveals that ring C houses one homoannular diene component, so we add 39 nm to the ledger. Careful scrutiny also reveals two occurrences of exocyclic double bonds: both the α and β and the ε and ζ olefins termi-nate in ring B. We add 5 nm for each occurrence.

The accounting of substituents is sometimes tricky, particularly for cyclic molecules. First, we must recognize that the substituent connected to the carbonyl group is already accounted for, so we do not double-count it. We start instead with the methoxy substit-uent in the α-position, which adds 35 nm to the chromophore. The rest of the substitu-ents are dealt with in the same manner. To help sort out what are bona fide substituents, imagine the chromophore is a hallway we could walk through—how many doorways

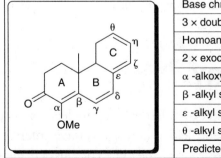

Base chromophore (6-ring enone)	215
3 × double bond extensions	+ 90
Homoannular diene (in ring C)	+ 39
2 × exocyclic double bonds	+ 10
α -alkoxy substituent	+ 35
β -alkyl substituent	+ 12
ε -alkyl substituent (same as γ)	+ 18
θ -alkyl substituent (same as γ)	+ 18
Predicted λ_{max}	437

FIGURE 26.2 Example in the application of predictive UV-Vis rules.

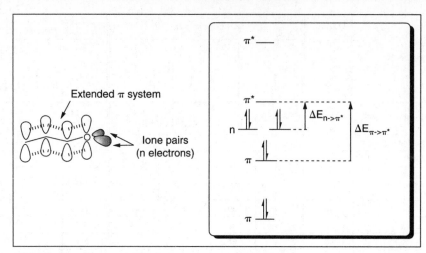

FIGURE 26.3   Two possible electronic transitions in enones.

would we see and in what positions? Thus, starting from the carbonyl, we would see a door to our right at the α-position, one on our left at the β-position, another left door at ε, and finally a left door at θ. For accounting purposes, it matters not that there are substituents attached to those substituents (it is also inconsequential whether the "doors" are on the right or left—it simply helps us visualize the virtual corridor).

The intensity of the absorbance can also be diagnostic. For example, in the tricyclic enone in Figure 26.2, we would expect to see at least two bands in the UV-Vis spectrum. The absorbance in Figure 26.3 corresponds to the π→π* transition from the HOMO to the LUMO. However, the lone pair electrons on oxygen can also undergo excitation. Since they are technically not connected to the extended π system, they are neither bonding nor antibonding; therefore, they are considered nonbonding (n) electrons. The absorption is thus designated an n→π* transition (Figure 26.3). Because the energy gap is smaller, this absorption occurs at higher wavelengths than the π→π* transitions.

The two types of excitation events differ not only in the maximum wavelength, but also in intensity. Since the lone pairs are essentially orthogonal to the extended π system, it would seem difficult to imagine how electrons could be promoted from one to the other. Indeed, these n→π* events are known as symmetry-forbidden electronic transitions. Like so many other forbidden things, they still happen, but the quantum efficiency is much lower; therefore, the intensity of the absorption is considerably weaker than the π→π* absorption.

MASS SPECTROMETRY

Mass spectrometry is based on the principle of differentiating molecules by accelerating charged species through a strong magnetic field or across a voltage potential, in which behavior is dictated by the charge-to-mass ratio of the ions. The classical method for ion generation is known as EI, or electron impact. Here a sample is bombarded with very high-energy electrons, which transfer energy into the molecules, much as photons of

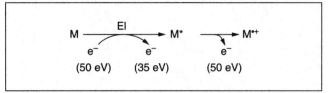

FIGURE 26.4 Formation of a molecular ion by electron impact (EI).

visible light induce the formation of an excited state in UV-Vis spectroscopy. However, these excited species are so energetic that the only way for them to relax is to release an electron, thereby forming a radical cation, as shown in Figure 26.4.

Once formed, these ions are accelerated through some differentiating field. The classical approach for differentiation is to pass the beam of charged particles through a magnetic field, which refracts the ions based on their charge-to-mass ratios and velocities. If we assume that only one electron is lost (that is, the charge of all species is +1), then the time of flight can be directly correlated to mass—thus, the name *mass spectrometry*.

Indeed, some of the most useful information from this technique derives from the mass of the molecular ion. For example, while combustion analysis gives information about the atomic ratios within a molecule, it does not provide a definitive value for the molecular weight. In other words, a compound with molecular formula $C_6H_{12}O_6$ would give the same elemental analysis results as a $C_{12}H_{24}O_{12}$ compound. However, mass spectrometry can provide this missing information: a molecular ion peak at 200 amu is very strong evidence for the latter molecular formula. Thus the combination of elemental analysis and low-resolution mass spectrometry can be used to establish the molecular formula of an unknown compound or help to prove the identity of a synthesized molecule—elemental analysis provides the ratio of elements, and mass spectrometry fixes the total weight.

Moreover, the very decomposition processes that diminish the molecular ion peak can themselves provide important structural information about the substrate. As one example, radical cations derived from ketones undergo fragmentation in the vicinity of the carbonyl. Figure 26.5 shows two such processes for 2-methylhexan-3-one. The first involves σ bond cleavage, in which the isopropyl radical and an acyl cation are formed from the initial radical cation. The molecular ion can also undergo the McLafferty rearrangement, a six-electron process that liberates ethene and a lower molecular weight radical cation. Keep in mind that only charged species are detected, although the lost pieces can be inferred from the difference between the molecular ion peaks and the fragment peaks. Without a rigorous analysis, it is at least intuitively straightforward that knowledge about these fragmentation processes can be useful in piecing together the structure of the original compound. Indeed, the painstaking interpretation of fragmentation patterns was once *de rigeur* for structure proof; however, the increasingly

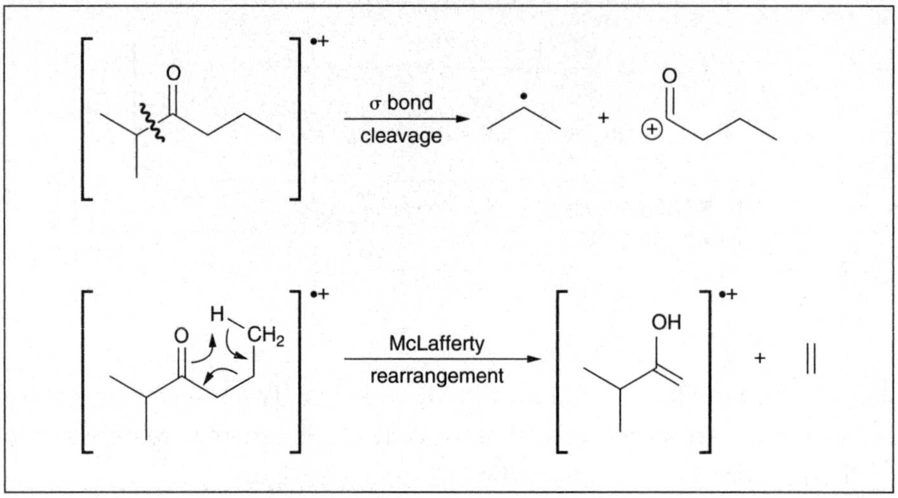

FIGURE 26.5 Two fragmentation processes for 2-methylhexan-3-one radical cation.

powerful (and more convenient) technique of NMR has provided an alternative source of structural knowledge available previously only from MS data.

Another very diagnostic feature in mass spectroscopy is the isotopic fingerprint left by bromine and chlorine. Unlike carbon, hydrogen, nitrogen, and oxygen, which have one overwhelmingly predominant isotope (^{1}H, 99.98%; ^{12}C, 98.93%; ^{14}N, 99.62%; ^{16}O, 99.76%), bromine has two almost equally abundant natural isotopes (^{79}Br, 50.51%; ^{81}Br, 49.49%), and chlorine has a roughly 3:1 ratio of isomers in nature (^{35}Cl, 75.47%; ^{37}Cl, 24.53%). The practical result of this phenomenon is that molecules containing chlorine or bromine leave characteristic M + 2 patterns in a ratio of 1:1 or 3:1, depending upon which halogen is present.

In addition to the patterns seen for chlorine and bromine atoms, there are certain patterns for the functional groups. Keep in mind that, to help keep this simple, the rearrangements of some of the fragments will be overlooked. Instead, we will look at the structures and their m/z ratio without any rearrangements. Also, keep in mind that these are possible structures for common ion fragments only and not every functional group will be covered.

➤ **Hydrocarbons:** fragments of 15, 29, 43, 57, and 71 m/z (methyl, ethyl, propyl, butyl, and pentyl)
➤ **Aromatics:** fragments of 77, 91, 94, and 105 m/z (benzene, benzyl, C_6H_5-O-, and C_6H_5-C=O-)
➤ **Primary alcohols:** 31 m/z (CH_2=OH$^+$)
➤ **Ketones:** fragments of 43, 57, and 71 m/z (CH_3-C≡O+, etc.)
➤ **Aldehydes:** fragments of 29, 44, 58, or 72 m/z (CHO+, etc.)
➤ **Carboxylic acids:** fragments of 45 and 60 m/z (CO_2H+, CH_2=C(OH)$_2$$^+$)

PROBLEM: What will be the similarities and differences in the mass spectra of toluene and ethyl benzene?

SOLUTION: The following table summarizes the answer to this question:

Compound	Similarities	Differences
Toluene	Shows a base ion peak at 91 m/z, indicating benzyl group.	M+ peak of 92 m/z.
Ethyl benzene	Shows a base ion peak at 91 m/z, indicating benzyl group.	M+ peak of 106 m/z. Shows loss of 15 m/z, indicating loss of methyl group.

PROBLEM: What will be the similarities and differences in the mass spectra of chlorobenzene and bromobenzene?

SOLUTION: The following table summarizes the answer to this question:

Compound	Similarities	Differences
Chlorobenzene	Shows a peak at 77 m/z, indicating benzene ring.	M+ peak of 112 m/z. M+2 peak of 114 m/z.
Bromobenzene	Shows a peak at 77 m/z, indicating benzene ring.	M+ peak of 156. M+2 peak of 158 of equal height as M+ peak.

INFRARED SPECTROSCOPY

Just like the electronic transitions, movement among vibrational energy levels is quantized and can be studied through spectrophotometric methods. For most vibrational excitations, absorption occurs in the infrared region of the spectrum. Although governed by quantum considerations, many vibrational modes can be modeled using classical physics. For example, a stretching vibration between two nuclei can be characterized using Hooke's law, which predicts that the frequency of an absorbance is given by the relationship:

$$\bar{v} = k \sqrt{\frac{f}{\left(\dfrac{m_1 m_2}{m_1 + m_2}\right)}}$$

where v is the frequency in wavenumbers (equal to $1/\lambda$), m_1 and m_2 are the masses of the two nuclei in amu units, and f is the force constant, which can be roughly correlated to bond strength.

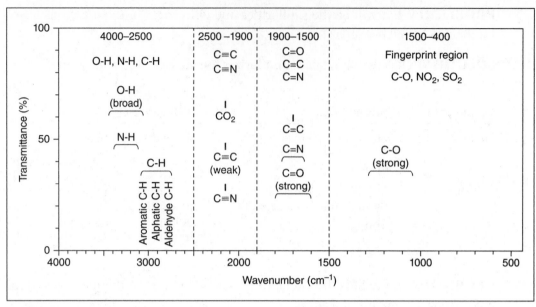

FIGURE 26.6 Overview of infrared absorbance ranges and fingerprint regions.

According to Hooke's law, then, there are two influential parameters for the frequency of molecular vibrations: the force constant and the reduced mass, which is given by $m_1 m_2 / (m_1 + m_2)$. Therefore, the C=C bond is predicted to absorb at a higher wavenumber than the C-C bond, and the C≡C bond higher still. Likewise, heavier atoms give rise to lower-frequency vibration. With this understanding, the IR spectrum can be broken into four very broad categories (Figure 26.6): at very high frequencies (2500–4000 cm⁻¹) we see what can be dubbed the X-H stretches; the region between 1900 and 2500 cm⁻¹ is home to the triple bonds; the region between 1500 and 1900 cm⁻¹ houses many of the doubly bonded species, including alkene and carbonyl stretches; and the portion of the spectrum bounded by 400 and 1500cm⁻¹ is known as the fingerprint region.

We complete this section with an overview of some of the wavenumbers and fingerprint regions of certain functional groups and structures. Taking a look at the functional groups with broad peaks (alcohols, carboxylic acids, amides, amines) we notice that these functional groups are able to make hydrogen bonds.

Functional Group/Structure	Peak Range cm⁻¹	Peak Types
Alcohol and ether C-O stretch phenol/Ar-O	1250	Strong
Alcohol and ether C-O stretch primary C	1050	Strong
Alcohol and ether C-O stretch secondary C	1100	Strong
Alcohol and ether C-O stretch tertiary C	1150	Strong
Alcohol O-H stretch	3600–3200	Strong, broad

Functional Group/Structure	Peak Range cm^{-1}	Peak Types
Aldehyde and ketone C=O	1720	Strong, sharp
Aldehyde C=O to H stretch	2800–2700	Moderate, sharp
Alkane C-H stretch	3000–2850	Strong, sharp
Alkane methyl	1375	Moderate, sharp
Alkane methylene	1450	Moderate, sharp
Alkane methylene chain rocking	720	Very weak
Alkene =C-H stretch	3100–3050	Moderate, sharp
Alkene C=C stretch	1680–1640	Moderate, sharp
Alkyne C≡C stretch (internal/terminal alkyne)	2150	Moderate, sharp
Alkyne terminal ≡C-H bending	630	Strong, broad
Alkyne terminal ≡C-H stretch	3300	Strong, sharp
Amide I and II bands (C=O) and (N-H)	1680 and 1600	Strong, broad
Amine or amide N-H bend	900–650	Moderate, broad
Amine or amide N-H stretch secondary	3500–3400	Moderate, broad
Amine or amide N-H stretch primary	3600–3500 and 3400–3300	Moderate, broad
Aromatic Ar-H stretch	3050	Moderate, sharp
Aromatic C to C stretch	1600–1450	Moderate, sharp
Aromatic overtones	2000–1600	Weak
Carboxylic acid C=O	1720	Strong, sharp
Carboxylic acid O-H bend	950–900	Strong, broad
Carboxylic acid O-H stretch	3600–2800	Strong, broad
Disubstituted benzene meta	820 and 700	Moderate, sharp
Disubstituted benzene ortho	700	Strong, sharp
Disubstituted benzene para	820	Strong, sharp
Ester C=O	1760	Strong, sharp
Ester C-O stretch	1300–1200	Strong
Mercaptans S-H	2600–2550	Weak
Monosubstituted benzene	770 and 700	Strong, sharp
Nitrile	2250–2000	Moderate, sharp
Nitro	1530 and 1350	Strong, sharp

PROBLEM: How can IR be used to distinguish between toluene and p-xylene?

SOLUTION: Toluene is monosubstituted, while p-xylene has two methyl groups positioned on carbon atoms 1 and 4. The toluene will show two strong sharp peaks at 770 and 700 cm^{-1} showing monosubstitution. The p-xylene will show just one strong sharp peak at 820 cm^{-1}. Both compounds will show a moderate, sharp peak at 3050 cm^{-1} and show peaks between 3000 and 2850 cm^{-1}.

PROBLEM: How can IR be used to distinguish between 1-hexyne and 2-hexyne?

SOLUTION: Both alkynes will show a moderate, sharp peak at 2150 cm^{-1}. Because the 1-hexyne is a terminal alkyne, it will also show a strong peak at 3300 cm^{-1}. This terminal alkyne peak will not be present in 2-hexyne.

PROTON NMR SPECTROSCOPY

When nuclei are placed in a strong magnetic field, the spin states become nondegenerate; nuclei in the lower-energy spin state can then be promoted to the next level by the absorption of electromagnetic radiation of the appropriate energy, as depicted in Figure 26.7.

In a local environment in which the electron cloud has been impoverished (by the inductive effect of an electronegative atom, for example), the nucleus is shielded less and thus experiences a stronger effective magnetic field (H_{eff}) (Figure 26.8). Consequently, the energy is enhanced and the resonance occurs at correspondingly higher frequency. This phenomenon of higher-frequency absorbances in electron-poor regions is known as deshielding.

Since the resonance frequency is field dependent, no two spectrometers will yield exactly the same resonance values. To alleviate this issue, spectroscopists historically have used an internal standard, against which all other signals are measured. The choice of tetramethylsilane as an NMR standard was driven by a few practical considerations. First, it is thermally stable and liquid at room temperature; second, it has 12 protons that are identical, so the intensity of absorption is high; and finally, the protons in TMS are quite shielded (silicon is not particularly electronegative), so almost all other proton resonances we observe occur at higher frequencies relative to TMS.

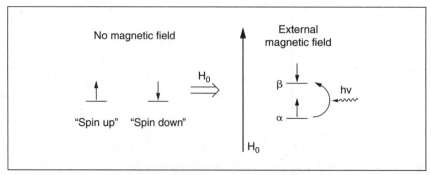

FIGURE 26.7 The splitting of degenerate nuclear spin states.

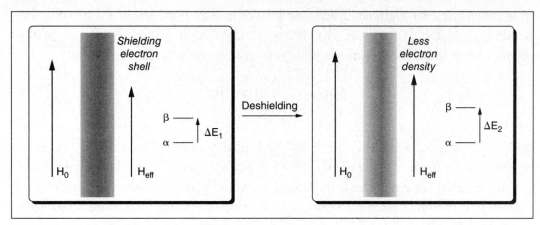

FIGURE 26.8 The shielding effect and deshielding.

Instruments are characterized by the resonance frequency of TMS in the magnetic field of that instrument. For example, a 400 MHz NMR spectrometer incorporates a superconducting magnet in which TMS resonates at 400 MHz. Stronger magnets lead to higher values (for example, 600 MHz and 900 MHz); in fact, magnets are so often specified by their TMS frequencies that we sometimes forget that the unit of MHz is a meaningless dimension for a magnetic field. That is, a 400 MHz NMR has a magnetic field strength of about 9.3 Tesla, yet for whatever reason this parameter is almost never mentioned.

Nevertheless, we can use the TMS resonance to talk about the general landscape of the NMR spectrum. Figure 26.9 shows a typical measurement domain for a 400 MHz spectrometer, which is bounded on the right by the resonance frequency of TMS (400,000,000 Hz). The range through which most organic molecules absorb extends to about 400,004,000 Hz, or 4000 Hz relative to TMS. However, these values change

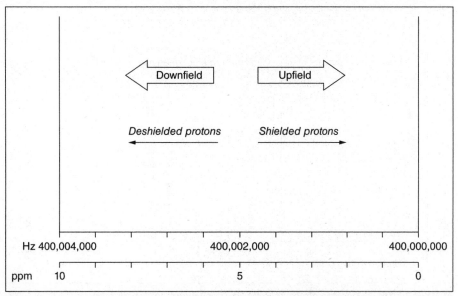

FIGURE 26.9 Important architectural features of the ^{1}H NMR spectrum.

as magnetic field strength is altered—an absorbance at 2000 Hz on a 400 MHz NMR would absorb at 1000 Hz on a 200 MHz NMR. To normalize these values, we instead report signals in terms of parts per million (ppm), which is defined as:

$$\text{ppm} = \nu/R = \text{Hz/MHz}$$

where ν is the signal frequency (in Hz) relative to TMS and R is the base resonance frequency of TMS (in MHz). Thus, on a 400 MHz instrument a signal at 2,000 Hz would be reported as 5 ppm (2,000 Hz / 400 MHz). This allows us to establish a universal scale for proton NMR ranging from 0 to about 10 ppm—although it is not terribly uncommon to find protons that absorb outside that range. Carboxylic acids are an excellent example of this (10–12 ppm).

Working within this framework, it is important to understand certain features and terminology related to position in the NMR spectrum. First, the ppm scale obscures the fact that frequency increases to the left, so this must be borne in mind. Thus, as protons are deshielded, they are shifted to the left—spectroscopists have dubbed this a downfield shift. Similarly, migrating to the right of the spectrum is said to be moving upfield. Phenomenologically, a downfield shift is evidence of deshielding, and this understanding will help us interpret NMR data.

Using this idea, we can establish general regions in the NMR spectrum where various proton types tend to congregate (Figure 26.10). For example, most purely aliphatic compounds (hexane, etc.) absorb far upfield in the vicinity of 1 ppm. The attachment of electron-withdrawing groups (e.g., carbonyls) tends to pull resonances downfield.

Thus, the protons on acetone show up at around 2.2 ppm. In general, the region between 0 and 2.5 ppm can be thought of as home to protons attached to carbons attached to carbon (H-C-C). This is also where terminal alkyne protons absorb.

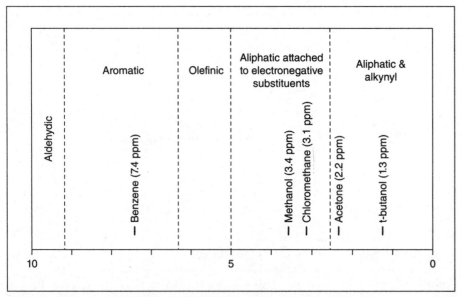

FIGURE 26.10 General regions of the ^{1}H NMR spectrum, with benchmarks.

As electronegative elements are attached, however, resonances are shifted even farther downfield. Thus, the methyl protons on methanol resonate at about 3.4 ppm, and the protons on chloromethane appear at about 3.1 ppm. Multiple electronegative elements have an additive effect: compared to chloromethane, dichloromethane resonates at 5.35 ppm, and chloroform (trichloromethane) absorbs at 7.25 ppm. As a rough guideline, the region between 2.5 and 5 ppm belongs to protons attached to carbons that are attached to an electronegative element (H-C-X).

Moving farther downfield, we encounter protons attached to sp^2 carbons, starting with the olefinic (alkenyl) variety, which absorb in the region between about 5 and 6.5 ppm. Next come the aromatic protons, which range from about 6.5 to 9 ppm. As a benchmark, benzene—the prototypical aromatic compound—absorbs at 7.4 ppm. Just like their aliphatic cousins, the olefinic and aromatic protons are shifted downfield as electron-withdrawing groups are attached to the systems. Finally, signals in the region between about 9 and 10 ppm tend to be very diagnostic for aldehydic protons—that is, the protons connected directly to the carbonyl carbon.

Additional information can be derived from a phenomenon known as scalar (or spin-spin) coupling, through which a proton is influenced by its nearest neighbors. For example, consider a proton (H_x) that is vicinal to a pair of protons (H_a and H_b). The latter two protons are either spin up or spin down, and in fact we can imagine four permutations (2^2) of two nuclei with two states to choose from. If both H_a and H_b are aligned with the external magnetic field, they will serve to enhance H_{eff}, thereby increasing the energy gap between the H_x α and β states, which in turn leads to a higher frequency absorbance (a downfield shift). Conversely, the situation in which both H_a and H_b oppose the external magnetic field diminishes the H_{eff}, leading to an upfield shift. The two remaining permutations have one spin up and the other spin down, thereby cancelling each other out. The result is a pattern known as a triplet, in which the three prongs of the signal are present in a 1:2:1 ratio. In other words, the pattern exhibited (or *multiplicity*) has one more prong than the number of neighboring protons. Patterns of this type are said to obey the "n+1 rule," where n = the number of neighboring protons, and n + 1 = the multiplicity of the signal. The most common splitting patterns and their abbreviations are summarized in Table 26.1.

Table 26.1 Some Common Splitting Patterns	
Abbreviation	**Pattern**
s	Singlet
d	Doublet
t	Triplet
q	Quartet
quint	Quintet
m	Multiplet

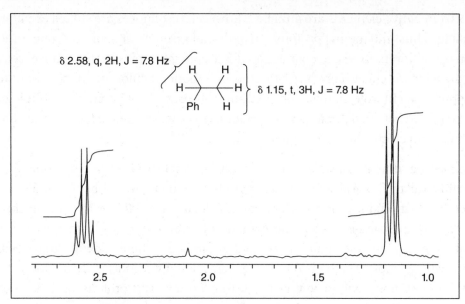

FIGURE 26.11 The ethyl moiety of ethyl benzene.

So the chemical shift tells us about a proton's electronic environment, and splitting patterns tell us about the number of neighboring protons—but still the spectrum has further information to yield. It turns out that the area under each signal is proportional to the number of protons giving rise to that signal. Therefore, integrating the area under the curves allows us to establish a ratio for all chemically distinct protons in the NMR. As an illustration, Figure 26.11 presents a portion of the NMR spectrum of ethylbenzene corresponding to the ethyl moiety. There are two signals (at 1.15 ppm and 2.58 ppm), corresponding to the two sets of chemically distinct protons on the ethyl substituent (a methyl and methylene group, respectively). The downfield shift of the methylene group is an indication of its being closer to the slightly electron-withdrawing benzene ring. The splitting patterns tell us that the protons resonating at 1.15 (the triplet) are next to two other protons, and the protons at 2.58 (the quartet) are adjacent to three other protons. Furthermore, the integral traces reveal that the two sets of protons are present in a 3:2 ratio.

Generally speaking, protons connected to the same carbon (geminal protons) do not split each other—with one significant exception. Figure 26.12 shows three types of geminal protons: homeotopic, enantiotopic, and diastereotopic. To better understand the terminology, consider the imaginary products formed by replacing each of the two geminal protons with another atom, say a chlorine substituent. In the homotopic

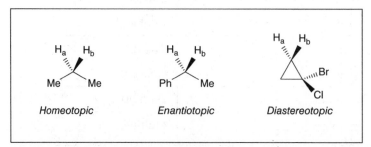

FIGURE 26.12 Three types of geminal protons.

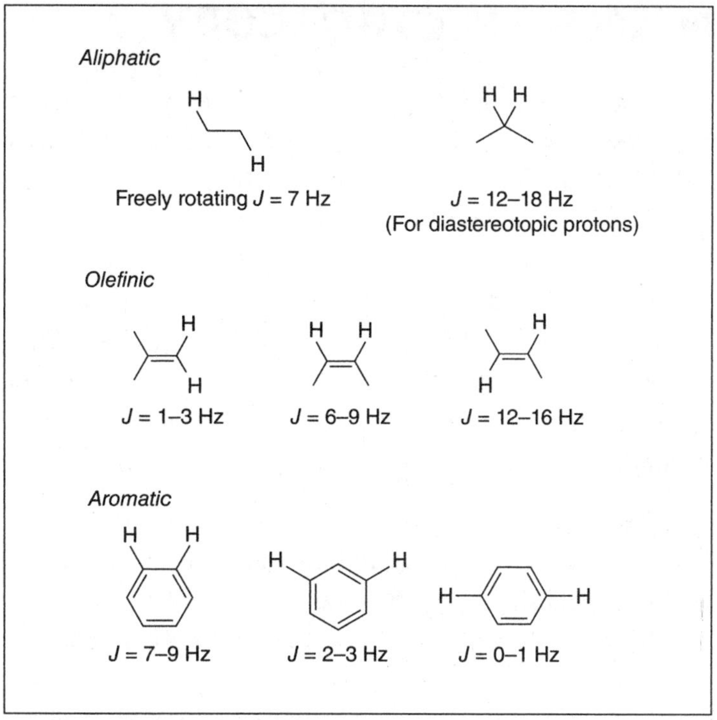

Aliphatic

H

H

Freely rotating $J = 7$ Hz

H H

$J = 12–18$ Hz
(For diastereotopic protons)

Olefinic

H

H

$J = 1–3$ Hz

H H

$J = 6–9$ Hz

H

H

$J = 12–16$ Hz

Aromatic

H H

$J = 7–9$ Hz

H H

$J = 2–3$ Hz

H H

$J = 0–1$ Hz

FIGURE 26.13 Some representative coupling constants.

example, enantiomeric "products" are formed [*R*- and *S*-(1-chloroethyl)benzene]; and replacing H_a with H_b in the cyclopropane derivative gives diastereomers (*cis*-dichloro vs. *trans*dichloro).

Homotopic and enantiotopic geminal protons do not split each other because they are chemically equivalent. In other words, they are identical through a plane of symmetry (the plane of this page). However, diastereotopic protons are not chemically equivalent—in the preceding example, H_a is in proximity to the chloro substituent, whereas H_b is close to the bromine. In short, they are in different worlds and therefore behave as individuals. Therefore, in these special cases, geminal protons do split each other, and the magnitude of the *J*-value is relatively large. Figure 26.13 lists this value, along with other representative coupling constants. This summary will be useful for the interpretation of spectra.

Finally, we end with a brief summary of where the chemical shifts will be for protons in certain chemical environments. This will be handy when answering the questions presented in the exams in this book.

R-C-H	δ 0.9–1.5	O-C-H	δ 3.5–4
C=C-H	δ 4.5–6.0	C(=O)-H	δ 9–10
C≡C-H	δ 2.0–3.0	C-O-H	δ 5.0
Ar-H	δ 7.0–8.0	C(=O)-O-H	δ 10–12
X-C-H	δ 2.5–4	C(=O)-C-H	δ 2.0–2.5

CARBON NMR SPECTROSCOPY

The principle of ^{13}C NMR is identical to that of ^{1}H NMR; however, there are a few practical differences that deserve mention. First, while the natural abundance of ^{1}H is almost 100 percent, the ^{13}C isotope makes up only slightly over 1 percent of carbon found in nature. This means that the NMR-active carbon nucleus is quite dilute in the typical molecule. As a result, signal-to-noise ratios tend to be lower and data collection times are usually longer. Moreover, although scalar coupling can exist (in principle) between two ^{13}C nuclei, the statistical likelihood that a pair of this species will be situated adjacent to each other is vanishingly small. Carbon can also couple to ^{1}H nuclei, which are plentiful, but most experimental methods wipe out this interaction with a technique known as off-resonance decoupling in order to simplify the spectrum.

Figure 26.14 provides a broad overview of ^{13}C resonances. In the 0–50 ppm range are mostly aliphatic carbons attached to nothing in particular. When π systems are introduced, a dramatic downfield shift occurs through an effect known as anisotropy—areas above and below the π bonds tend to be shielded, while the middle areas tend to be strongly deshielded. Thus, alkenes and aromatic carbons show up in the general region of 100–150 ppm. In alkynes an opposite anisotropic effect occurs: the barrel-like π structure of the alkyne sets up an electronic current whose field lines actually shield at the ends of the triple bond. Therefore, acetylenic carbons resonate in the 50–100 ppm range. When carbons of any type (sp, sp^2, sp^3) are attached to electronegative elements, a downfield shift occurs. Thus, aliphatics are moved into the 50–100 ppm region, acetylenics (nitriles) are moved into the 100–150 range, and olefinics (carbonyls) migrate to the 150–200 ppm region.

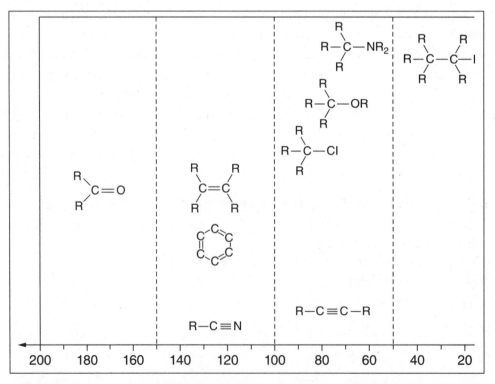

FIGURE 26.14 General landscape of ^{13}C NMR.

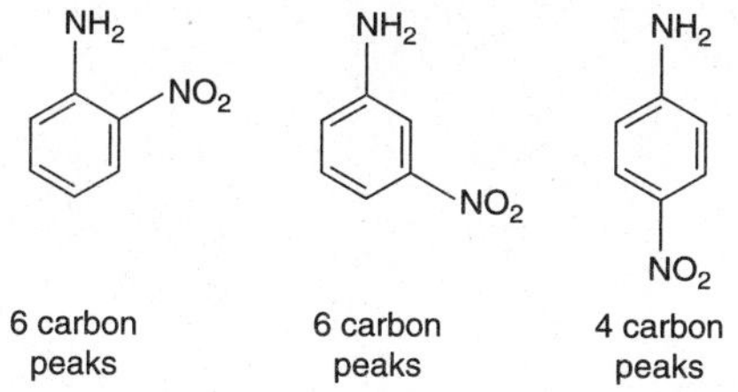

FIGURE 26.15 Impact of symmetry on ^{13}C NMR spectrum.

The combination of this wide landscape with the sharp singlet signals means that every unique carbon in a molecule usually can be resolved in a ^{13}C spectrum. This is useful because it can reveal important information about symmetry within a molecule. For example, 2-nitroaniline and 3-nitroaniline (Figure 26.15) exhibit six carbon peaks, as we would expect. However, 4-nitroaniline only has four carbon signals because of its inherent symmetry.

Much like we did for the other spectrometric methods, a summary chart for chemical shifts follows:

Alkanes C-C	0–60 ppm	C-O/C-N	30–80 ppm
Alkenes C=C	100–150 ppm	C=O acid, esters, amides	15–180 ppm
Alkynes C≡C	75–100 ppm	C=O aldehydes, ketones	190–220 ppm
Arenes	110–140 ppm		

PROBLEM: What will be the chemical shifts and splitting for the hydrogen atoms in a molecule of isopropyl benzene, C_6H_5-$CH(CH_3)_2$? How does this contrast to the 13-CNMR?

SOLUTION: The HNMR will feature a:

➤ Doublet at 1.1 ppm (6H)
➤ Septet at 2.7 ppm (1H)
➤ Multiplet at 7.2 ppm (5H)

The 13-CNMR will feature six peaks. There will be doublets in the arene range showing C-H. One peak will be a singlet in the arene region showing a carbon with no hydrogen atoms on it. The upfield region of the 13-CNMR will show a quartet peak that is twice the height of the other peaks. Finally, the upfield region will show a doublet indicating the C-H of the isopropyl group.

PART IV
PERCEPTUAL ABILITY

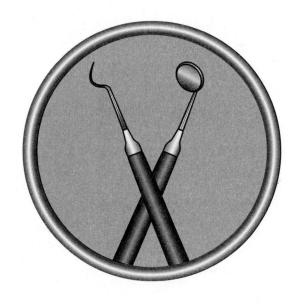

CHAPTER 27

Keyhole

Read This Chapter to Learn About

➤ The Keyhole Part of the Perceptual Ability Test
➤ Strategies for Answering Keyhole Questions

THE KEYHOLE PART OF THE PERCEPTUAL ABILITY TEST

These questions present a three-dimensional object and ask you to predict which of five apertures (keyholes) the object will be able to pass through. The object and the apertures are drawn to the same scale (Figure 27.1).

In order to perform well on this section, you need to become totally comfortable with the rules. Once you understand the task and its parameters, you will not need to waste valuable testing time reading the instructions on test day and you can go straight to the questions. Here are the rules:

1. The irregular solid object may be turned in any direction before it is passed through the aperture. It does not have to start through the aperture on the side shown; any side may be introduced first.

    A three-dimensional object may be viewed from any of six sides: front, back, top, bottom, left side, or right side. However, since if you introduce the object from the

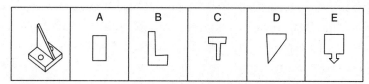

FIGURE 27.1 A question from the keyhole part of the perceptual ability test.

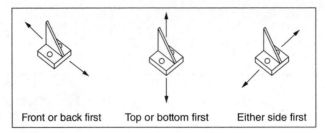

Front or back first   Top or bottom first   Either side first

FIGURE 27.2 Possible orientations of object in keyhole questions.

back first, the front must also fit, you may think of the object as having only three ways it can pass through the aperture (Figure 27.2):
➤ Front or back first
➤ Either side first
➤ Top or bottom first
You may mentally turn the object in any of these ways before inserting it.

2. Once the object has started passing through the aperture, it may not be turned or twisted. The object must pass completely through the aperture, which is always the exact shape of the appropriate external outline of the object.

This means that once you have turned the object in the desired direction and begun to insert the object into the keyhole, it must pass completely through the keyhole without being rotated or turned. If you introduce the object from the top, you cannot turn it halfway through in order to make it fit; it must go straight through without turning.

3. Both the apertures and the objects are drawn to the same scale. It is possible for an aperture to be the correct shape but too small for the object. Differences are large enough to judge with the eye.

This means that you can't always just go by shape. If the front view of the object is a rectangle, then you could pass it through a rectangular keyhole. But don't just immediately choose an answer that shows a rectangle. It must also be the right size rectangle. Pay attention to scale.

4. There are no irregularities in any part of the object not shown. However, if the figure has symmetric indentations, the part shown is symmetric with the hidden portion.

This means that there are no hidden parts that you cannot see that might get in the way when passing the object through the keyhole. You can only see three sides, but the fourth side has no surprises. You will be given enough information to determine which keyhole can accept the object.

5. There is only one correct aperture for each object.

Keep this in mind if you get confused when choosing an answer. If two apertures seem similar, then focus on what exactly is different. If the object seems like it will fit into two different apertures, then you probably missed some detail on the object that would rule one of them out. Go back and check it.

STRATEGIES FOR ANSWERING KEYHOLE QUESTIONS

In order to figure out what keyhole is correct, you first need to identify what the object will look like in each of the three entry positions. Use your erasable note board to sketch a silhouette of the object from each entry position. A silhouette is a two-dimensional representation of the outside of an object. It is a contour outline on a single plane; it does not show depth, just the outside edges. Consider the following when making your silhouettes:

➤ What is the basic shape of the object in this view?
➤ Does the object have any protrusions that will be visible from this view?
➤ Does the object have any indentations that will be visible from this view?
➤ If there are multiple protrusions in this view, which one sticks out the most?
➤ Is the object symmetrical in this view? If not, which side or feature is larger?
➤ Are the lines of the object in this view straight, slanted, or curved?

Using our previous example, the orientations of the object shown in the following figures would produce the silhouette shown to the right of each orientation:

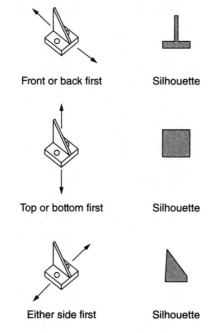

Front or back first   Silhouette

Top or bottom first   Silhouette

Either side first   Silhouette

By drawing these three silhouettes on your note board, you will save time when you go to compare answer choices. If you compare the silhouettes in the preceding figures to the answer choices for this question shown in the following figure, you can see quickly see that choices A, B, and E are incorrect. Choice C looks like the front- or back-first silhouette, and choice D looks like the side-first silhouette. Upon closer inspection, you can see that choice C does not have the proper dimensions. Therefore, the answer is D.

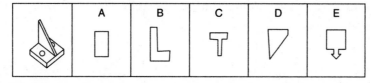

Working with Orientation

The orientation of the object as it is presented is probably not the one you will need in order to pass the object through the keyhole. You will most likely need to turn the object before introducing it. Therefore, you can start by trying the side-first introduction or the top- or bottom-first introduction. If neither of those orientations work, then try the front- or back-first orientation.

Let's look at another object. First, draw each of the three silhouettes in the spaces provided:

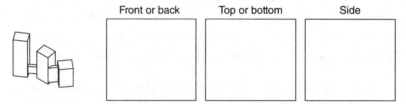

Now compare your silhouettes to the answer choices shown in the following figure:

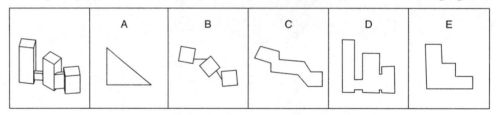

Your silhouette for the front or back view should match choice D.

Keyhole questions can be quite difficult, especially if the object is complex. If you run across a question that has you stumped, mark it and move on. Do not waste time on especially difficult questions. You can always come back to it at the end, if time permits. Focus on your goal: to gather as many correct answers as possible as quickly as you can.

Tips for Keyhole Questions

➤ The object can be inserted front or back first, side first, or top or bottom first. It will most likely need to be turned in a different direction than what is originally presented.

➤ Once the object enters the keyhole, it cannot be turned or twisted. It must fit straight through.

➤ Study the shape carefully, noting any protrusions or indentations.

➤ Sketch the three silhouettes of the object from the three different views.

➤ Compare your silhouettes to the answer choices.

➤ If there is more than one choice that seems to fit, compare them and go back to reconsider the object.

CHAPTER 28

Top/Front/End Projection

Read This Chapter to Learn About

➤ The Top/Front/End Projection Part of the Perceptual Ability Test

➤ Strategies for Answering Projection Questions

THE TOP/FRONT/END PROJECTION PART OF THE PERCEPTUAL ABILITY TEST

The second section of the Perceptual Ability Test (PAT) is top/front/end projections. In this section, you will be shown two of the following views of an object: top view, front view, end view. You must identify the third view of the object from four choices. All of these views are two-dimensional and are rendered without perspective. These views are similar to the three silhouettes you draw for keyhole questions. The front view is what you would see if you were looking directly at the front of the object. The end view is what you would see if you were looking directly at the right side of the object. The top view is what you would see if you were above the object and looking directly down on it. For example, see Figure 28.1.

The Projection Grid

A three-dimensional disk like the one shown in Figure 28.1 would look like the views shown in Figure 28.2 in a top/front/end projection.

If you looked directly down on the disk, all you would see is a circle. If you looked at it from the front, it would look like a rectangle. Since it is circular, the same view would present from the sides.

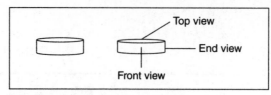

FIGURE 28.1 Top, front, and end views of a
three-dimensional object.

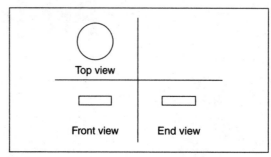

FIGURE 28.2 Top, front, and end projections of the
object shown in Figure 28.1.

If there was a hole in the disk and it looked more like a tire, the views would look like the
projections shown in Figure 28.3.

Lines for parts of an object that cannot be seen on the surface in a particular view are
dotted in that view, so in Figure 28.3 you can see little dotted lines in the front and end
views where the hole in the disk is located, though you cannot see the hole directly from
either view.

All the top/front/end projection questions on the PAT will use this same grid, shown in
Figure 28.4.

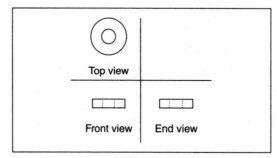

FIGURE 28.3 Projections of a disk with a hole in
the center.

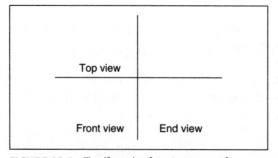

FIGURE 28.4 Top/front/end projection grid.

The views will always be in the order shown in Figure 28.4. For a question, only two of the three views will appear in the grid and the third missing view will be indicated with a question mark. Your job is to choose this missing third view from the four answer choices.

Visible Versus Invisible Lines

As shown in Figure 28.3, in which the disk had a center cutout, some parts of objects in the projections will be indicated with dotted lines, which means that those parts are not visible from the view but are within or on the other side of the object. While you would not see the hole in the object in Figure 28.3 from the front view, knowing that it is there would help you identify the top view of the object. All the lines that are visible in a particular view are indicated with solid lines. All the lines that are invisible in a particular view are indicated with dotted lines, as shown in the following figure.

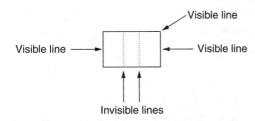

These dotted lines are very important. They indicate edges that are inside or behind the object and cannot be seen in that particular view but are essential to your understanding of what the object looks like. You will need them to understand the object's depth. For example, consider the object shown in the following figure:

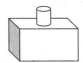

This object would have the projections shown in the following grid:

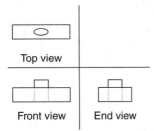

The front view and end view show you that the cylinder on top extends through the block. On the test, you will not be given a three-dimensional view, as you were given on the last example. However, given the two views that you will see, you will know certain things about the third view of the object. You will probably not know enough to picture the object in three dimensions, but each view gives you some clues, and when taken together, you can eliminate wrong answers and find the third view.

The questions do not always ask you to supply the same missing view. You should expect to see about five of each missing view: front, top, or end.

STRATEGIES FOR ANSWERING PROJECTION QUESTIONS

First, use the views you are given to identify how many visible and invisible lines make up the figure. What are the outside dimensions like? Are there internal or hidden parts? Consider the object outlined in the Figure 28.5.

In this view, you can see that there are five edges along the top of the figure and five edges on the side (though not all would be visible from that view). The top and bottom lines and the lines on the far left and right are always exterior lines and are always visible. There are no invisible lines in the end view shown in Figure 28.5. The edges marked with arrows can be seen as marking off four sections of the figure in this view. You can use this information to eliminate some of the answer choices. Let's say that you are asked to find the top view of this object. The two views you would be presented are shown in Figure 28.6.

What additional information can you see from the front view in Figure 28.6? How many edges are visible and invisible? From the front view, only two of the horizontal edges (top and bottom) are visible. The rest appear as invisible dotted lines. These lines mark off four sections in the front view. In the end view, you can see that if the figure were viewed from the top, the four sections would be narrow, wide, narrow, narrow (remember, the end view is from the right side).

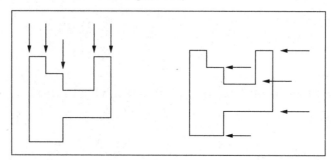

FIGURE 28.5   End view of an object.

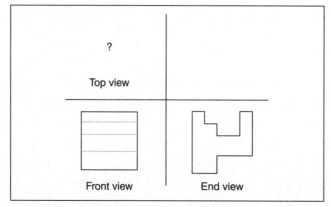

FIGURE 28.6   Test question for the object shown in Figure 28.5.

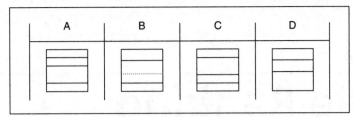

FIGURE 28.7   Answer choices for question in Figure 28.6.

The answer choices are shown in Figure 28.7.

From the top, all the edges would be visible, so eliminate choice B. Choice D only has three sections, and this figure has four, so eliminate D. Choices A and C have the correct number of lines, and all are visible. Now it's time to check placement. The top view should show narrow, wide, narrow, narrow sections, and choice A does not do that. Choice C is the correct answer.

Remember, if you encounter a tough figure that you do not understand, mark it and move on. Do not waste time on especially difficult questions. You can always come back to it at the end, if time permits. Focus on your goal: to gather as many correct answers as quickly as you can.

Tips for Top/Front/End Projection Questions

➤ There are three views of the object: the top view, the end view (right end), and the front view.
➤ You are given two of the three and asked to find the third.
➤ Visible lines are solid and invisible lines are dotted.
➤ In each view shown, note the number of visible and invisible lines. Count how many sections are formed by these lines.
➤ In each view shown, note the position and order of the visible and invisible lines.
➤ Project how many sections will be in the missing view. Eliminate answers that do not match.
➤ Project how many visible and invisible lines will be in the missing view. Eliminate answers that do not match.
➤ If you have more than one choice with the correct number and order of visible and invisible lines, check their relative positions and lengths.

Angle Ranking

THE ANGLE RANKING PART OF THE PERCEPTUAL ABILITY TEST

The third section of the PAT is angle ranking. In this section, you will be shown four angles and asked to rank them by size from smallest to largest. Compared to the other sections of the PAT, this is a relatively uncomplicated task, though it can be tricky to discriminate between similar angles. Despite the occasional trickiness, this section will probably take the least amount of time to complete.

Compare the angles in the following figure. Which one is larger?

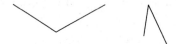

You probably have no trouble seeing that the one on the left is larger, right? What about the pair of angles in Figure 29.1?

This one is a bit more difficult. The one on the left is larger, but it is harder to see that immediately. Here are three strategies you can use to help you determine which of two angles is larger:

1. Compare each angle to a 90-degree angle. Most people can picture a right angle, so compare your mental 90-degree angle to the angles shown. The one on the left in Figure 29.1 is definitely larger than 90 degrees. The one on the right is close to 90 degrees. Therefore, the left one is larger.

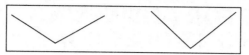

FIGURE 29.1 Sample pair of angles.

2. Mentally superimpose one angle on top of the other. This takes more skill, but with practice, you will improve at it. This method is easiest if the angles are near each other on the computer screen or if they are facing in the same direction. If the angles in Figure 29.1 were superimposed, they would look like the following figure:

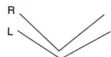

The right angle fits within the left one, so the left angle is larger.

3. You can mentally measure the angles to compare them if you do so at a set point fairly close to the vertexes of the angles. Measure off a quarter inch from the vertex and learn what that looks like so you can picture it in your mind. Then compare two angles at that same point to see which is larger. This is not easy to do accurately, but if you practice, you will improve at it. If the two angles in Figure 29.1 were measured this way, you could see that the left one is larger, as shown in the following figure.

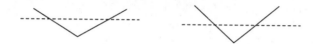

Which of the following angles appears larger?

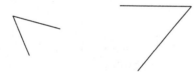

If you said that the one on the right appears larger, you are not alone. However, these angles are exactly the same size. Many people get tricked by looking at the length of the sides of the angles. Longer sides do not indicate a larger angle. You must measure each angle at the same spot in order to compare them properly. That's why if you can learn to compare angles at one-quarter inch from their vertexes, you can improve your score on this section.

You may also encounter an angle that has two legs of different lengths. This should not change how you view the angles to compare them. Try ranking the following angles:

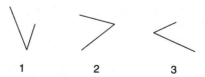

The correct ranking, from smallest to largest, is 1-3-2.

STRATEGIES FOR ANSWERING ANGLE RANKING QUESTIONS

First, identify the smallest and largest angles. If only one of them is clear, just identify that one for now. Write them down on your note board, but leave room in between to add the middle ones.

Next, eliminate any answer choices that do not match the sequence you have identified so far. If you identified both the smallest and the largest angles, this may be all you have to do to answer the question.

If more than one choice remains, compare the remaining two angles to each other (or if you have three remaining, compare the two that are positioned closest to each other on the computer screen). Rank them from smallest to largest and write them on your note board in your sequence. Eliminate answers that do not match.

Now try the following set of angles with answer choices:

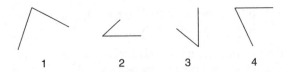

1   2   3   4

A. 2-3-1-4
B. 3-4-2-1
C. 1-4-3-2
D. 2-3-4-1

Perhaps the easiest first step here is to identify the largest angle: number 1. That means that 1 should be last in the ranking. Eliminate choices A and C. The smallest is harder to determine, but you can probably tell that 4 is the second largest. Therefore the ranking is __, __, 4, 1. The correct answer must be D. The correct ranking of the angles from small to large is 2-3-4-1. Using this strategy helps you avoid some tough calls, as on this question. You don't actually need to be able to compare angles 2 and 3, which are very similar.

Tips for Answering Angle Ranking Questions

➤ You must rank the four angles from smallest to largest.
➤ Do not be fooled by longer leg length or by angles with differing leg lengths. Only the angle measure matters.
➤ Identify the largest or smallest, or both. Eliminate answers based on this.
➤ Compare remaining angles using one of the three methods:
   ➤ Compare to 90 degrees
   ➤ Superimpose
   ➤ Measure one-quarter inch from vertexes
➤ Place more angles into the sequence and eliminate again.

CHAPTER 30

Paper Folding

Read This Chapter to Learn About

➤ The Paper Folding Part of the Percepual Ability Test
➤ Strategies for Answering Paper Folding Questions

THE PAPER FOLDING PART OF THE PERCEPTUAL ABILITY TEST

The fourth section of the PAT is paper folding. In this section, you are shown a square piece of paper that is folded one or more times in various ways. Once the paper is folded, a hole is punched in the paper and you are shown the location of this hole. Your job is to identify what the paper will look like once it is unfolded. Here are the rules:

➤ The paper is never turned. It is kept in the same orientation and simply folded.
➤ The paper is never twisted or torn.
➤ None of the folds will result in a shape that goes outside the original parameters of the square.
➤ Only one hole will be punched.
➤ Depending on where it is punched, the hole may go through one or more layers of the paper.

As the paper is folded, the original shape of the square will continue to be shown as a dashed line if the paper no longer conforms to that shape, as shown in the following figure:

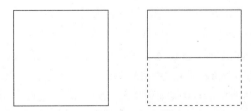

The original square paper is shown at left. On the right is what the paper looks like after the bottom half has been folded up to the top edge. The bottom of the original square is now shown with dashed lines.

If the paper is folded a second time, another figure will be shown, as in the following example:

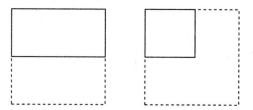

This second figure shows that the rectangle on top has been folded again, the right side over the left. The original outline of the square is still shown by the dashed lines.

To make this process easier to visualize, the following figure shows the sequence with arrows to show how the paper has been folded. There will *not* be arrows on the actual questions.

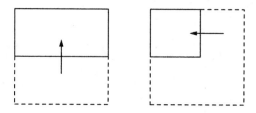

When the hole is punched, the paper might look like the following figure:

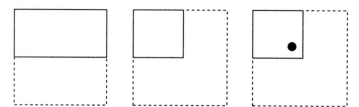

The black dot shows the location of the punched hole. In this figure, the hole will go through four layers of paper, resulting in four holes.

The answer choices are presented as punch grids, as shown here:

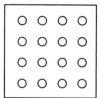

There are 16 possible holes in the punch grid, evenly arranged in rows and columns. The location of punched holes will be shown by blackening holes in this grid. Since the answers are always shown on these punch grids, there is no paper that is folded and hole-punched in a way that would result in a hole in a location different from the

16 spots shown. For the previous example, the correct answer punch grid is shown in the following figure:

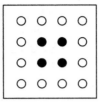

STRATEGIES FOR ANSWERING PAPER FOLDING QUESTIONS

First look at how many times the paper has been folded and the location of the hole. How many layers of paper does the hole go through? The resulting punch grid will have the same number of blackened circles. You can usually eliminate a choice or two simply by counting the number of holes. Be sure you are counting the layers where the hole is punched. Look at the example in the following figure.

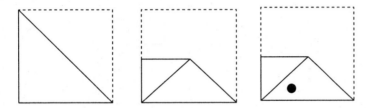

The paper is folded twice, but the hole is punched where the paper is only folded once, so there will only be two holes.

Also be careful to note the way in which the paper is folded. Sometimes a second fold may cover up a first fold, as shown in the following figure:

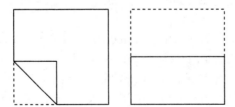

When the second fold is made, the top half of the paper is folded down over the bottom and covers up the left corner that was folded in.

Suppose the hole is punched as shown in the following figure:

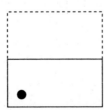

This hole will only go through one layer. Alternatively, suppose the hole is punched as shown in the following figure:

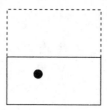

The hole will now go through three layers.

The best way to practice for this section is to actually perform the paper folding and hole punching. At the end of this chapter you will find templates of the punch grids that you can copy, cut out, and use to practice. Make one or more folds of the square, and then punch a hole through one of the circles on the grid. Use a second punch grid to predict the result by coloring in the circles you think will have holes in them. Unfold your original punched paper and check your results.

Try a complete example with answer choices, as shown in the following figure:

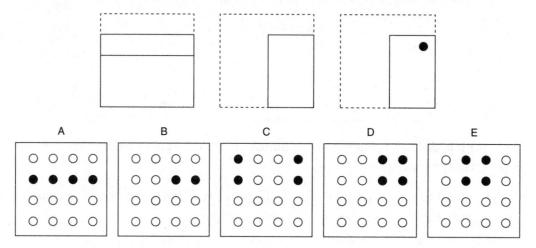

The top quarter of the square is folded once toward the center, and then the paper is folded in half from left to right. The hole is punched in the top right corner of the folded part. This means that the hole goes through four layers of paper and there will be four holes. You can eliminate choice B. Since the hole is punched in the far right side, there should be a hole on the far right side in the second circle down from the top. Eliminate choice E. Since the paper is folded symmetrically, there should also be a hole in the second circle down from the top on the left side. Eliminate choice D. Since the paper was originally folded down from the top, the hole will go through the top left and right circles as well as the second circles down on the left and right sides. Only choice C has holes in those positions, so the correct answer is C.

Tips for Paper Folding Questions

➤ The paper is always a square. It may be folded one or more times, but only in ways that remain inside the area of the original square.

➤ Only one hole is punched, and it can only be punched through an area that results in holes in the circles on the punch grid.

➤ Determine how many layers of paper the hole goes through. Eliminate choices that do not have the correct number of holes.

➤ Identify the location of one punched hole. Eliminate choices that do not have that hole punched.

➤ The corresponding hole on the other side of the fold will also be punched. Eliminate choices that do not have that hole punched.

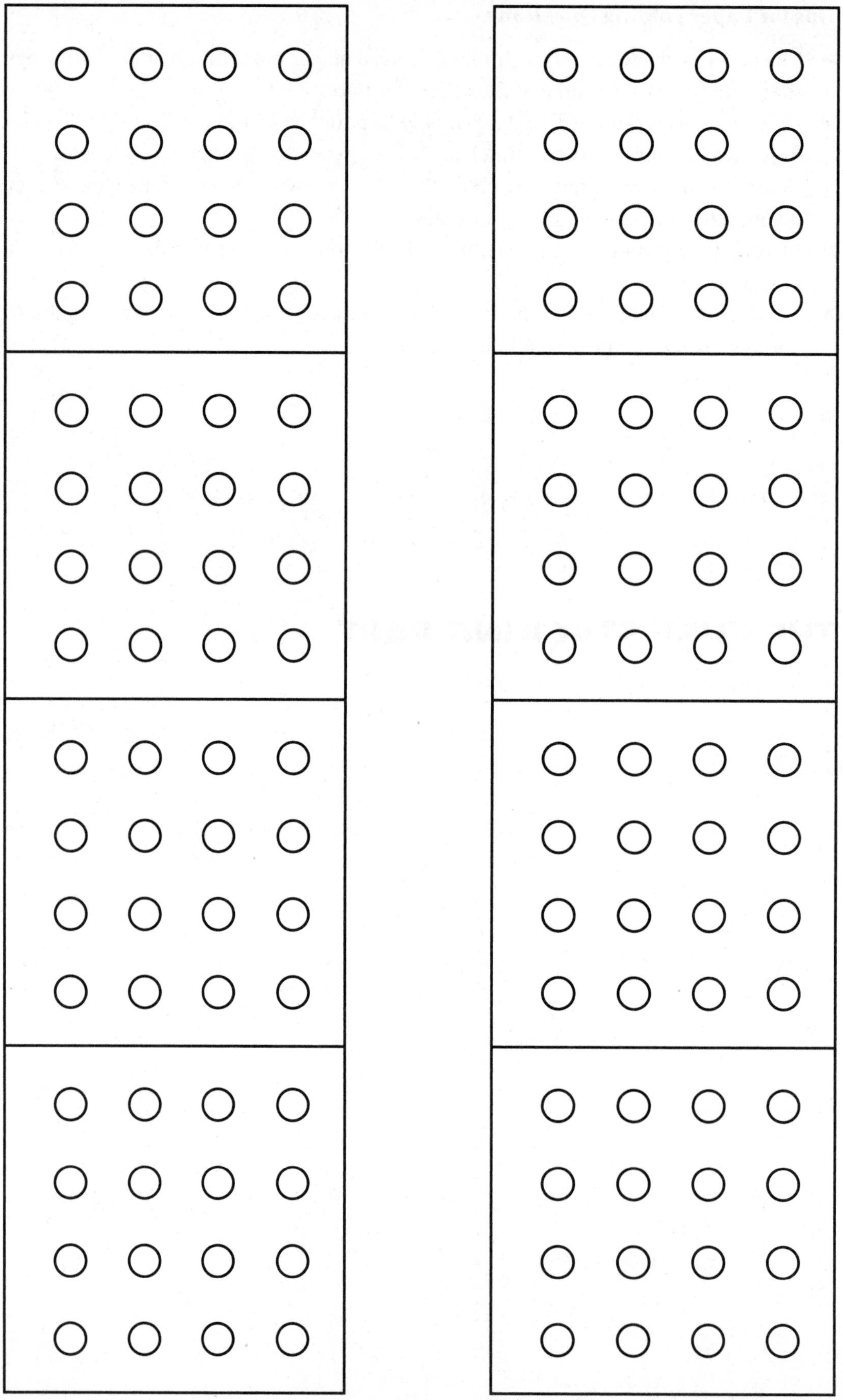

Cube Stacking

THE CUBE STACKING PART OF THE PERCEPTUAL ABILITY TEST

The fifth section of the PAT is cube stacking. In this section, you are shown sets of stacked cubes that have been cemented together. The stacks are then painted on all sides except the bottom. Your job is to figure out how many sides of each cube are painted. There are several questions for each stack of cubes shown. Once you get the hang of this, it should be one of the easier sections of the PAT and one of the quickest to complete. If you pay careful attention to this section and learn the strategies, you can really rack up some points on the PAT with cube stacking.

A basic cube stack looks like the following figure:

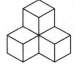

This stack is made up of four cubes: three visible cubes and one invisible hidden cube that supports the top cube. You will need to consider all the cubes in a stack, not just the visible ones. There will be no cubes that are unsupported, so pay attention to the location of invisible support cubes.

How many cubes are in the following figure?

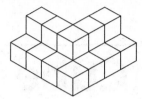

If you counted 17, you are correct. There are 5 in the top level, which must be supported by 5 more (invisible) cubes underneath. Then there are 7 cubes in the front bottom level. There could theoretically be another hidden cube on the bottom level center, as indicated in the following figure,

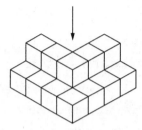

but this will not be the case on the PAT. The *only* cubes that are invisible are those that directly support visible cubes.

Count the cubes in the following stack:

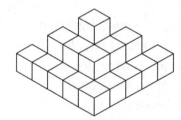

If you counted 22, you are correct. There are 15 in the bottom level, 6 in the middle level, and 1 on top. These include 6 invisible cubes on the bottom level supporting the middle level and 1 invisible cube on the middle level supporting the top cube.

STRATEGIES FOR ANSWERING CUBE STACKING QUESTIONS

An easy way to count cubes and their painted sides is to disassemble the levels of cubes. You can draw each level separately (in two dimensions) on your note board and then count how many cubes there are and how many sides each one has painted. You can disassemble cube stacks like this:

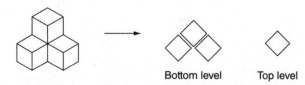

Bottom level   Top level

Now label each cube according to how many sides it has painted, as in the following drawing:

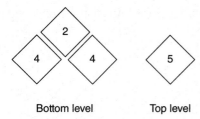

Bottom level   Top level

Try the more complicated stack in the following figure:

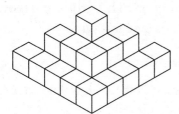

You should get a drawing like the following one:

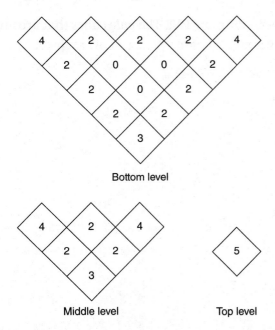

Bottom level

Middle level   Top level

Now make a chart on your note board to record how many cubes have each number of sides painted, like this:

	0 Sides	1 Side	2 Sides	3 Sides	4 Sides	5 Sides
Number of cubes	3	0	12	2	4	1

Once you have done this, answering the questions will be a snap. The questions typically look like this:

1. In figure A, how many cubes have four of their exposed sides painted?
   A. 1 cube
   B. 2 cubes
   C. 3 cubes
   D. 4 cubes
   E. 5 cubes

Once you have done the separation of layers and counting of painted sides, just mark the correct answer for each question in the group and move on to the next figure. There are usually three to six questions for each figure.

Tips for Cube Stacking Questions

➤ Stacks are made up of both visible and invisible cubes. The only invisible cubes are those required to support visible cubes.
➤ Disassemble the levels of cubes. Draw each level separately (in two dimensions) on your note board.
➤ Label each cube according to how many sides it has painted.
➤ Make a chart on your note board to record how many cubes have each number of sides painted.

Form Creation

THE FORM CREATION PART OF THE PERCEPTUAL ABILITY TEST

The sixth and final section of the PAT is form creation. In this section, you are shown a flat two-dimensional pattern that is folded and manipulated into a three-dimensional shape. You might see a flat shape like this:

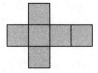

This pattern will become a cube when folded, as in the following figure:

You will be given four three-dimensional objects from which to choose. Your job is to choose the three-dimensional object that would be created from the pattern. This section requires careful observation and good visual dexterity. It will likely be one of the most time-consuming sections of the PAT, so be sure you allocate your time on the test wisely. Do not hesitate to skip a difficult question. Mark it and you can return to it at the end of the test if time allows. Focus on your goal: gather as many correct answers as you can as quickly as possible.

Pace Yourself

You will have 60 minutes to answer 90 questions. That gives you 10 minutes for each of the six sections and works out to an average of only 40 seconds per question. Of course, you may find that you are faster at one question type than at another. For example, if you are able to do 15 cube stacking questions in only seven minutes, then you can have three extra minutes for those nasty keyhole questions.

Time yourself as you practice so that you know how long it will take you to do each of the six sections. Make sure you average 15 questions in only 10 minutes so that you can do the whole 90 questions in 60 minutes. Reserve a few minutes at the end of your 60 minutes to go back to questions you skipped. Fill in any answer choice for those questions; there is no penalty for guessing. Keep an eye on the clock and be sure to mark an answer for every question.

Here are the rules for the form creation section:

1. The flat pattern forms only one of the three-dimensional objects shown in the four answer choices. This means that three of the four answer choices have something wrong with them.
2. The three-dimensional objects shown in the answer choices are rendered to scale with the flat pattern. This means that you might see the correct shape as an answer choice, but the object shown might be too small or too big to have been actually made from the pattern.
3. Each line in the flat pattern drawing represents an edge of the object, a fold in the pattern, or the border of a shaded region. Use these lines to help you imagine what the object will look like.
4. After the form is constructed, it may be turned in any direction. This makes your job harder. The object can be rotated or flipped upside down, and so on. It cannot, however, be changed from the shape created by the flat pattern; that is, it cannot be compressed, torn, etc. The following flat pattern matches both of the three-dimensional renderings, though they are in different rotations:

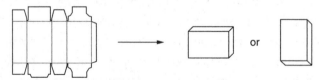

5. If a portion of the flat pattern is shaded or marked, you must find an answer choice that has the same shading or marking in the same location as on the pattern. Some questions have specific markings on the pattern, and you need to choose an answer that keeps those markings in the same relative position. For example, here is the flat pattern of an alphabet block:

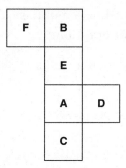

When the three-dimensional rendering is constructed, the relative positions of the letters must remain the same as in the flat pattern. You could eliminate a choice that had the letter A adjacent to the letter B. According to the flat pattern, these letters must be on opposite sides of the cube. Similarly, as you can see from the flat pattern, the letters F and B are adjacent and are in the same orientation. You could eliminate any choice that had them on opposite sides of the cube, or any choice that had them in a different orientation, such as with the F upside down in relation to the B. These details can help you quickly eliminate some wrong answer choices.

STRATEGIES FOR ANSWERING FORM CREATION QUESTIONS

Some of the flat patterns may be very complex, with multiple folding or an unusual shape. Do not get frustrated with these figures. Focus on finding one shape in the flat pattern that you can use to eliminate answer choices. Find one side of the object, perhaps the base of the object, and then eliminate answers that do not have this same shape. For example, consider the following pattern:

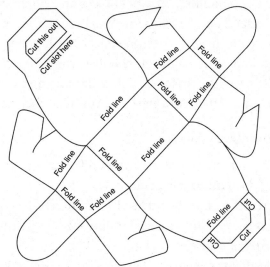

This is a weird shape that may remind you of a bird. But focus on one shape in the pattern. Look at the top left of the pattern. There is a cutout here that looks like it forms a handle. The same is shown on the bottom right of the pattern. Focus on that feature and eliminate any choices that do not have a handle with a cutout. That may be all you need to do to answer the question.

Features that are good for identification include:

➤ Large features
➤ Features that are mirrored on the opposite side of the pattern
➤ The base of the object
➤ Distinctive shapes, such as triangles, circles, and so on

Let's consider the following example:

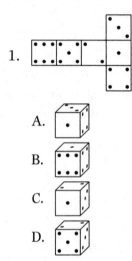

Focus on one thing in the flat pattern. The sides with three and four dots will be folded in, so they will be on opposite sides, with the one in between. That eliminates choice A. Now find another detail you can use. Since this is a cube, it may be easier to test the position of the dots on the remaining answer choices and eliminate that way. Let's look at choice B. Could the six and four be adjacent? Yes, though the six side would be turned in a different direction with three dots on the edge that touches the four side. In any case, with the six and four sides adjacent, the five would be on top, not the one, so eliminate choice B. Let's look at choice C. Could the one and three be adjacent? Yes. Would the two be on top in that orientation? Yes. You've found the correct answer, C.

Tips for Form Creation Questions

➤ A two-dimensional flat pattern is shown, and you are to choose what three-dimensional object the pattern will create.
➤ After the form is created, it may be turned in any direction.
➤ Each line in the flat pattern drawing represents an edge of the object, a fold in the pattern, or the border of a shaded region.
➤ Find one distinctive feature that you can use for identification. Eliminate choices that do not have that feature or do not have it in the proper location.

➤ Use your answer grid to eliminate choices.

➤ If there are markings or shadings on the flat pattern, they must also be on the object in three dimensions. Eliminate choices that do not have markings or shadings where they should appear.

➤ Do not hesitate to mark a difficult question and come back to it at the end, if time allows.

PART V
READING COMPREHENSION

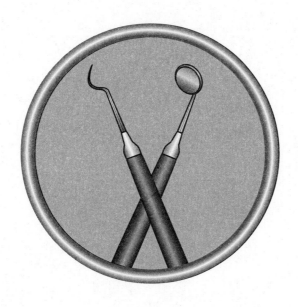

Preparing for the Reading Comprehension Test

Read This Chapter to Learn About

➤ What the Reading Comprehension Section Tests

➤ Reading Better by Reading More

➤ Active Reading Strategies

➤ Speed-Reading Strategies

WHAT THE READING COMPREHENSION SECTION TESTS

By this stage in your educational career, you should have a pretty good sense of your test-taking skills. If you have achieved solid scores on reading comprehension tests in the past, the DAT Reading Comprehension Test should be no different. You can work quickly through this chapter, work a practice test, and be confident in your performance on the actual exam. If your reading comprehension skills are subpar, if you freeze when faced with difficult reading passages, if you read very slowly, or if English is not your first language, you should take the time to work carefully through this section of the book.

In contrast to the sections on chemistry or biology, the Reading Comprehension Test does not test specific knowledge. Instead, it assesses your ability to comprehend, analyze, and evaluate information from an unfamiliar written text. Its format will be familiar to anyone who has attended school in the United States. Most reading comprehension tests look similar to this one, though the DAT Reading Comprehension Test is longer than most standardized reading comprehension tests.

The DAT Reading Comprehension Test consists of three passages of about 1,300 to 1,500 words, each of which is followed by a set of 16 or 17 multiple-choice questions. The passages are nonfiction and are usually on areas of natural or physical sciences. The passages are written by dental school professors and are representative of the type of reading material you will be presented with in your first year of dental school. You are not expected to be familiar with the content of a given passage.

Since you do not know in advance what the topics will be, it is not possible to *study* for the Reading Comprehension Test. It is also not necessary to do so. However, you do need to *prepare* for the Reading Comprehension Test. By learning certain strategies and methods for reading comprehension and practicing those strategies, you can significantly increase your score on this section of the DAT.

READING BETTER BY READING MORE

The best way to learn to read better and faster is simply to read *more*. The passages you will see on the DAT are written by dental school professors and represent the type of materials you will be reading in dental school. They are often dry and may contain terminology with which you are not familiar. You will need to practice reading materials that do not, at first glance, hold much appeal for you. You must learn to focus your attention on what you are reading and deal with difficult material. Pick up a scholarly journal in a scientific field that relates to dentistry. Better yet, read journal articles online. Reading on a computer screen is different from reading on paper, and you should practice reading on a computer as much as possible. Here is a brief list of journals available online that may provide you with relevant practice material:

➤ *Contemporary Clinical Dentistry*
➤ *Dental History Magazine*
➤ *Journal of Dentistry*
➤ *Journal of Dentistry and Oral Hygiene*
➤ *Journal of Esthetic and Restorative Dentistry*
➤ *Journal of Public Health Dentistry*
➤ *Open Dentistry Journal*
➤ *Special Care in Dentistry*

Once you have found a journal, locate an appropriate article. DAT passages are approximately 1,300 to 1,500 words in length. This is about three full pages in a paper journal. Read the article as quickly as you can, and then try to answer the following questions:

➤ What are the key ideas?
➤ What is the author's purpose?
➤ If the author is making an argument, does it make sense to you? Is it logically sound?
➤ Where might the author go next with this article?
➤ What is the author's tone?
➤ Who is the audience for this article?

All of this may sound like a chore, but it is the key to teaching yourself to read actively. An active reader interacts with a text rather than skimming over it. Success on the DAT Reading Comprehension Test requires active reading.

ACTIVE READING STRATEGIES

You can use any of the following strategies to focus your attention on your reading. You may use many of them already, quite automatically. Others may be just what you need to shift your reading comprehension into high gear.

> **Monitor your understanding.** When faced with a difficult text, it is all too easy to zone out and skip through challenging information. You will not have that luxury when the text you are reading is followed by 16 or 17 questions that require your understanding. Pay attention to how you are feeling about a text. Are you getting the author's main points? Is there something that makes little or no sense? Are there words that you do not know? Figuring out what makes a passage hard for you is the first step toward correcting the problem. Once you figure it out, you can use one of the following strategies to improve your connection to the text.

> **Predict.** Your ability to make predictions is surprisingly important to your ability to read well. If a passage is well organized, you should be able to read the introductory paragraph and have a pretty good sense of where the author is going with the text. Practice predicting the main idea by reading newspaper articles, in which the main idea should appear in the first paragraph. Then move on to more difficult reading, such as science magazine articles and then scholarly journal articles. See whether your expectation of a text holds up through the reading of the text. Making predictions about what you are about to read is an immediate way to engage with the text and to keep yourself engaged throughout your reading.

> **Ask questions.** Keep a running dialogue with yourself as you read. You do not have to stop reading; just pause to consider, "What does this mean? Why did the author use this word? Where is he or she going with this argument? Why is this important?" This will become second nature after a while. When you become acclimated to asking yourself questions as you read a test passage, you may discover that some of the questions you asked appear in different forms on the test itself.

> **Summarize.** You do this when you take notes in class or when you prepare an outline as you study for an exam. Try doing it as you read unfamiliar materials to prepare for the DAT. You will be given an erasable note board on which to take notes. Use it well for reading passages! At the end of each paragraph, try to reduce the author's verbiage to a single, cogent phrase that states the main idea of that paragraph. Number your notes by paragraph so that you can quickly find information again when you need it. At the end of the passage, write down the overall theme or message in a phrase or two.

> **Connect.** Every piece of writing is a communication between the author and the reader. You connect to a text first by bringing your prior knowledge to that text and

last by applying what you learn from the text to some area of your life. Even if you know nothing at all about architecture or archaeology, your lifetime of experience in the world carries a lot of weight as you read an article about those topics. Connecting to a text can lead to "Aha!" moments as you say to yourself, "I knew that!" or even "I never knew that!" If you are barreling through a text passively, you will not give yourself time to connect. You might as well record the passage and play it under your pillow as you sleep. As you read, try to make connections to your prior knowledge and relate to what you are reading.

SPEED-READING STRATEGIES

The following strategies are ones that speed-readers use to move quickly through reading material while gathering the main ideas of the passage:

➤ **Avoid subvocalizing.** It is unlikely that you move your lips while you read, but you may find yourself "saying" the text in your head. This slows you down significantly, because you are slowing down to speech speed instead of revving up to reading speed. You do not need to "say" the words; the connection between your eyes and your brain is perfectly able to bypass that step.

➤ **Do not regress.** If you do not understand something, you may stop and "reread" it. What you are really doing is simply running your eyes back and forth and back and forth over it. Speed-readers know this as *regression*, and it is a big drag on reading speed. It is unlikely that reading the same word, sentence, or paragraph twice in a row will increase your comprehension of it. It is better to read the entire passage once all the way through and then reread a section that caused you confusion. By reading a little further, the confusion may be cleared up anyway.

➤ **Bundle ideas.** Read phrases rather than words. Speed-readers refer to this as *chunking*. Remember, you are being tested on overall meaning, which is not derived from single words but rather from phrases, sentences, and paragraphs. If you read word by word, your eye stops constantly, and that slows you down. Read bundles of meaning, and your eyes will flow over the page, improving both reading speed and comprehension.

➤ **Focus on key points.** When you learn to read, you are taught to read every word from left to right and give everything equal weight. Reading comprehension passages are organized with the main point at the beginning of each paragraph. The first sentence and the last sentence of each paragraph are likely to be more important than the details in the middle. Actively find the main point of each paragraph and let your eyes skip over the supporting examples, anecdotes, metaphors, or experiments. Take notes only on points that seem important, not on details.

➤ **Review.** After each paragraph, ask yourself, "What was the main point of that paragraph?" "How does that fit into the big picture?" Note it. When you finish the passage, ask yourself what the big picture is—what is the author's argument, and how is it supported? Note it.

443

**CHAPTER 33:
PREPARING FOR
THE READING
COMPREHENSION
TEST**

Once you have practiced using these methods, you will become a much faster reader and will be able to quickly focus on the most important ideas in a passage. These skills are necessary for success on the DAT Reading Comprehension Test (and will also help you with the readings you will have in dental school). Practice on general materials from scholarly journals until you have become comfortable using these techniques and then start working practice DAT passages with questions.

Approaching Questions on the Reading Comprehension Test

> **Read This Chapter to Learn About**
>
> ➤ Types of Questions
> ➤ Strategy for Reading Comprehension Questions

TYPES OF QUESTIONS

When it comes to taking tests, knowing what to expect is half the battle. The DAT assesses a variety of reading skills, from the most basic comprehension skills to the higher-level analysis and evaluation skills. The Reading Comprehension Test questions may ask you to do any of the following:

➤ Identify the main idea of the passage
➤ Analyze an argument presented in the passage and judge its validity
➤ Use information from the passage to solve a given problem
➤ Determine cause-and-effect relationships for events or conditions described in the passage
➤ Evaluate a claim made in the passage based on the strength of the evidence or argument provided to support that claim
➤ Identify the reasons or evidence offered in support of a particular viewpoint
➤ Recognize stated or unstated assumptions that underlie a viewpoint presented in the passage

445

**CHAPTER 34:
APPROACHING
QUESTIONS ON
THE READING
COMPREHENSION
TEST**

➤ Identify new facts or results that might undermine a conclusion presented in the passage

➤ Apply information from the passage to a new situation

➤ Determine the meaning of an unfamiliar word based on its context

There are three types of questions on the Reading Comprehension Test: they address comprehension, analysis, and evaluation of the reading passage.

Comprehension

These questions deal with the author's main idea and the support given for his or her hypothesis. Expect questions on finding the main idea, locating supporting details or evidence, and interpreting vocabulary. Comprehension questions make up approximately 75 percent of the reading comprehension questions on the DAT.

➤ **Main idea.** DAT passages are scientific in nature and may seem complex, but they all have an underlying structure. The main idea will be presented in the first paragraph and then refined throughout the rest of the passage. When you do your initial reading, you should be actively looking for the main idea. The first paragraph, along with the first sentence of each subsequent paragraph and the last sentence of the passage, should give you a fairly good grasp of the main idea. Be sure to ask yourself active reading questions along the way (see Chapter 33) and some review questions at the end. If you do this, you will have the main idea.

➤ **Supporting details or evidence.** Some questions will ask you about supporting details or evidence that the author uses to support his or her argument. It is unlikely that you will have retained these details from your initial reading, so be sure you go back to the passage to answer these questions. Do not reread the entire passage! Focus only on the small part of the passage that discusses the question topic. Use key words in the question to help you find the place in the passage that you need to read. For example, if the question says, "The author mentions microboard collaboration as a source of ...," then skim the passage for the phrase *microboard collaboration*. Once you find the phrase, read several lines before and after the phrase to get the entire context.

➤ **Interpreting vocabulary.** You may be asked the meaning of a specific word used in the passage. You will need to use the context of the sentence and paragraph to determine which of the five answer choices presents the best definition of the given word. Often, several answer choices will be similar; but always, only one will fit the context used in the passage. The best method for dealing with this question type is to read the sentence in the passage and make sure you understand what the word means. Then focus on the details in the answer choices, eliminating any that do not fit the context of the passage. If more than one choice is still close, try to replace the underlined word with the answer choices that seemed close to find the one that works best in context.

Analysis

These questions deal with the purpose and structure of the passage. Expect questions on making predictions and drawing conclusions, recognizing or analyzing organization, and identifying the author's purpose. Analysis questions make up approximately 20 percent of the Reading Comprehension Test.

➤ **Making predictions and drawing conclusions.** Some questions may ask you what would be the result if certain conditions are met or are not met. There will always be clues in the passage to tell you what that result would be. Read the sentences before and after the area of the passage in which the topic is discussed so that you get the full context.

➤ **Analyzing organization.** A paragraph or passage may be organized in a number of different ways. Some modes of organization support an author's purpose better than others. On the DAT, paragraphs are numbered, and those numbers are often referred to in questions to make it easier for you to scan or skim the passage and find out what you need to know. Some organizational modes frequently used in nonfiction passages include time order or sequence; spatial order; order of importance; and organization by causes and effects, opinion and reasons, thesis statement and examples, or comparisons and contrasts.

➤ **Purpose.** Some questions will ask you why the author used a certain method or mentioned a certain detail. Focus on the function of the method or detail. Does it support a point, describe a detail, illustrate a point, or provide an example or counterexample? State the purpose in your own words before you look at the answer choices.

Analysis Sample Question Stems

➤ Based on the passage, you can tell that...
➤ The passage implies that...
➤ The purpose of X is to...
➤ The ideas in the first and second paragraphs relate by...
➤ The author's purpose in the third paragraph is...
➤ The author includes X to show...

447

**CHAPTER 34:
APPROACHING
QUESTIONS ON
THE READING
COMPREHENSION
TEST**

Evaluation

These questions deal with your understanding of the author's assumptions and viewpoints. These questions are relatively rare and make up only about 5 percent of the Reading Comprehension Test. They may ask you to analyze an argument, judge credibility, assess evidence, distinguish between fact and opinion, or evaluate tone.

Evaluation Sample Question Stems

➤ Which of the following statements provides the *least* support...

➤ Which of the following assertions does the author support...

➤ The author's claim that X is supported by...

➤ The tone of the passage suggests that...

➤ What evidence could the author have added to show...

Pace Yourself

The Reading Comprehension Test is timed. If you are a slow reader, you are at a decided disadvantage. You will have 60 minutes to read three long passages and answer 50 questions. That gives you 20 minutes for each question set. Time yourself as you practice so that you get used to doing a passage and its 16 or 17 questions in only 20 minutes. Keep an eye on the clock and be sure to mark an answer for every question since there is no penalty for guessing.

You do not need to speed-read to perform well on the Reading Comprehension Test, but you might benefit from some techniques that speed-readers use. Since the DAT reading passages are so long, it is essential that you be able to move through the passages quickly while getting the information that you need in order to answer the questions correctly.

STRATEGY FOR READING COMPREHENSION QUESTIONS

Your task on reading comprehension questions is to choose the *best* answer among the choices. This often means choosing the answer that is the least bad. When you look at the choices, you will probably be able to eliminate one or two very quickly, but if you try to do that in your head, you will forget which ones you eliminated and cause yourself to duplicate your efforts. The best way to keep track of which answer choices you want to eliminate is to use an answer grid. An answer grid is a simple chart like the following:

	A	B	C	D	E
1	X		X	X	
2		X			X
3	X	X		X	

You will need 16 to 17 rows in the grid to match the number of questions in the passage. The first thing you should do when you encounter a reading passage is to set up an answer grid on your note board.

Since the majority of the questions are comprehension questions that ask about specific details from the passage, you will need to be able to locate such information quickly. When you read a question, identify what the question is asking you to do and then focus in on what key detail you will need to find. Each question contains a key word or phrase that tells you what to look for in the passage. For example, in this question, "According to the passage, ether was originally used for . . . ," the key word is *ether* and you are asked for its *original use.* You should quickly scan the passage for the word *ether*. Do not read. Simply scan for the word until you find it. If necessary, start at the end of the passage and scan backward to prevent yourself from reading anything. You don't want to get sucked back into reading the passage at this time; you want to quickly identify the relevant part for this particular question.

For practice, circle the key words in the following questions:

1. Based on the information in the third paragraph, you can conclude that most microscopes . . .
2. All of these are typical studies at Arecibo *except* . . .
3. The remote-control command center will most likely be used to . . .
4. Based on information in the passage, about how many gorillas have survived Ebola in regions where the virus is prevalent?
5. What has been the result of investigations of distant asteroids?

You should have identified the following:

1. third paragraph / most microscopes
2. typical studies at Arecibo
3. remote-control command center
4. gorillas / survived Ebola
5. investigations of distant asteroids

Once you have located the key words in the passage, read a sentence or two before and after the key words to get the context. Do not go into a different paragraph. Answer the question in your own words before you look at the answer choices. Once you have answered the question in your own words, compare your answer to the answer choices. If more than one choice is close, refer back to the section of the passage to confirm one choice over the other.

If you have practiced the methods outlined here and in Chapter 33 and are ready to try out your skills, move on to the sample Reading Comprehension Test in the next chapter. Don't forget to set up an answer grid so that you can eliminate answers you know are incorrect.

Reading Comprehension Practice

SAMPLE READING COMPREHENSION TEST

It is certainly true that the more you practice reading comprehension, the better you are likely to perform on the DAT Reading Comprehension Test. Here is a practice passage followed by a question set and explanatory answers. Practice using your active reading strategies as you read the passage. Do not time yourself on this passage and question set. Learn to use the strategies without the pressure of a clock, and then work on your speed by using the full-length practice test in this book.

Ether

1. The use of inhaled anesthetics can be traced back as far as the medieval Moors, who used narcotic-soaked sponges placed over the nostrils of patients. Some 300 years later, in 1275, Majorcan alchemist Raymundus Lullus is supposed to have discovered the chemical compound later called ether. The compound, which would later have a brief but important run as the anesthetic of choice in Western medicine, was synthesized by German physician Valerius Cordus in 1540. Adding sulfuric acid, known at the time as oil of vitriol, to ethyl alcohol resulted in the compound Cordus called sweet vitriol.

2. During the next few centuries, ether was used by physicians for a variety of purposes. Its effectiveness as a hypnotic agent was well known, and a favorite pastime of medical students in the early nineteenth century was the "ether frolic," an early version of the drunken frat party. Nevertheless, no record of ether's being used as an anesthetic in surgery appears until the 1840s.

3. Dr. Crawford Williamson Long of Jefferson, Georgia, removed neck tumors from a patient under ether anesthesia on March 30, 1842. However, he failed to publish the record of his experiment until 1848, by which time Dr. William Thomas Green Morton, a dentist in Hartford, Connecticut, had conducted a variety of experiments with ether on animals and himself, culminating in the painless extraction of a tooth from a patient under ether on September 30, 1846. William T. G. Morton participated in a public demonstration of ether anesthesia on October 16, 1846, at the Ether Dome in Boston, Massachusetts. The Ether Dome is an amphitheater in the Bulfinch Building at Massachusetts General Hospital in Boston. It served as the hospital's operating room from its opening in 1821 until 1867. It was the site of the first use of inhaled ether as a surgical anesthetic. William T. G. Morton used ether to anesthetize Edward Gilbert Abbott. John Collins Warren, the first dean of Harvard Medical School, then painlessly removed a tumor from Abbott's neck. After Warren had finished and Abbott regained consciousness, Warren asked the patient how he felt. Reportedly, Abbott said, "Feels as if my neck's been scratched." Warren then turned to his medical audience and uttered, "Gentlemen, this is no Humbug." This was presumably a reference to the unsuccessful demonstration of nitrous oxide anesthesia by Horace Wells in the same theater the previous year, which was ended by cries of "Humbug!" after the patient groaned with pain. The operation is recorded in several paintings of the era, indicating its critical importance. Despite its volatility and side effects, ether continued to be used as an anesthetic until it was overtaken by less harmful potions. Because of its associations with Boston, the use of ether became known as the "Yankee Dodge." Morton, meanwhile, struggled unsuccessfully to be granted a patent for his "discovery" and then, when that failed, for his "technique." After years of litigation, he died penniless at age 49.

4. However, Crawford Williamson Long, M.D., is now known to have demonstrated its use privately as a general anesthetic in surgery to officials in Georgia, as early as March 30, 1842, and Long publicly demonstrated ether's use as a surgical anesthetic on numerous occasions before 1846. British doctors were aware of the anesthetic properties of ether as early as 1840, and it was widely prescribed in conjunction with opium.

5. Diethyl ether was formerly sometimes used in place of chloroform because it had a higher therapeutic index, a larger difference between the recommended dosage and a toxic overdose. Diethyl ether, also known simply as ether or Et_2O, is the organic compound with the formula $(C_2H_5)_2O$. It is a colorless and highly flammable liquid with a low boiling point and a characteristic odor. It is the most common member of a class of chemical compounds known generically as ethers. Ether is

sparingly soluble in water (6.9 g/100 mL). Diethyl ether depresses the myocardium and also increases tracheobronchial secretions. A cytochrome P450 enzyme is proposed to metabolize diethyl ether. Diethyl ether inhibits alcohol dehydrogenase and thus slows the metabolism of ethanol. It also inhibits metabolism of other drugs requiring oxidative metabolism. Diethyl ether could also be mixed with other anesthetic agents such as chloroform to make C.E. mixture, or chloroform and alcohol to make A.C.E. mixture.

6. Today, ether is rarely used. The use of flammable ether was displaced by nonflammable anesthetics such as halothane. Additionally, diethyl ether had many undesirable side effects, such as postanesthetic nausea and vomiting. Modern anesthetic agents, such as methyl propyl ether (Neothyl) and methoxyflurane (Penthrane) reduce these side effects.

1. The statement in the first paragraph that ether would "have a brief but important run as the anesthetic of choice in Western medicine" implies that the author believes that
    A. ether was not a particularly good anesthetic
    B. ether was not used long enough to judge its effectiveness
    C. ether was effective during the period when it was used
    D. ether was a noteworthy import from the East to the West
    E. ether was not used in Eastern medicine

2. In the context of the second paragraph, the word *agent* is used to mean
    A. manager
    B. negotiator
    C. instrument
    D. arbitrator
    E. official

3. Which of these would be the best title for the passage?
    A. "Inhaled Anesthetics"
    B. "An Important Anesthetic"
    C. "How Anesthetics Have Changed"
    D. "Our Debt to Ancient Physicians"
    E. "Why Ether Is No Longer Used"

4. Which of the following statements from the passage provides the *least* support for the author's claim that ether was an important discovery for physicians at the time?
    A. "Dr. Crawford Williamson Long of Jefferson, Georgia, removed neck tumors from a patient under ether anesthesia on March 30, 1842."
    B. "Warren then turned to his medical audience and uttered, 'Gentlemen, this is no Humbug.'"
    C. "The operation is recorded in several paintings of the era, indicating its critical importance."

D. "Nevertheless, no record of ether's being used as an anesthetic in surgery appears until the 1840s."

E. "British doctors were aware of the anesthetic properties of ether as early as 1840, and it was widely prescribed in conjunction with opium."

5. In the first paragraph, the author probably writes that Lullus "is supposed to have discovered" ether because
   A. there is conflicting evidence about his discovery
   B. Lullus did not really discover ether at all
   C. although Lullus was meant to discover it, someone else did
   D. no one can really "discover" a chemical compound
   E. Lullus is credited with ether's discovery

6. How is the information in the third paragraph organized?
   A. By reasons and examples
   B. Using comparisons and contrasts
   C. In time order
   D. Using cause-and-effect relationships
   E. Setting up a hypothesis and then testing it

7. What evidence could the author have included that would best support the contention that ether was important to the history of medicine?
   A. The chemical makeup of diethyl ether—CH_3-CH_2-O-CH_2-CH_3
   B. Names and occupations of the patients on whom Long and Morton worked
   C. A comparison of chloroform to nitrous oxide when used as anesthesia
   D. Examples of how ether was used in battlefield medicine during the Civil War
   E. A list of the positive benefits of using halothane

8. The author probably includes information about Dr. Long in the third paragraph to show that
   A. Morton was not the first to use ether in a surgical procedure
   B. publishing results can mean the difference between fortune and penury
   C. both dentists and doctors used ether to good effect
   D. doctors in the Northeast often received more attention than Southern doctors
   E. Long publicly demonstrated the use of ether

ANSWERS AND EXPLANATIONS FOR THE SAMPLE TEST

1. **C** Ether's run is described as "brief but important," implying that despite its short reign as the anesthetic of choice, it was an effective choice. There is no support in the passage for any of the other answer choices.

2. **C** The word *agent* has multiple meanings, but only one works in context here. The author speaks of ether's use as "a hypnotic agent," meaning an instrument that causes hypnosis. Only choice C is a synonym that works in the context given.

3. **B** Choice A is far too broad for the six-paragraph passage given here, which really focuses on a single anesthetic. Choice C is not relevant to the passage, which focuses more on how anesthetics have been similar from century to century than on how they have changed. Although the passage opens with reference to ancient physicians (choice D), this is not the main idea of the passage. Choice E is also too narrow to be the main idea.

4. **D** Your answer will be the statement that least indicates that ether was important. To find it, you must read each statement with that key idea in mind. Choice A supports the idea by showing how one doctor used ether. Choice B supports the idea by showing that Warren considered the discovery to be important. Choice C supports the idea by showing that artists of the day captured the important event. Choice E shows that ether was popularly used by British doctors. Only choice D does not fit; it states only that the usefulness of ether had not been discovered for many years.

5. **A** "Supposed to have discovered" means that Lullus is "said to have discovered." This might make you want to choose choice E, but "supposed to have discovered" also implies that there is not a lot of corroborating evidence; if there were, the author would have simply said "discovered." Choice B may be true, but for the time being, the author is implying that Lullus may or may not have made the discovery. The best answer is A.

6. **C** The third paragraph is a narrative that tells about Morton's demonstration, followed by his attempts to win a patent. It is told in story form, in the order in which events occurred.

7. **D** If ether was truly important to the history of medicine, it would be nice to see some examples of its use that support that claim. Of the suggestions given, only choice D provides such examples. Ether's chemical makeup (choice A) has nothing to do with its importance. The names and occupations of patients (choice B) are unlikely to offer evidence of this kind—unless they proved to be famous historical figures. Since there is no evidence that they were, choice B is not the best answer. A comparison of two other anesthetic agents (choice C) would not add or subtract useful evidence about ether's importance. Choice E is not about the history or use of ether. The best answer is choice D.

8. **A** Use what is given to you in the passage to answer this question. The inclusion of information about Long may in part be a cautionary tale about the importance of publishing results (choice B), but since Morton himself died in penury, it is not a very good cautionary tale. Choices C and E are true, but neither is the primary reason the author included this information. There is no evidence to support choice D; in fact, the author makes clear that Long's being overlooked was largely his own fault. The best answer is choice A; Long performed an operation using ether before Morton did.

Tips for Reading Comprehension Questions

➤ Set up an answer grid on your note board.

➤ Read the passage quickly, using your active reading strategies.

➤ Identify the question type. Is this a comprehension question, an analysis question, or an evaluation question? What are you asked to do?

➤ Find the key words in the question. Scan the passage to find the key words.

➤ Read one sentence before and after the key words to get the full context for the question.

➤ Answer the question in your own words.

➤ Compare your answer to the answer choices. Eliminate choices that do not match on your answer grid.

➤ If more than one choice is close, compare the choices to see how they differ. Go back to the passage to confirm one choice over the other.

Now that you have done a practice section, review any questions you missed as well as any questions you guessed on. If you were down to two choices and picked the wrong one, what made you choose the one you did? Look closely at the two options and see how they are different. You can learn a lot from your mistakes so that you do not make them again in the future.

PART VI

QUANTITATIVE REASONING

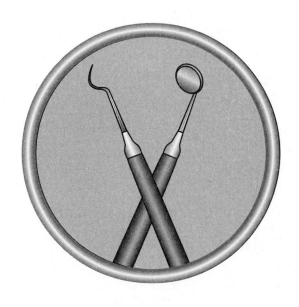

Mathematics: A Basic Review

DECIMALS

Addition of decimal numbers is done in the same way as addition of ordinary numbers. However, in this case, each number should be written such that all of the decimal points are lined up vertically. For example, the numbers 23.467 and 2.589 are added by:

$$\begin{array}{r} 23.467 \\ + 2.589 \\ \hline 26.056 \end{array}$$

Subtraction of decimal numbers is done in a manner similar to addition in that the numbers are positioned with the decimal point lined up. Also, as in the subtraction of ordinary numbers, the smaller decimal number must be subtracted from the larger decimal number. For example, subtracting the number 6.821 from 37.49 can be done as shown:

$$37.490$$
$$-6.821$$
$$\overline{30.669}$$

Note that the zero added at the end of 37.940 does not alter the value of the number and just serves as a placeholder in the subtraction operation.

You multiply two decimal numbers just as you would multiply two ordinary numbers. In this case, however, the decimal points do not have to be lined up. Knowing where to put the decimal point is important, but you can deal with it after you finish multiplying the two numbers. For example, when the two decimal numbers 7.4 and 3.6 are multiplied, the two numbers are multiplied without regard to the decimal point, yielding the following result:

$$7.4$$
$$\times 3.6$$
$$\overline{2664}\text{ (prior to placement of the decimal point)}$$

To determine the placement of the decimal point in the product, you must first determine the position of the decimal point in each of the two numbers being multiplied. There is one decimal place for the 7.4 and one for the 3.6. Therefore, one must add the two and realize that there are two decimal places in the answer, making it 26.64.

Division of decimal numbers requires a little bit of manipulation before calculating the answer. In this case one must first move the decimal places of both numbers to the right until one of the numbers is no longer a decimal. From there one can then proceed with long division as needed. For example, $483.84 \div 38.4$ is the same as $4838.4 \div 384$ where 4838.4 is called the dividend and the 384 is the divisor. The answer now becomes 12.6 because of the use of three significant figures. Keep in mind that when multiplying or dividing with significant figures, the answer has the same number of significant figures as the number in the calculation with the fewest number of significant figures.

To round decimal numbers to the nearest place, follow these steps, considering the decimal number 3.4925 as an example.

1. Identify the digit in the decimal number to be rounded.
    ➤ If asked to round to the nearest tenth, the digit is 4.
    ➤ If asked to round to the nearest hundredth, the digit is 9.
    ➤ If asked to round to the nearest thousandth, the digit is 2.
2. Then identify the digit immediately to the right of the number that is being rounded.
    ➤ The digit immediately to the right of the tenth position is 9.
    ➤ The digit immediately to the right of the hundredth position is 2.
    ➤ The digit immediately to the right of the thousandth position is 5.

3. Depending on the result of Step 2, there are two possibilities.
   ➤ If the digit identified in Step 2 is 0 to 4 (0, 1, 2, 3, 4), then the digit being rounded remains the same.
   ➤ If the digit identified in Step 2 is 5 to 9 (5, 6, 7, 8, 9), then the digit being rounded increases by 1.
4. Apply the result of Step 3 as follows:
   ➤ If asked to round 3.4925 to the nearest tenth, the result is 3.5.
   ➤ If asked to round 3.4925 to the nearest hundredth, the result is 3.49.
   ➤ If asked to round 3.4925 to the nearest thousandth, the result is 3.493.

FRACTIONS

Fractions represent a part or portion of a whole and consist of two numbers with one written above the other with a line or rule between them. If a and b are numbers, then a fraction can be written as $\frac{a}{b}$ with b not equal to 0. The top number, a, is known as the numerator, and the bottom number, b, is known as the denominator. All of the major arithmetic operations (addition, subtraction, multiplication, and division) can be applied to fractions.

Two or more fractions can be added only if they have a common denominator. To find a common denominator, the two denominators are multiplied. Then, each fraction must be converted into a new fraction with the same value yet having a denominator different from its original denominator. Once the fractions have a common denominator, the numerators of the fractions are added and written over the common denominator. For example:

$\frac{1}{3}+\frac{2}{4}$ needs to be arranged so that the common denominator is 12:

$$\frac{4}{12}+\frac{6}{12}=\frac{10}{12} \text{, which can be reduced to } \frac{5}{6}$$

Just as is the case with addition, fractions can be subtracted only if they have a common denominator. Once the fractions have a common denominator, the numerators of the fractions are subtracted and written over the common denominator. For example, the following problem needs to be arranged so that the common denominator is 14:

$$\frac{5}{7}-\frac{1}{2}=\frac{10}{14}-\frac{7}{14}=\frac{3}{14}$$

Two fractions can be multiplied by multiplying the numerators and denominators. For example:

$$\frac{1}{2}\times\frac{3}{4}=\frac{3}{8}$$

When dividing two fractions, one must rationalize the denominator. To simplify this process, remember to "keep, switch, flip"—that is, keep the first fraction as it is, switch the division sign to a multiplication sign, and then flip or reciprocate the second fraction. For example:

$\frac{3}{4}$ divided by $\frac{5}{6}$ becomes $\frac{3}{4} \times \frac{6}{5} = \frac{18}{20}$. Once reduced, this becomes $\frac{9}{10}$.

When reducing fractions, one must find a number that evenly divides both the numerator and the denominator. For example, let us reduce the fraction $\frac{96}{60}$. Both the 96 and 60 are divisible by 3. Doing so makes the fraction $\frac{32}{20}$. Looking further, we see that both numbers can be divided by 4, making the fraction $\frac{8}{5}$. This could also have been done in one step if we recognized that the number 12 (which equals 3×4) evenly divides both 96 and 60. The choice is yours. Breaking down the math into multiple steps takes longer, but it might allow you to easily work with numbers in your head—without the use of a calculator.

Mixed Fractions

At times one will come across a fraction that accompanies a whole number. This is called a mixed fraction. An example is $5\frac{1}{3}$. What this really means is that the number 3 "went into" another number 5 times and there is 1 left over. In order to get the original fraction back, we must multiply the whole number (5) by the denominator (3) and then add the numerator (1). Doing so gives $5 \times 3 = 15, + 1 = 16$. This means that the final answer is $\frac{16}{3}$. Looking at the following fraction, $\frac{25}{4}$, the 25 is not evenly divided by the 4, but the 4 can "go into" the numerator 6 times. The whole number will be 6. There is 1 remaining, and this will be the numerator of the remaining fraction. The mixed fraction will be $6\frac{1}{4}$.

RATIOS AND PROPORTIONS

The setting of two fractions equal to each other can help one solve for an unknown value. The technique used to solve a problem of this nature is to cross multiply and then divide. For example, to solve for x in the problem $\frac{2}{3} = \frac{4}{x}$ one can easily see that $\frac{2}{3}$ and $\frac{4}{6}$ are in the same ratio and that the value of x would be 6. If one wanted to check, one could cross multiply $3 \times 4 = 2x$, which gives $12 = 2x$, in which $x = 6$. What happens when the problems are not so easy is that one must use the cross multiplication method, along with other algebraic manipulation.

PROBLEM: Solve for x:

$$\frac{1}{x+3} = \frac{5}{x}$$

SOLUTION: Cross multiplication and the distributive property of mathematics gives:

$$1x = 5(x+3) \text{ and then}$$
$$x = 5x + 15$$

Subtracting $5x$ from both sides gives:

$$-4x = 15$$

Dividing both sides by -4 gives a final answer of:

$$x = \frac{15}{-4}$$

which can be reduced to the mixed fraction:

$$x = -3\frac{3}{4}$$

PERCENTAGES

Remembering that fractions mean that the numerator is divided by the denominator, one can find a percentage by dividing a numerator by the denominator and then multiplying the result by 100%. For example, two-thirds is $\frac{2}{3}$, which means 2 divided by 3. This gives a value of 0.67. Multiplying by 100% we get: $0.67 \times 100\% = 67\%$.

A *percent*, a word meaning "of one hundred," is a ratio with a denominator equal to 100. Percentages are represented by the symbol %. Because a percent is a ratio, it can easily be converted into a fraction or a decimal number. Percents can be converted to fractions by removing the % symbol and dividing by 100. Some examples are $4\% = \frac{4}{100} = 0.04$, $52\% = \frac{52}{100} = 0.52$, $84\% = \frac{84}{100} = 0.84$. (The zero is generally used before a decimal to make clear that the result is not a whole number.)

Finding the percentage of a number involves the use of a decimal. For example, to find 20% of the number 35, we must convert the percentage back to a decimal. This is done by dividing the percentage by 100% and then multiplying by the number in question: 20% divided by $100\% = 0.20$. Multiplying gives: $0.20 \times 35 = 7$. Therefore, 20% of 35 is 7.

APPROXIMATIONS

We have all encountered a situation in life, usually when shopping, when approximating numbers comes into play. Sometimes it is easier to round off numbers and then perform a calculation—again, allowing us to work with numbers that are easier to manipulate. This skill allows us to get a general idea of where an answer or calculation should be in value to check or get a feel for what a result should look like.

> **PROBLEM:** A person goes shopping and buys items priced as follows: $1.79, $2.99, $5.39, and three for a dollar. About how much money does the person need for the purchase?

> **SOLUTION:** To tackle this, start rounding off to numbers that are easier to work with. This comes out to be, respectively, $2 + $3 + $5 + $1 = $11. So just to be sure, the shopper would first need to make sure that he or she has a minimum of $12 before making the purchase.

SCIENTIFIC NOTATION

Scientific notation is a means of expressing numbers, regardless of their size, in powers of 10. Any nonzero number can be expressed in scientific notation when written in the form $a \times 10^b$ where a is a real number such that $1 \le a < 10$ (or $-10 < a \le -1$) (a is referred to as the coefficient) and b is an integer that describes the power of the exponent. To convert a number into scientific notation, follow the steps below. The number 397 serves as an example.

1. Express the number in terms of a real number such that $1 \le a < 10$.

$$397 \text{ would change to } 3.97$$

2. Determine the value of b, the integer that is the power of the exponent. In order to perform Step 1, you divided 397 by 100. Thus, in order to retain the original number, you also need to multiply by 100, which, in terms of exponents, is 10^2. The integer b in this case is 2. Thus 397 expressed in scientific notation would be:

$$397 = 3.97 \times 100 = 3.97 \times 10^2$$

Multiplication of Numbers Expressed in Scientific Notation

To multiply numbers expressed in scientific notation, you multiply the coefficients to reveal the new coefficient and multiply the exponents to reveal the new exponent. However, when exponents are multiplied, the powers add. For example, suppose you want to multiply the following numbers:

$$1.36 \times 10^2 \text{ and } 4.6 \times 10^4$$
$$(1.36 \times 10^2) \times (4.6 \times 10^4) = (1.36 \times 4.6) \times (10^2 \times 10^4) = 6.256 \times 10^6$$

CONVERSIONS

When learning to do conversions, it is easiest to learn using everyday conversions that you make—probably without even being conscious that you are doing it. The factor-label method can be used to cancel out undesired units to obtain the desired unit, as in the following example.

PROBLEM: How many minutes are in one hour?

SOLUTION: Because we want minutes to remain and hours to be canceled out, the unit of hours must be in the denominator and be canceled out by multiplying by hours. We must also put in the number of minutes that are equivalent to one hour, 60 minutes:

$$(1 \text{ hour}) \times \frac{60 \text{min}}{1 \text{ hour}}$$

Now cancel the hours unit and complete the calculation:

$$(1 \ \cancel{\text{hour}}) \times \frac{60 \text{min}}{1 \ \cancel{\text{hour}}} = 60 \text{ minutes}$$

PROBLEM: Convert 6 pounds to grams.

SOLUTION: Set up the problem knowing that 1 kg = 2.2 lbs and that 1 kg = 1,000 g. The units of pounds and kilograms must be in the numerator and denominator an equal number of times so that they cancel out and disappear from the calculation:

$$6 \ \cancel{\text{lbs}} \times \frac{1.0 \ \cancel{\text{kg}}}{2.2 \ \cancel{\text{lbs}}} \times \frac{1,000 \text{ g}}{1.0 \ \cancel{\text{kg}}} = 6 \times \frac{1.0}{2.0} \times \frac{1,000 \text{ g}}{1.0} = 2,727.3 \text{ grams}$$

PROBLEM: Convert 50 degrees Fahrenheit to degrees Celsius.

SOLUTION: This calculation requires a simple equation, $C = \frac{5}{9} (F - 32)$, which gives:

$$C = \frac{5}{9} (50 - 32)$$

$$C = (0.56)(18) = 10 \text{ degrees C (rounded)}$$

Temperature Conversions

A little trick in converting the degrees C back to Fahrenheit is the following:

1. Double the degrees C: 10 becomes 20

2. Subtract 10%:   20 − 2 = 18

3. Add 32:   18 + 32 = 50 degrees Fahrenheit

Algebra

EXPONENTIAL NOTATION

In science, numbers can be very small or very large, too small or large to be written out. Consider Avagadro's number, 6.02×10^{23}. Would you really want to write out the number 602,200,000,000,000,000,000,000 every time you did a mole calculation? Also, when covering a topic such as the Richter magnitude scale or the pH of a solution, one will need powers of 10 to understand that a pH of 4 is 100 times more acidic than a pH of 6 or that an earthquake of 5.0 on the Richter scale is 10 times more powerful than an earthquake of 4.0.

Some simple examples of changing numbers to scientific notation include $1 \times 10^3 = 1,000$ and $2.4 \times 10^4 = 24,000$. Things can get a little tricky when the power of 10 has a negative exponent. This requires a little manipulation before the calculation is made. An example is 1×10^{-2}. The negative exponent means that the number can be rewritten as: $\dfrac{1}{1 \times 10^2}$. Yes, the exponent is now positive, but that positive exponent is now in the denominator. Carrying out the calculation, we see that the fraction is now $\dfrac{1}{100} = 0.01$. This is easy when we are multiplying the power of 10 by the number 1. There is another method, as shown here:

PROBLEM: What is the value of 2×10^{-5}? Of 1.8×10^{-3}?

SOLUTION: We can solve by moving decimal places to the left for each negative value of 10. The value of 2×10^{-5} is 0.00002, and 1.8×10^{-3} is equal to 0.0018.

When multiplying or dividing exponents, we follow these rules:

1. $x^m \cdot x^n = x^{m+n}$

2. $\dfrac{x^m}{x^n} = x^{m-n}$ when $x \neq 0$.

3. $(x^m)^n = x^{mn}$

4. $(xy)^m = x^m y^m$

5. $\left(\dfrac{x}{y}\right)^m = \dfrac{x^m}{y^m}$

6. $x^{-m} = \dfrac{1}{x^m}$

PROBLEM:

Solve for each:

$3^2 \cdot 3^3$

$\dfrac{5^5}{5^2}$

$(2^2)^4$

$\left(\dfrac{5}{3}\right)^2$

6^{-2}

SOLUTION:

$3^2 \cdot 3^3 = 3^{2+3} = 3^5 = 243$

$\dfrac{5^5}{5^2} = 5^{5-2} = 5^3 = 125$

$(2^2)^4 = 2^{2 \times 4} = 2^8 = 256$

$\left(\dfrac{5}{3}\right)^2 = \left(\dfrac{5^2}{3^2}\right) = \dfrac{25}{9} = 2\dfrac{7}{9}$

$6^{-2} = \dfrac{1}{6^2} = \dfrac{1}{36}$

ALGEBRAIC EXPRESSIONS

An algebraic expression is a collection of ordinary numbers, letters, and operational signs. Examples of algebraic expressions include $3t^2$, $4x^2 + 2y$, $6a^4 - 8b^3 - 10c^2$, and $7(4t - s)$. Each individual collection of numbers and letters that are separated by + or − signs is referred to as a term. Considering the algebraic expression $4x^2 + 2y$ listed previously, $4x^2$ and $2y$ are both terms.

PROBLEM: Identify the terms in the algebraic expressions $6a^4 - 8b^3 - 10c^2$ and $7(4t - s)$.

SOLUTION: The expression $6a^4 - 8b^3 - 10c^2$ has three terms: $6a^4$, $8b^3$, and $10c^2$, and the expression $7(4t - s) = 28t - 7s$ has two terms (found by multiplying the terms in parentheses by 7), 28t and 7s.

If an algebraic expression has one term, it is known as a monomial. Examples of monomials are: $4rs^2t^3$, $7a$, and $\dfrac{5x^2}{y^4}$. If an algebraic expression has more than one term, it is referred to as a polynomial. Examples of polynomials are: $3a + 4b$, $x^2 - 4y^5 - 8z^9$, and $9(4m - n) = 36m - 9n$. A polynomial with two terms is called a binomial, and a polynomial with three terms is called a trinomial.

Two or more polynomials can be added by combining like terms. The process can be simplified by arranging the polynomials with like terms aligned in the same column. The sum can be found by adding each column.

PROBLEM: Add the following polynomials: $3x - 2xy + 4y^2$, $5xy + y^2 - 2x$, and $-3y^2 + 7x + 10xy$.

SOLUTION: Arrange the three polynomials for addition such that like terms are in the same column.

$$3x - 2xy + 4y^2$$
$$-2x + 5xy + y^2$$
$$+7x + 10xy - 3y^2$$
$$\overline{8x + 13xy + 2y^2}$$

The result is $8x + 13xy + 2y^2$.

Two or more polynomials can be subtracted by first changing the sign of every term in the polynomial being subtracted. Like terms between the polynomials undergoing subtraction are then added to provide the difference.

PROBLEM: Subtract $3a^2 - 2ab - 4b^2$ from $9a^2 - 5ab + 6b^2$.

SOLUTION: First, change the sign of each term in the polynomial being subtracted, which in this problem is $3a^2 - 2ab - 4b^2$. So, $3a^2 - 2ab - 4b^2$ becomes $-3a^2 + 2ab + 4b^2$. Then, arrange the two polynomials for addition such that like terms are in the same column:

$$9a^2 - 5ab + 6b^2$$
$$-3a^2 + 2ab + 4b^2$$
$$\overline{6a^2 - 3ab + 10b^2}$$

The result is $6a^2 - 3ab + 10b^2$.

Algebraic expressions can be multiplied by multiplying the terms in each expression using the laws of exponents (covered earlier in the chapter), the rules of signs, and the commutative and associative properties of multiplication. Let us consider some special cases of multiplication of algebraic expressions.

PROBLEM: Multiply $4a^2b^4c$ by $-7a^5b^3$.

SOLUTION:

1. Write the product of the two monomials as $(4a^2b^4c)(-7a^5b^3)$
2. Arrange the terms according to the commutative and associative properties: $[(4)(-7)][(a^2)(a^5)][(b^4)(b^3)][(c)]$.
3. Use the rules of signs and laws of exponents to obtain the product of the two monomials: $-28a^7b^7c$.

PROBLEM: Multiply $5x^2 - 2xy + 7xy^2 + 8y^2$ by $4x^3y^5$

SOLUTION:

1. Write the product of the polynomial and monomial as: $(4x^3y^5)(5x^2 - 2xy + 7xy^2 + 8y^2)$.
2. Multiply each term of the polynomial by the monomial: $(4x^3y^5)(5x^2) - (4x^3y^5)(2xy) + (4x^3y^5)(7xy^2) + (4x^3y^5)(8y^2)$.
3. Use the rules of signs and laws of exponents to obtain the product of each term: $(20x^5y^5) - (8x^4y^6) + (28x^4y^7) + (32x^3y^7)$.

The product is $20x^5y^5 - 8x^4y^6 + 28x^4y^7 + 32x^3y^7$.

Division of monomials requires one monomial to be in the numerator and one in the denominator. One must be careful of the quotient of the variables and numerical coefficients. It is helpful to break down these types of problems into multiple calculations to avoid confusion.

PROBLEM: Divide $36x^5y^3z^2$ by $-9xz^4$.

SOLUTION: Set up the calculation:

$$\frac{36x^5y^3z^2}{-9xz^4} =$$

Separate the like terms (recall that $x = x^1$ and $y^0 = 1$ in order to be able to divide by subtracting the exponent of each term in the denominator from the exponent of the same term in the numerator):

$$\frac{(36)(x^5)(y^3)(z^2)}{-9(x^1)(z^4)} =$$
$$-4x^{5-1}y^{3-0}z^{2-4} =$$
$$-4x^4y^3z^{-2}$$

Because the exponent of -2 on z indicates division, this is equal to:

$$\frac{-4x^4y^3}{z^2}$$

ABSOLUTE VALUE AND INEQUALITIES

Let us begin by defining the absolute value of a quantity. The absolute value of a real number, written as $|x|$, is defined as the distance between that number and zero on the number line. That distance can be in the positive direction, that is, $+x$, or in the negative direction, that is, $-x$. The formal definition of an absolute value of a real number is:

$$|x| = -x \text{ if } x < 0 \text{ or } +x \text{ if } x \geq 0$$

When an absolute value is present in an equation, it becomes helpful to consider the single equation as two equations. For example, the equation $|x + 10| = 5$ can be rewritten as $x + 10 = +5$ and $x + 10 = -5$. Thus, the solutions of the equation $|x + 10| = 5$ are $x = -15$ and -5.

Next, let us discuss inequalities. An inequality is a mathematical equation in which the two sides are unequal—one side of the equation is either greater than or less than the other side of the equation. Inequalities are represented with the following symbols:

$a > b$	a is greater than b	or b is less than a
$a \geq b$	a is greater than or equal to b	or b is less than or equal to a
$a < b$	a is less than b	or b is greater than a
$a \leq b$	a is less than or equal to b	or b is greater than or equal to a

For example:

$$0 < x < 4 \text{ means } x \text{ is greater than 0 but less than 4}$$

$$-5 \leq x < 8 \text{ means } x \text{ is greater than or equal to } -5 \text{ but less than 8}$$

In a problem involving absolute value inequalities, the goal is to solve the inequality for the unknown variable.

PROBLEM: Solve the inequality $|x + 4| < 7$ for x.

SOLUTION: The inequality can be rewritten as $-7 < x + 4 < + 7$. To isolate x, you must eliminate 4, which means you will have to subtract 4 from all terms of the inequality. The solution becomes:

$$-7 - 4 < x + 4 - 4 < + 7 - 4$$

$$-11 < x < 3$$

The solution interval is written as $(-11, 3)$.

When solving inequalities, there are a few rules to follow. For example, if given the inequality, $2x + 5 < 7$, subtracting 5 from both sides gives:

$$2x < 2$$

Dividing both sides by 2 gives:

$$x < 1$$

Consider the following problem:

$$7 - x \leq 8$$

Subtracting 7 from both sides gives:

$$-x \leq 1$$

If we multiply both sides by -1 to rid the x of the negative sign, however, we must switch the $\leq$ to a $\geq$:

$$x \geq -1$$

Remember that you need to return to your answers and double-check your work. You can also use your answer and work backward to perform calculations to give back a number in the original problem.

CHAPTER 38

Geometry and Trigonometry

Read This Chapter to Learn About

➤ Line Segments
➤ Quadrilaterals
➤ Triangles
➤ Circles
➤ Functions
➤ Logarithms
➤ Graphical Analysis
➤ Trigonometric Functions

LINE SEGMENTS

A line segment is a line with definite endpoints. The word *segment* is used because a line continues in two directions without an end. The endpoints are given coordinates to determine the position of those points. These coordinates can be determining the x-coordinate and y-coordinate values for the points. These points can be written in the form (x, y).

Knowing the coordinates of the endpoints of a line can help one determine the slope of a line. This can be calculated looking at the change in values of the y coordinates divided by the change in values of the x coordinates:

$$\frac{\Delta y}{\Delta x} \text{ or } \frac{y_2 - y_1}{x_2 - x_1}$$

PROBLEM: Given the two points A(3, 8) and B(5, 12), what is the slope of the line segment that these points form?

SOLUTION:

$$\frac{y_2 - y_1}{x_2 - x_1} = \frac{12 - 8}{5 - 3} = \frac{4}{2} = 2$$

The slope of the line can also be found by using the equation of a straight line, $y = mx + b$, where m is the slope of the line. For example, if an equation of a straight line is $y = -3x + 4$, the slope of the line would be -3. While on the topic, it is also worth noting that the value of b is $+4$, indicating that the y-intercept is $+4$.

Parallel lines are lines that lie in the same plane and are the same distance apart over their entire length. The reason that parallel lines do not meet is because they have the same slope.

PROBLEM: Will the following two line equations produce lines that are parallel?

$$y = 2x + 4 \text{ and } y = -\frac{1}{2}x + 3$$

SOLUTION: These lines have different values for m and will *not* be parallel. Instead they will be perpendicular.

Perpendicular lines meet each other to form a right, 90-degree, angle. The slopes of two perpendicular lines will be negative reciprocals of each other as demonstrated in the previous problem where the line equations were $y = 2x + 4$ and $y = -\frac{1}{2}x + 3$. (The slopes of the two lines are 2 and $-\frac{1}{2}$.)

PROBLEM: The lines represented by the equations: $y + \frac{1}{2}x = 4$ and $3x + 6y = 12$ are:

A. the same line
B. parallel
C. perpendicular
D. none of the above

SOLUTION: Both equations need to be written in the form $y = mx + b$. In the equation on the right, we must divide by 6 so that the y is no longer being multiplied by a number. This gives: $\frac{1}{2}x + y = 2$. Subtracting $\frac{1}{2}x$ from the left side of both equations one gets: $y = -\frac{1}{2}x + 4$ and $y = -\frac{1}{2}x + 2$. These lines are parallel, so B is the correct answer.

The two endpoints of a line segment also have a point that is called the midpoint. This point is equidistant from the two endpoints and lies on the line segment. The midpoint is calculated by taking the average of the x coordinates and the y coordinates: $\left(\frac{x_2 + x_1}{2}, \frac{y_2 + y_1}{2} \right)$.

PROBLEM: What is the midpoint of a line whose coordinates are $(-4, 5)$ and $(0, 13)$?

SOLUTION: Substitution leads to the following:

$$\left(\frac{x_2 + x_1}{2}, \frac{y_2 + y_1}{2}\right) =$$

$$\left(\frac{-4 + 0}{2}, \frac{5 + 13}{2}\right) = \left(\frac{-4}{2}, \frac{18}{2}\right) = (-2, 9)$$

PROBLEM: A line segment has two endpoints, A and B. If the coordinates of A are $(0, 6)$ and the midpoint is $(4, 9)$, then what are the coordinates for B?

SOLUTION: The values of the x-coordinates are 0 and 4, meaning that 4 is the midpoint of 0 and another number. Since 0 is 4 less than 4, the other number must be 4 more than 4, or 8. The values of the y-coordinates are 6 and 9. Since 6 is 3 less than 9, the other number must be 3 more than 9—in other words, 9 is the midpoint of 6 and 12. The coordinates of B are $(8, 12)$.

The distance between two endpoints can be calculated using the distance formula:

$$d = \sqrt{(x_2 - x_1)^2 + (y_2 - y_1)^2}.$$

PROBLEM: What is the distance between the points $(-2, -3)$ and $(-4, 4)$?

SOLUTION: Stay organized while you solve:

$$d = \sqrt{(-4 - -2)^2 + (4 - -3)^2}$$
$$d = \sqrt{(-2)^2 + (7)^2}$$
$$d = \sqrt{4 + 49}$$
$$d = \sqrt{53} = 7.3$$

PROBLEM: What is the length of the line segment with endpoints $A(-6, 4)$ and $B(2, -5)$?

A. $\sqrt{13}$

B. $\sqrt{17}$

C. $\sqrt{72}$

D. $\sqrt{145}$

SOLUTION:

$$d = \sqrt{(2 - -6)^2 + (-5 - 4)^2}$$
$$d = \sqrt{(8)^2 + (-9)^2}$$
$$d = \sqrt{64 + 81}$$
$$d = \sqrt{145}$$

QUADRILATERALS

Quadrilaterals are shapes that have four sides to them. Quadrilaterals include squares, rectangles, trapezoids, and, isosceles trapezoids. The sum of the angles of a quadrilateral must be 360°. The perimeter of each shape is the sum of the lengths of all four sides. The properties of these shapes can be summarized as follows:

➤ The square has four right angles and sides that are equal in length. The diagonals bisect each other perpendicularly. The area is calculated by squaring the length of a side.

➤ The rectangle is much like the square except that only the opposite sides of the rectangle need to be equal in length. The diagonals bisect each other in equal length. The area is calculated by multiplying the length by the width.

➤ The trapezoid has one pair of parallel bases that are not equal in length. The legs are not parallel to each other. An isosceles trapezoid must have the legs of equal length. The area of the trapezoid is calculated using $A = \frac{1}{2}(a+b)h$ where a and b are the lengths of the the bases and h is the height.

PROBLEM: Calculate the area of a trapezoid that has a base of 6 cm, a base of 11 cm, and a height of 8 cm.

SOLUTION: Substituting into $A = \frac{1}{2}(a+b)h$ gives $A = \frac{1}{2}(6+11)(8)$. Remember the order of operations calls for the addition to take place first, $A = \frac{1}{2}(17)(8) = 68$ cm^2.

PROBLEM: Two adjacent sides of a rectangle are represented by $x+6$ and $2x$. In terms of x, what is the area of the rectangle? What is the perimeter of the rectangle?

SOLUTION: To find the area we multiply the distance of the two adjacent sides. $2x(x+6) = 2x^2 + 12x$. The perimeter is equal to the sum of all four sides, $2x + 2x + (x+6) + (x+6) = 6x + 12$.

TRIANGLES

Triangles are three-sided figures that contain three straight sides in addition to three angles. The sum of the angles in a triangle is 180 degrees. Triangles can be defined as equilateral, isosceles, and scalene, where these triangles have three, two, and no sides equal, respectively. Referring to the angles within a triangle, they can be one of the following: a right triangle with one 90-degree angle, equiangular with all angles measuring 60 degrees, obtuse with one angle greater than 90 degrees, and acute with all angles measuring less than 90 degrees.

The Pythagorean theorem allows one to calculate a side of a right triangle, given the value of the lengths of the other two sides of a triangle. This can be accomplished with the use of the following equation: $a^2 + b^2 = c^2$ where c is the length of the hypotenuse (the longest side of the right triangle). There are situations where one does not have to worry about calculating the length of the hypotenuse. Two examples are when the legs have lengths of 3 and 4, the hypotenuse will be equal to 5, and when the legs are lengths of 5 and 12, the hypotenuse will be equal to a length of 13. These triangles are called 3:4:5 and 5:12:13 triangles.

PROBLEM: A right triangle has an angle equal to 35 degrees. If the third angle has a value of $5x$, what is the value of x?

SOLUTION: The sum of the angles is $180°$. One angle is $90°$ and the other is $35°$. This means that the third angle is $55°$ in measure. If $5x = 55$, then dividing both sides by 5, we find that the value of x is 11.

PROBLEM: In the following figure, the vertices of triangle DEF are the midpoints of the sides of the equilateral triangle ABC, and the perimeter of triangle ABC is 36 cm. What is the length of segment EF?

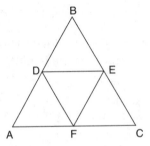

SOLUTION: The perimeter of the triangle is 36 cm. Because all sides are equal in length, each side is 12 cm. The midpoints of the larger triangle create a smaller, yet still equilateral triangle, with sides that are 6 cm each. Segments EF, FC, and, CE will all be 6 cm.

The area of a triangle can be calculated by using the equation $A = \frac{1}{2}bh$, where b and h are the base and height of the triangle respectively. Remember that your units for area must reflect that they are "squared" because two units for distance are being multiplied.

PROBLEM: A rectangle with sides 5 cm and 12 cm in length has a diagonal drawn from one corner to another. What is the area of the triangle that is made once this diagonal is drawn? What is the length of this diagonal?

SOLUTION: The diagonal drawn from one corner to another corner of the rectangle creates two right triangles. If one of the legs of the triangles is 5 cm and the other is 12 cm, then the area of each triangle is $A = \frac{1}{2}bh$, or $A = \frac{1}{2}(5)(12)$, which equals 30 cm^2. Answering the second part of this problem, if the legs of a right triangle (remember that rectangles have four $90°$ angles) are 5 and 12, the hypotenuse must have a length of 13, or in this case 13 cm.

CIRCLES

Circles can be considered to be a line that is bent around until the ends join, making a perfectly circular loop where all points are equidistant from the center. The radius is the distance from the center to a point on the circle. The diameter is the length of any chord (line segment joining two points on the circle) that passes through the center. The value of the diameter will be twice that of the radius, d = 2r.

There are two important calculations that one should know regarding the circle, the circumference (distance around the circle) and the area. These two equations are, respectively, $C = 2\pi r$ and $A = \pi r^2$, where $\pi = 3.14$. Keep in mind that the units for area will be units squared but not so for the circumference.

> **PROBLEM:** A circle as a diameter of 4 meters. What is the circumference of the circle? The area?

> **SOLUTION:** To solve this problem, one needs the radius. The radius is half of the diameter so, r = 2 m. Knowing the radius, we can now calculate the circumference: $C = 2\pi r$, C = 2(3.14)(2) = 12.56 m. The area is $A = \pi r^2$, $A = (3.14)(2)^2$. Remember to square the 2 first, so A = (3.14)(4) = 12.56 m². Keep in mind that while the values for these answers are the same, the units are not.

FUNCTIONS

A function is a mathematical relationship between a quantity called input and a value calculated, called an output. An example of a function is $f(x) = 3x$. Because a function has one value calculated per input, the resulting graph of a function can pass the vertical line test and show that each value for x has just one y value.

> **PROBLEM:** Which of the following graphs does not represent a function?

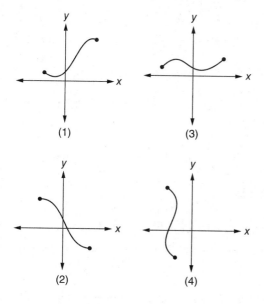

(1)　　　(3)

(2)　　　(4)

> **SOLUTION:** Taking the time to draw a vertical line through the curve of each graph, one can see that choice 4 has multiple y values for one x value, so it is not a function.

PROBLEM: If $f(x) = x^2 - 5$ and $g(x) = 6x$, then what is the value of $g(f(x))$?

SOLUTION: Being careful to substitute the value of $f(x)$ into $g(x)$, one gets: $6(x^2 - 5) = 6x^2 - 30$. If one were not careful and accidentally substituted incorrectly, the solution could have been: $(6x)^2 - 5 = 36x^2 - 5$, which would have been the answer to $f(g(x))$.

TRIGONOMETRIC FUNCTIONS

When studying right triangles, the three most important trigonometric functions to know are sine, cosine, and tangent (abbreviated sin, cos, and tan). From these trigonometric functions, one can then calculate their reciprocal trigonometric functions: cosecant, secant, and cotangent (abbreviated csc, sec, and cot). These can be summarized by examining the following right triangle and one of its acute angles, θ.

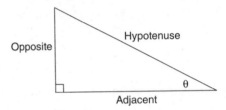

Sine θ	Cosine θ	Tangent θ	Cosecant θ	Secant θ	Cotangent θ
$\dfrac{\text{side opposite}}{\text{hypotenuse}}$	$\dfrac{\text{side adjacent}}{\text{hypotenuse}}$	$\dfrac{\text{side opposite}}{\text{side adjacent}}$	$\dfrac{\text{hypotenuse}}{\text{side opposite}}$	$\dfrac{\text{hypotenuse}}{\text{side adjacent}}$	$\dfrac{\text{side adjacent}}{\text{side opposite}}$

PROBLEM: In a 5, 12, 13 right triangle, the $\sin \theta = \dfrac{5}{13}$. What is the value of $\sec \theta$?

SOLUTION: If the $\sin \theta = \dfrac{5}{13}$, that means that the side opposite θ is 5 and that the hypotenuse is 13. Therefore, the $\cos \theta$ must be $\dfrac{\text{side adjacent } \theta}{\text{hypotenuse}} = \dfrac{12}{13}$. Because we are looking for $\sec \theta$, which is the reciprocal of $\cos \theta$, the value of $\sec \theta$ must be $\dfrac{13}{12}$.

LOGARITHMS

Logarithmic functions are the inverse function of exponential functions. That is, if one had the equation $x = a^y$, then it can be rearranged to show that $y = \log_a x$. For example, the equivalent logarithmic function of $y = 4^x$ would be $x = \log_4 y$.

PROBLEM: Evaluate the logarithmic expression $\log_4 256$.

SOLUTION: This is equivalent to $n = \log_4 256$. Converting this to $4^n = 256$, $n = 4$.

PROBLEM: What is the value of the expression $\log_5\left(\frac{1}{25}\right)$?

SOLUTION: This is equivalent to $x = \log_5\left(\frac{1}{25}\right)$, which is $5^x = \frac{1}{25}$. A value of $x = -2$ makes for a correct answer.

GRAPHICAL ANALYSIS

Graphs are useful in that they can help us find trends that occur over time. Also, A graph can tell us which type of mathematical equation was used in plotting it. Let us look back at two graphs that we examined while studying the gas laws:

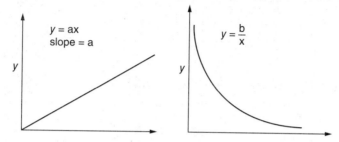

The graph on the left indicates a direct relationship in that as one variable increases in value, the other increases as well. The one on the right demonstrates an inverse relationship, as one variable increases in value, the other decreases.

There are other graphs we can examine for these types of relationships. For example, the graph on the left in the following figure shows a relationship where one of the variables was squared ($y = x^2$) while the one on the right shows a constant value for y no matter what the value of x is.

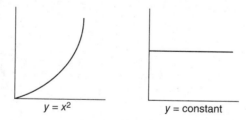

The graph of a circle, shown here, follows the equation $(x - h)^2 + (y - k)^2 = r^2$, where the center of the circle lies at (h, k). The equation for the circle below is $(x - 3)^2 + (y + 4)^2 = 18$ as $(3, -4)$ is the center and the radius has a value of $\sqrt{18}$.

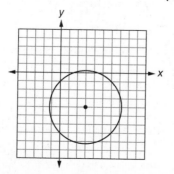

There is also the general shape of a parabola, whose graph (see the following figure) comes about from the equation $ax^2 + bx + c$. Depending upon the signs of b and c, the parabola can be drawn in a number of directions.

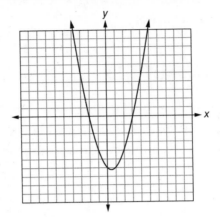

Finally, we examine the graphs of sin x, cos x, and tan x, shown consecutively.

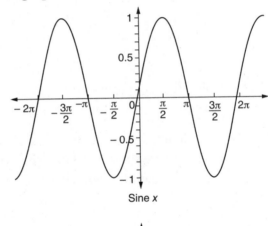

Sine x

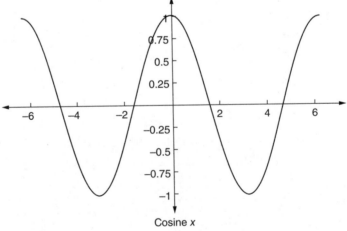

Cosine x

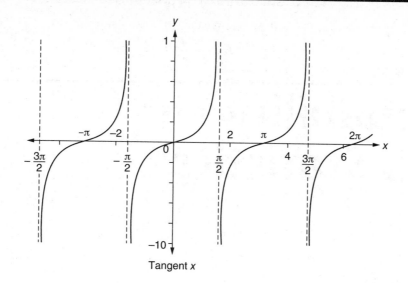

Tangent x

A review and memorization of the graphs here will be of utmost importance to avoid confusion during the test.

Probability
and Statistics

PROBABILITY

A flip of the coin, a roll of the dice, or a card picked from a deck are just three examples of probability. The probability of an event is a numerical measure of the likelihood that the given event will occur. The calculations involving probability depend on how many and in what order are the successful outcomes and the total number of desired outcomes. If you assume that there are n different but equally possible outcomes of an event, with a number s of these outcomes considered successes and a number $f = n - s$ considered failures, then the probability of success for a given event is $p = \dfrac{s}{n}$ and the probability of failure for a given event, q, is $q = \dfrac{f}{n}$.

Single-event probability is the probability of a single event occurring within a given set of possible outcomes. If you were to apply this to the probability of obtaining heads in a coin flip, there is one successful outcome (heads) and two possible outcomes (heads or tails). So the probability of obtaining heads in a coin flip is: $p = \dfrac{s}{n} = \dfrac{1}{2}$.

Since the probability is a fraction, it can be expressed as a percentage, with the probability of obtaining heads in a coin flip being 50 percent. Single-event probability can also be applied to a single playing card drawn from a standard deck of 52 cards. To determine the probability that a selected card is of a black suit, you first note that a card can be selected from a deck in n = 52 different ways. Since there are two black suits (clubs and spades) with 13 cards per suit, a card of a black suit can be drawn from the deck in s = 26 different ways. Thus, the probability that the selected card is a card of a black suit is:

$$p = \frac{s}{n} = \frac{26}{52} = \frac{1}{2}$$

PROBLEM: What is the probability of not selecting the king of hearts from a deck of cards?

SOLUTION: To determine the probability of not selecting the king of hearts, let's determine the probability of selecting the king of hearts. Since the king of hearts is but one of 52 cards, the probability of selecting the king of hearts is $p = \frac{s}{n} = \frac{1}{52}$.

Thus, the probability, q, of *not* selecting the king of hearts is q = 1 − p or

$$\frac{52}{52} - \frac{1}{52} = \frac{51}{52}$$

In single-event probability, you seek to determine the probability or likelihood of a single successful outcome out of a set of possible outcomes. In multiple-event probability, you seek to determine the probability or likelihood of any of two or more successful outcomes occurring, but not at the same time (referred to as mutually exclusive events), or the probability of one outcome occurring without influencing another outcome (referred to as independent events).

Let us say that the probability of one successful event is P(A), the probability of another is P(B), and the two events have no common outcomes. Then the probability that either of these events will occur, P(A or B), is the sum of their individual probabilities, P(A) + P(B) or P(A or B) = P(A) + P(B).

PROBLEM: Upon rolling a pair of dice, what is the probability that the sum of the two numbers on the dice is either 6 or 12?

SOLUTION: The number of total possible outcomes from the roll of two dice is 36. In other words, there are 36 different pairs of numbers that can be obtained. You first need to determine the number of possible outcomes yielding a sum of 6 or 12 from the two dice. The number of possible outcomes yielding a sum of 6 is 5 or {(1, 5), (2, 4), (3, 3), (4, 2), (5, 1)}. The probability of yielding a sum of 6 between the two dice is

$$P(A) = P(6) = \frac{5}{36}$$

The number of possible outcomes yielding a sum of 12 is 1 or {(6, 6)}. The probability of yielding a sum of 12 between the two dice is

$$P(B) = P(12) = \frac{1}{36}$$

Upon the roll of two dice, you cannot obtain a sum of 6 and a sum of 12 at the same time; the two successful outcomes thus are mutually exclusive. The probability that the sum of the two dice is either 6 or 12 is:

$$P(A \text{ or } B) = P(A) + P(B) = P(6) + P(12) = \frac{5}{36} + \frac{1}{36} = \frac{6}{36} = \frac{1}{6}$$

In the case of probability involving independent events, one is being asked to determine the probability of two events that occur in sequence. Two events are independent if the success of one event does not influence the success of the second event. The probability of two independent events, $P(A \text{ and } B)$, can be determined by first calculating the probability of each event occurring separately, $P(A)$ and $P(B)$, then multiplying these probabilities, $P(A) \times P(B)$, or

$$P(A \text{ and } B) = P(A) \times P(B)$$

PROBLEM: What is the probability that two cards drawn from a deck of cards are face cards (king, queen, or jack) if the first card drawn is replaced before the second card is drawn?

SOLUTION: Because the two drawings are both made from a full deck of cards, the two events are independent of one another. You first need to determine the probability of drawing a face card from a deck of cards. Out of a total of 52 cards, there are 3 face cards in each of the four suits, resulting in 12 face cards in a deck. The probability of drawing a face card, $P(A)$, is therefore $\frac{12}{52}$. Because the first card is replaced before the second drawing, the probability of again drawing a face card, $P(B)$, is also $\frac{12}{52}$. Thus, the probability of drawing two face cards is:

$$P(A \text{ and } B) = P(A) \times P(B) = \frac{12}{52} \times \frac{12}{52} = \frac{144}{2704}$$

Because both the numerator and the denominator are divisible by 16, the probability fraction can be simplified to $P(A \text{ and } B) = \frac{9}{169}$.

STATISTICS

Statistics is a branch of mathematics that reveals important information about variables and their relationships from groups or sets of data. Some statistical terms that are used in describing an individual variable from a data set include *mean*, *median*, *mode*, and *range*. As these terms are explained and discussed, consider the example of a student who has received the 11 following classroom grades for a certain grading period:

$$\{72, 86, 97, 95, 81, 79, 81, 67, 70, 65, 83\}$$

The *mean* is the average value of the data set. To determine the mean, the terms in the data set are added and then divided by the number of terms in the set. The sum of all of the data is 876, and the number of values in the data set is 11. Dividing 876 by 11 gives a mean of 79.6, which rounds to 80.

The *median* is the middle term in a data set. In order to identify the median, it is helpful to arrange the terms of the data set in ascending order. If there is an odd number of terms in the data set, the single term in the middle is the median. However, if there is an even number of terms in the data set, the median is the average of the two terms that are in the middle of the data set. The median of the data set given earlier can be found by first arranging the terms of the data set in ascending order:

$$\{65, 67, 70, 72, 79, 81, 81, 83, 86, 95, 97\}$$

The middle term of the data set, the median, is 81.

The *mode* is the term that occurs most frequently in the data set. Referring to the aforementioned data set, the term 81 occurs twice and is therefore the mode of the data set. The *range* is the difference between the largest and smallest terms in the data set. The largest term of the data set is 97, and the smallest term is 65. Thus, the range of the data set is:

$$\text{Range} = 97 - 65 = 32$$